Introduction to
Clinical
Methods
in
Communication
Disorders
SECOND EDITION

Introduction to
Clinical
Methods
in
Communication
Disorders

SECOND EDITION

edited by

Rhea Paul, Ph.D.
and
Paul W. Cascella, Ph.D.
Southern Connecticut State University, New Haven

with invited contributors

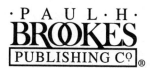
·P·A·U·L·H·
BROOKES
PUBLISHING C?®

Baltimore • London • Sydney

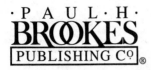

Paul H. Brookes Publishing Co.
Post Office Box 10624
Baltimore, Maryland 21285-0624

www.brookespublishing.com

Production and composition services by
Hearthside Publishing Services.
Manufactured in the United States of America by
Victor Graphics, Inc., Baltimore, Maryland.

The case studies appearing in this book are composites based on the authors' experiences; these case studies do not represent the lives or experiences of specific individuals, and no implications should be inferred.

Several of the definitions in the glossary are from Dirckx, J. (Ed.). (1997). *Stedman's concise medical dictionary* (3rd ed.). Baltimore: Lippincott Williams & Wilkins; reprinted by permission.

Second printing, January 2008.
Third printing, March 2010.
Fourth printing, December 2011.

Library of Congress Cataloging-in-Publication Data

Introduction to clinical methods in communication disorders / edited by Rhea Paul and
  Paul W. Cascella ; with invited contributors.—2nd ed.
     p.   ; cm.
  Includes bibliographical references and index.
  ISBN-13: 978-1-55766-879-0 (pbk.)
  ISBN-10: 1-55766-879-5 (pbk.)
  1. Speech therapy. 2. Audiology. I. Paul, Rhea. II. Cascella, Paul W.
     [DNLM: 1. Communication Disorders—therapy. 2. Clinical Medicine—methods.
     3. Speech-Language Pathology—methods.   WL 340.2 I618 2007]
  RC423.I545 2007
  616.85'506-dc22   2006027675

British Library Cataloguing in Publication data are available from the British Library.

Contents

About the Editors

Rhea Paul, Ph.D., Professor, Department of Communication Disorders, Southern Connecticut State University, Davis Hall, 501 Crescent Street, New Haven, Connecticut, 06515

Rhea Paul received her bachelor's degree from Brandeis University in Waltham, Massachusetts, in 1971; her master's degree from Harvard Graduate School of Education in 1975; and her doctoral degree in communication disorders from the University of Wisconsin–Madison in 1981. Dr. Paul has published more than 70 journal articles and has authored six books. Her research on language development in toddlers with delayed language acquisition was funded by the National Institutes of Health. She has also held grants from the Meyer Memorial Trust, the American Speech-Language-Hearing Association (ASHA) Foundation, the Medical Research Foundation, and the National Association for Autism Research. Dr. Paul has been a fellow of ASHA since 1991 and received the 1996 Editor's Award from the *American Journal of Speech-Language Pathology.* In September 1997, she accepted a faculty appointment in the Communication Disorders Department at Southern Connecticut State University and a research appointment at the Yale Child Study Center. She spent the summer of 1998 as a visiting professor at the University of Sydney in Australia. Dr. Paul received a Yale Mellon Fellowship for 1998–1999 and the Southern Connecticut State University Faculty Scholar Award for 1999. She was awarded an Erskine Fellowship to spend a semester as a visiting scholar at Canterbury University in Christchurch, New Zealand, in 2002 and was a Visiting Scholar at the Department of Experimental Psychology at Oxford University in 2005. The third edition of her textbook, *Language Disorders from Infancy Through Adolescence: Assessment and Intervention,* will be published in 2007 by Mosby. Dr. Paul has been teaching child language development and disorders courses for 25 years.

Paul W. Cascella, Ph.D., Professor, Department of Communication Disorders, Southern Connecticut State University, Davis Hall, 501 Crescent Street, New Haven, Connecticut, 06515

Paul W. Cascella received his bachelor's degree from Marquette University in Milwaukee, Wisconsin; his master's degree from the State University of New York at Buffalo; and his doctoral degree in special education from the University of Connecticut. Dr. Cascella is a speech-language pathologist whose primary interests are communication services and supports for individuals with severe and low-incidence disabilities. He has published more than 20 journal articles and book chapters, and his research specifically focuses on functional assessment of and intervention strategies for individuals with intellectual disability and autism spectrum disorders. Dr. Cascella also has clinical expertise in pediatric phonology and fluency, and he is an active clinician who routinely collaborates with public school districts throughout Connecticut. Dr. Cascella is the speech-language pathologist for the Hamden Transition Academy, a high school program on the campus of Southern Connecticut State University aimed at meeting the educational needs of older high school students as they make the transition to adult living and employment. Dr. Cascella was a Mellon Fellow at the Yale Child Study Center (2000–2001) and is an editorial consultant for *Mosby's Medical, Nursing, & Allied Health Dictionary, Seventh Edition* (Mosby Harcourt, in press). He currently serves on the Board of Directors for Vantage, Inc., a community agency providing residential and vocational supports to adults with disabilities.

Contributors

Michele A. Anderson
Doctoral Student
Western Michigan University
1903 West Michigan Avenue
Kalamazoo, Michigan 49008

G. Robert Buckendorf, Ph.D.
Speech-Language Pathology Discipline
  Director
Assistant Professor of Pediatrics
Child Development and Rehabilitation
  Center
Oregon Health & Science University
Post Office Box 574
Portland, Oregon 97207

James J. Dempsey, Ph.D.
Professor, Chair
Department of Communication
  Disorders
Southern Connecticut State University
501 Crescent Street
New Haven, Connecticut 06515

Marc E. Fey, Ph.D.
Professor
Hearing and Speech Department
University of Kansas Medical Center
3901 Rainbow Boulevard
Kansas City, Kansas 66160

Melanie Fried-Oken, Ph.D.
Director
Assistive Technology Program
Associate Professor
Neurology, Biomedical Engineering,
  and Otolaryngology
Oregon Health & Science University
Post Office Box 574
Portland, Oregon 97207

Brian Goldstein, Ph.D.
Associate Professor, Acting Chair
Communication Sciences
Temple University
109 Weiss Hall
Philadelphia, Pennsylvania 19122

Allyson Goodwyn-Craine, M.S.
Director
Children's Clinical Services
Hearing and Speech Institute
1675 Southwest Marlow
Suite 200
Portland, Oregon 97225

Jane Hindenlang, M.S.
Clinical Instructor, Adjunct Faculty
Department of Communication
  Disorders
Southern Connecticut State University
501 Crescent Street
New Haven, Connecticut 06515

Yvette D. Hyter, Ph.D.
Associate Professor
Department of Speech Pathology
  and Audiology
Western Michigan University
1903 West Michigan Avenue
Kalamazoo, Michigan 49008

Aquiles Iglesias, Ph.D.
Dean
Graduate School
Temple University
501 Carnell Hall
Philadelphia, Pennsylvania 19122

Laura M. Justice, Ph.D.
Associate Professor
Curry School of Education
University of Virginia
Post Office Box 400873
Charlottesville, Virginia 22904

Marianne Kennedy, Ph.D.
Professor
Department of Communication
  Disorders
Southern Connecticut State University
501 Crescent Street
New Haven, Connecticut 06515

Kevin M. McNamara, M.A.
Clinic Director, Adjunct Faculty
Southern Connecticut State University
501 Crescent Street
New Haven, Connecticut 06515

Nickola W. Nelson, Ph.D.
Charles Van Riper Professor
Department of Speech Pathology
  and Audiology
Western Michigan University
1903 West Michigan Avenue
Kalamazoo, Michigan 49008

Mary H. Purdy, Ph.D.
Associate Professor
Department of Communication
  Disorders
Southern Connecticut State University
501 Crescent Street
New Haven, Connecticut 06515

Ellen Reuler, M.A.
Clinic Director, Senior Instructor
Speech and Hearing Sciences
Portland State University
Post Office Box 751
Portland, Oregon 97207

Denise LaPrade Rini, M.A.
Clinical Instructor, Adjunct Faculty
Department of Communication
  Disorders
Southern Connecticut State University
501 Crescent Street
New Haven, Connecticut 06515

Froma Roth, Ph.D.
Professor
Department of Hearing and Speech
  Sciences
University of Maryland
College Park, Maryland 20742

John Tetnowski, Ph.D.
Ben Blanco Endowed Professor
Communicative Disorders
University of Louisiana at Lafayette
Post Office Box 43170
Lafayette, Louisiana 70504

Acknowledgments

The completion of this book owes much to its outstanding contributors, who met deadlines and incorporated editorial suggestions with efficiency and good grace that are as rare as they are appreciated. To our colleagues at the Department of Communication Disorders at Southern Connecticut State University, we express thanks for their forbearance and support.

This book is dedicated to the loving memory of
Charles R. Isenberg and Elizabeth A. Cascella
with our gratitude for their pride and joy in our endeavors.

CHAPTER 1

Introduction to Clinical Practice in Communication Disorders

RHEA PAUL AND PAUL W. CASCELLA

CLINICAL ART AND SCIENCE

In thinking about the message we wanted to convey to our audience, the students reading this book, we editors found ourselves recalling some of our own clinical experiences. One of us remembered supervising a first-term student clinician by the name of Jane. Jane was working on articulation with Mike, a pixie-faced 3-year-old with almost completely unintelligible speech. Mike had lots to say, but Jane could understand almost none of it. He was trying to tell her something about the toy dinosaur he had brought from home and, try as she might, she just was not getting it. After attempting three or four times to get the same message across, poor little Mike burst into tears of frustration. Jane was, naturally, taken aback. Sitting behind the mirror, the supervisor saw Jane trying to "talk" the little boy into feeling better. Finally, unable to contain her own distress at seeing Mike so miserable, the supervisor went into the room and held him, rocking him until he finished crying. Mike was soon able to resume his work. In our conference following this incident, Jane remarked, "I was so glad when you came in and held him. I didn't think I was allowed to do that; it didn't seem like the kind of thing a clinician is supposed to do."

We also recalled clients who helped our students stretch their notions of what communication disorders professionals do in other ways, as well. Garrett, a 10-year-old boy with an autism spectrum disorder, had a tantrum every week in the hallway on his way to speech-language therapy. Although initially frustrated, our graduate student, Jamie, took only a few weeks to figure out the function of Garrett's behavior and how to replace his tantrums with communication. Another graduate student, Colin, spent a semester learning how to embed communication opportunities into the daily routines of adults with severe disabilities at a sheltered vocational workshop. Colin was challenged to see his professional role be one as a consultant instead of as a direct service provider, and this meant he had to evaluate communication patterns of the workshop

1

staff, not only the clients who attended the workshop. Kate, another graduate student, spent a semester learning how to assess students with severe and profound intellectual disability without any standardized tests so that the assessment was both functional and realistic.

This book is all about the kinds of things that clinicians are supposed to do and think about. In our first example, Jane learned something essential about clinical practice: Even the clinician with the highest level of technical training and the most scientific outlook sometimes has to remember that our clients are first and foremost **people**—people with complicated, sometimes conflicting feelings and needs; people who sometimes do not use their clinical time efficiently; people whose motivation to learn better communication skills is sometimes overwhelmed by their emotions or the broader circumstances of their lives. Jamie, Colin, and Kate faced unique circumstances in which they were challenged to critically evaluate their role as a speech-language pathologist and think out of the box about clinical services. These examples show that a good clinician must be part scientist, humanist, and philosopher, someone who is willing to carefully evaluate what professionals do (and do not do) as part of the clinical services.

But, you may be thinking, how can I learn to be a scientist, a humanist, a philosopher, and an expert on normal and disordered communication before I see my first client NEXT SEMESTER? Well, fortunately for all of us, there is one more thing that every clinician needs to be, and that is a human being. Neither your supervisor, your client, nor anyone else will expect you to be a fully evolved clinician your first term. With your first client, and probably with some of your later ones, too, you will make mistakes. Like any other human being you will have to make amends for these mistakes, try to learn from them, and do better the next time. Competent clinicians recognize and learn from their own mistakes. Still, the purpose of this book is to help you begin to make the transition from a student of communication disorders to a speech, language, and/or hearing clinician.

Being a clinician entails some qualities that probably cannot be taught by your professors. These are the qualities we identify with the humanist, and to some extent they arise out of your own beliefs, needs, desires, and personality. It is these qualities that probably brought you to consider a career in communication disorders. These qualities include

1. A desire to help others

2. Strengths in social interactions

3. Enjoyment of close contact with people

4. Strong communication skills

5. The ability to take pleasure in "just talking"

6. An interest in the various processes by which communication takes place

7. A level of comfort with people with disabilities

These qualities are not present in everyone, but as a starting point for becoming a clinician, they are essential. As you must know by now, although these qualities contribute to making you a good clinician, more is needed. You need an in-depth knowledge of the normal processes and development of communication and the characteristics, causes, and correlates of the various kinds of communication disorders. You also need knowledge of the information introduced in this book. Here you will learn about the kinds of behaviors and activities in which a clinician engages and about the contexts in which these behaviors and activities take place. The goal is that when you are through, you will have a better sense of what it is a clinician does; where he or she does it; and what general principles of ethics, public policy, cultural sensitivity, and respect for clients and families guide our behaviors and activities.

SCOPE OF PRACTICE

What do speech-language pathologists (SLPs) and audiologists do? Where do they do it? With and for whom? Why do they take this approach and not that one? These are the questions that define our scope of practice. SLPs and audiologists work with clients from birth through old age. Audiologists screen newborns for hearing loss; SLPs work with premature infants to develop feeding, swallowing, and early parent-child communication skills. Audiologists and SLPs work with infants and toddlers with a variety of developmental disabilities, including hearing impairment, intellectual disability, autism spectrum disorders, congenital anomalies such as cleft palate, congenital disorders such as cerebral palsy or fetal alcohol syndrome, and feeding and swallowing problems. We work with children with cochlear implants. Clinicians who work with very young children are often engaged in *secondary prevention* assessment and intervention aimed at limiting the impact of disorders on communication and development. SLPs and audiologists also work with preschool children who have these kinds of problems and speech and/or language delays that surface in early childhood. These include articulation disorders, fluency disorders, and specific language delays. We also, unfortunately, see children in this age range whose communication has been affected by abuse or neglect or whose development has been influenced by parental substance abuse.

SLPs and audiologists often work with school-age populations. In this age range, we see children such as those already described, as well as children who abuse their voices, have trouble producing fluent speech, or endanger their hearing through noise exposure. A large part of an SLP's practice in schools deals with students who have language-based learning disorders that affect their ability to master the academic curriculum. These students require support to enhance their language so they can use it more effectively to succeed in school. With impetus from the No Child Left Behind Act of 2001 (PL 103-82) and the Individuals with Disabilities Education Improvement Act of 2004 (PL 108-446), school-based SLPs provide communication intervention within the context of academic instruction. SLPs also sometimes provide management for students with emotional or social disorders that affect communication, such as Asperger syndrome, selective mutism, or children diagnosed with mental illness.

Many SLPs and audiologists work with adult clients as well. Adults with various developmental disabilities continue to require the services of communication specialists. Some young and middle-age adults experience communication disabilities as a result of illnesses or traumatic brain injury. Older adults are especially vulnerable to acquiring communication disorders. Many audiologists work with older adults experiencing age-related hearing loss. SLPs serve older clients who lose speech and language skills due to neurological diseases, such as strokes, Parkinson's disease, and amyotrophic lateral sclerosis (Lou Gehrig's disease).

Best practice for clients all along the spectrum of development includes close collaboration with their families and with other professionals involved in their care. When a client receives services from several professionals, it serves the client best if these professionals are aware of each other's goals and methods and can coordinate services for the client. Many professionals cross-train each other to help deliver services in a more integrated manner, so the client receives consistent feedback and reinforcement and has more opportunities for generalization. Clinical practice in communication disorders often involves collaboration with teachers and special educators; physical and occupational therapists; psychologists and social workers; recreational and vocational counselors; nurses and physicians; as well as with the staff of schools, residential centers, group homes, rehabilitation facilities, hospitals, and skilled nursing facilities.

SCOPE OF TEXT

In this book, we attempt to introduce you to the processes, settings, and issues involved in clinical practice in communication disorders. In Chapter 2, we talk about the Code of Ethics, disseminated by the American Speech-Language-Hearing Association (ASHA) and the American Academy of Audiology (AAA). This Code is central to the practice of our profession, because it lays out our obligations to our clients, our payers, and our colleagues and provides guidelines to help us in making sometimes difficult ethical decisions. In Chapter 3, you learn about basic principles of assessment. We discuss the properties that make standardized tests fair and accurate. We talk about the times when it is appropriate to use tests and when other methods of assessment come to the fore. Chapter 4 provides information on the physical examination of the speech mechanism, and the methods of assessing its functional status. SLPs and audiologists are the only professionals who do this examination, so it is especially important to be confident and capable in this aspect of our work. Chapter 5 addresses the issue of the assessment of samples of communicative behavior. These include samples of speech and language, nonverbal communication, and the use of augmentative and alternative modes such as sign language and picture boards. One of the most important functions of an SLP is the sampling of communicative behaviors in order to determine appropriate goals and methods for intervention.

Chapter 6 moves our discussion from assessment to the domain of intervention. Here we talk about the range of intervention procedures used to help people with communication disorders improve their functioning. We discuss a continuum of approaches and show how they apply across a variety of communication disorders. In Chapter 7, we address the issue of evidence-based practice and the steps a clinician can take to find support for specific assessment protocols and intervention strategies. In Chapter 8, we address the need for communication skills such as those used in interacting with clients, families, and other professionals. We learn about the various kinds of documentation that are professionally required and the importance of acquiring skills not only in conducting assessment and intervention but also in collaborating with families and colleagues to ensure our clients' progress. We are reminded, too, of our role as—not professional counselors—but as humanists: caring individuals who listen to concerns of clients and families, even when they extend beyond speech, hearing, and language issues. Chapter 9 provides information on the laws, rules, and regulations that govern SLP and audiologist practice. We find out about clients' rights, professional responsibilities, and the emerging public policies that affect practice. In Chapter 10, the varied settings in which communication disorders professionals practice is the topic. We present the kinds of practice options each provides, the kinds of documentation each requires, and the various roles of communication professionals in each one. This may give you a first sense of the setting in which you might like to start your own practice. Chapter 11 addresses the issues of helping clients communicate when they come from cultural and language backgrounds different from their clinician's. These issues have become increasingly important as the demographic trends in our society reflect greater numbers of citizens with cultural and linguistic differences, who, like everyone else, are vulnerable to disorders of communication. But, as you can imagine, facilitating communication is complicated when the client and clinician speak different languages or have different cultural rules for communicating. Chapter 12 reviews the many ways assistive technology affects our practice. Because many of these new technologies are *information* systems, it is not surprising that they will have a great impact on how to deliver services. Finally, in Chapter 13 we discuss the important role that clients and families play in the clinical process. We consider ways of including the perspectives of families at every stage of the clinical decision-making process so as to maximize the impact of treatments beyond the clinical setting, and into the real, integrated lives of the clients we serve.

Our hope is that after completing your studies with this book, you will have a greater sense of what a clinician does and does not do and a greater confidence that you will be able to make the correct choices with your first client and with every client thereafter. Although mastering both the science and the art of clinical practice will take much longer than the time you spend in school, your clinical education will provide you with the tools you need to continue learning and improving your service to clients. We hope you will consider this book a useful part of that education. Yet another part, though, will be the support you receive from your colleagues after you graduate and from the national organization that represents our professions in the United States of America. We would like to take the opportunity at this juncture to introduce you to this organization as well.

THE AMERICAN SPEECH-LANGUAGE-HEARING ASSOCIATION AND THE CLINICIAN

ASHA is the professional, scientific, and credentialing association for the nearly 118,000 communication disorders professionals around the world. Its mission is to "promote the interests of and provide the highest quality services for professionals in audiology, speech-language pathology, and speech and hearing science, and to advocate for people with communication disabilities" (see http://www.asha.org/about_asha.htm). ASHA disseminates standards of ethical conduct, publishes original research in its journals, and provides continuing education programs to its members. It advocates for our clients by monitoring and participating in the development and implementation of education and health care reform proposals and programs at the federal and state levels. The list following highlights many of the services ASHA provides to its members and the community. These include[1]

---

[1] © American Speech-Language-Hearing Association; adapted with permission.

Political advocacy: ASHA tracks issues of concern to our clients and colleagues in legislatures, courts, and regulatory agencies at state and federal levels.

Networking: ASHA provides opportunities for its members to shape the profession and effect changes that benefit clients and colleagues.

Continuing education: ASHA sponsors state and national conferences, distance learning opportunities, newsletters, journals, and audio- and videoconferences that enable members to keep up to date on clinical and professional issues.

Multicultural initiatives: ASHA provides support to members who need to deal with multicultural issues in their practice, from lists of tests and resources to educating citizens from minority groups about the importance of communicative health.

Research: ASHA supports basic and applied research in communication disorders, and it keeps an extensive database to help members write grants, business plans, and reports. ASHA also publishes several journals, including: the *Journal of Speech, Language and Hearing Research, Language, Speech, and Hearing Services in Schools, American Journal of Audiology,* and *American Journal of Speech-Language Pathology.*

Technical assistance: Members can receive information about funding agencies, developing proposals, and other professional issues by contacting ASHA at actioncenter@asha.org or by telephone (1-800-498-2071) or fax (301-571-0457).

Referral service: ASHA maintains a referral list of clinical programs and private practitioners who have asked to be listed. It is grouped by state and available to individuals who request referrals.

Employment service: Members seeking new positions may use ASHA's job placement services.

Specialty recognition: ASHA supports the credentialing of personnel with expertise in a particular disorder (e.g., child language or fluency disorders).

Special Interest Divisions: ASHA maintains 16 Special Interest Divisions (SIDs) that focus on particular aspects of practice, such as language learning and education, aural rehabilitation and its instrumentation, and augmentative and alternative communication, to name a few.

Contact the ASHA web site for further information (http://asha.org).

ASHA provides the standards for earning the clinical credential in our field, the Certificate of Clinical Competence (CCC), which can be earned in either speech-language pathology, audiology, or both. The standards for ASHA certification in speech-language pathology (as of 2005) and audiology (as of 2007) are outlined in Appendices A and B at the end of this chapter, but you should be aware that these standards change from time to time. In addition, many states require SLPs and audiologists to be licensed with the state board of health, certified with the state department of education, or both. In many cases, licensing and teacher certification requirements overlap with ASHA certification, but it is important to check on the licensing and certification requirements for the state in which you plan to practice and for the practice settings (e.g., schools, hospitals, home health agencies, birth-to-3 programs) in which you intend to participate.

MOVING FORWARD AND LOOKING BACK

We have begun to talk here about what it means to be a clinician. What it means for you personally will unfold as you consolidate your knowledge and test it in your practicum experiences. It is our hope that you will acquire some of that knowledge from your interactions with this book's authors and their chapters. But as you acquire this new knowledge, do not let yourself forget the things you have always known. When you begin to feel overwhelmed by all the new things you must learn, by all the facts you must amass, by the equipment you must master, by the papers and reports and lesson plans, remember to look back. Look back to the reasons you entered into this process, and remember what motivated you to go through such a long and rigorous training program in the first place. You do not need to leave your humane instincts behind. If you find yourself faced with a situation like the ones Jane, Jamie, Colin, or Kate encountered, trust your intuition. As you move forward in your clinical education, your newly gained knowledge will inform your actions, but it will never replace the humane motive of bringing the birthright of communication to every individual. This is the impulse that first set you on your present path, and it should continue to guide your steps throughout your career.

REFERENCES

Individuals with Disabilities Education Improvement Act of 2004, PL 108-446, 20 U.S.C. §§ 1400 *et seq.*
No Child Left Behind Act of 2001, PL 107-110, 115 Stat. 1425, 20 U.S.C. §§ 6301 *et seq.*

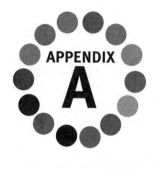

APPENDIX A

An Outline of Standards for the Certificate of Clinical Competence in Audiology

Effective January 1, 2007

STANDARD I: THE DEGREE

- Candidates must have a minimum of 75 semester credit hours of post-baccalaureate education culminating in a recognized graduate degree. Beginning in January 2012, applicants must have a doctoral degree.

STANDARD II: THE INSTITUTION

- The graduate degree must be obtained from an accredited institution of higher education.

- The graduate degree must be completed in a program accredited by the Council on Academic Accreditation in Audiology and Speech-language Pathology (CAA) of ASHA.

STANDARD III: PROGRAM OF STUDY

- Candidates must complete a minimum of 75 semester credit hours that includes academic coursework and a minimum of 12 months' full-time equivalent supervised clinical practicum. Supervision must be provided by an individual who holds the appropriate CCC.

The information in this appendix can be found at http://asha.org. ©American Speech-Language-Hearing Association; adapted with permission.

STANDARD IV: KNOWLEDGE AND SKILLS

- Candidates must have a foundation of prerequisite knowledge and skills
  - Oral and written communication
  - Knowledge and course work in
    - Life sciences
    - Physical sciences
    - Behavioral sciences
    - Mathematics
- Candidates must have acquired knowledge in
  - Foundations of practice
    - Professional codes of ethics and credentialing
    - Patient characteristics (e.g., age, demographics, cultural and linguistic diversity, medical history and status, cognitive status, physical and sensory abilities) and how they relate to clinical services
    - Educational, vocational, social, and psychological effects of hearing impairment and their impact on the development of a treatment program
    - Anatomy and physiology, pathophysiology, embryology, and development of the auditory and vestibular systems
    - Normal development of speech and language
    - Phonologic, morphologic, syntactic, and pragmatic aspects of human communication associated with hearing impairment
    - Normal processes of speech and language production and perception over the life span
    - Normal aspects of auditory physiology and behavior over the life span
    - Principles, methods, and applications of psychoacoustics
    - Effects of chemical agents on the auditory and vestibular systems
    - Instrumentation and bioelectrical hazards
    - Infectious and contagious diseases and universal precautions
    - Physical characteristics and measurement of acoustic stimuli
    - Physical characteristics and measurement of electric and other nonacoustic stimuli
    - Principles and practices of research, including experimental design, statistical methods, and application to clinical populations
    - Medical and surgical procedures for treatment of disorders affecting auditory and vestibular systems
    - Health care and educational delivery systems

- Ramifications of cultural diversity on professional practice
- Supervisory processes and procedures
- Laws, regulations, policies, and management practices relevant to the profession of audiology
- Manual communication, use of interpreters, and assistive technology
- Prevention and identification
  - Interact effectively with patients, families, professionals, and other appropriate individuals
  - Prevent the onset and minimize the development of communication disorders
  - Identify individuals at risk for hearing impairment
  - Screen individuals for hearing impairment and disability using clinically appropriate and culturally sensitive screening measures
  - Screen individuals for speech and language impairments and other factors affecting communication function using clinically appropriate and culturally sensitive screening measures
  - Administer conservation programs designed to reduce the effects of noise exposure and of agents that are toxic to the auditory and vestibular systems
- Evaluation
  - Interact effectively with patients, families, professionals, and other appropriate individuals
  - Evaluate information from appropriate sources to facilitate assessment planning
  - Obtain a case history
  - Perform an otoscopic examination
  - Determine the need for cerumen removal
  - Administer clinically appropriate and culturally sensitive assessment measures
  - Perform audiologic assessment using physiologic, psychophysical, and self-assessment measures
  - Perform electrodiagnostic test procedures
  - Perform balance system assessment and determine the need for balance rehabilitation
  - Perform aural rehabilitation assessment
  - Document evaluation procedures and results
  - Interpret results of the evaluation to establish type and severity of disorder

- Generate recommendations and referrals resulting from the evaluation process
- Provide counseling to facilitate understanding of the auditory or balance disorder
- Maintain records in a manner consistent with legal and professional standards
- Communicate results and recommendations orally and in writing to the patient and other appropriate individuals
- Use instrumentation according to manufacturer's specifications and recommendations
- Determine whether instrumentation is in calibration according to accepted standards

- Treatment
  - Interact effectively with patients, families, professionals, and other appropriate individuals
  - Develop and implement treatment plan using appropriate data
  - Discuss prognosis and treatment options with appropriate individuals
  - Counsel patients, families, and other appropriate individuals
  - Develop culturally sensitive and age-appropriate management strategies
  - Collaborate with other service providers in case coordination
  - Perform hearing aid, assistive listening device, and sensory aid assessment
  - Recommend, dispense, and service prosthetic and assistive devices
  - Provide hearing aid, assistive listening device, and sensory aid orientation
  - Conduct aural rehabilitation
  - Monitor and summarize treatment progress and outcomes
  - Assess efficacy of interventions for auditory and balance disorders
  - Establish treatment admission and discharge criteria
  - Serve as an advocate for patients, families, and other appropriate individuals
  - Document treatment procedures and results
  - Maintain records in a manner consistent with legal and professional standards
  - Communicate results, recommendations and progress to appropriate individuals.

- Use instrumentation according to manufacturers' specifications and recommendations
- Determine whether instrumentation is in calibration according to accepted standards

STANDARD V: OUTCOMES ASSESSMENT

- The candidate must successfully complete formative (ongoing) and summative (final) assessment of the knowledge and skills in Standard IV.

STANDARD VI: MAINTAINING CERTIFICATION

- As of January 1, 2003, audiologists must accumulate 3 continuing education credits (30 contact hours) from approved providers every 3 years.

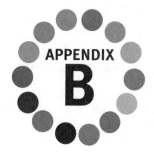

APPENDIX B

An Outline of Standards for the Certificate of Clinical Competence in Speech-Language Pathology

Effective January 1, 2005

STANDARD I: THE DEGREE

- Candidates must have a master's or doctoral degree.

- Graduate work must be in the area of certification and completed in a Council on Academic Accreditation (CAA) accredited program.

- A minimum of 75 semester credit hours of must be completed in speech-language pathology.

- A minimum of 36 semester credit hours must be earned at the graduate level.

STANDARD II: THE INSTITUTION

- The graduate degree must be obtained from an accredited institution of higher education.

- The graduate degree must be completed in a program accredited by the CAA of ASHA.

The information in this appendix can be found at http://asha.org. ©American Speech-Language-Hearing Association; adapted with permission.

STANDARD III: KNOWLEDGE OUTCOMES

- The candidate must present skills in oral and written communication sufficient for clinical practice.

- The candidate must demonstrate knowledge and show transcript credit in each of the following areas:

  - Biological sciences

  - Physical sciences

  - Mathematics

  - Social and behavioral sciences

- The candidate must demonstrate knowledge of human communication and swallowing processes.

- The candidate must demonstrate knowledge of the nature of speech, language, hearing, swallowing, and communication disorders, specifically in:

  - Articulation

  - Fluency

  - Voice and resonance

  - Receptive and expressive language in speaking, listening, reading, and writing modalities

  - Hearing

  - Swallowing

  - Cognitive aspects of communication (e.g., attention, memory, sequencing, problem solving, executive function)

  - Social aspects of communication (e.g., multicultural aspects, challenging behaviors, lack of communication opportunities

  - Nonoral communicative modalities

- The candidate must demonstrate knowledge of prevention, assessment, and intervention for communication and swallowing disorders.

- The candidate must demonstrate knowledge of standards of ethical conduct.

- The candidate must demonstrate knowledge of processes used in research and the integration of research principles in clinical practice.

- The candidate must demonstrate knowledge of contemporary professional issues.

- The candidate must demonstrate knowledge of certification, specialty recognition, licensure, and other professional credentials.

STANDARD IV: SKILL OUTCOMES

- The candidate must complete at least 400 clock hours of supervised clinical practicum. 25 of these hours must be spent in clinical observation, and the other 375 hours in client contact.

- At least 325 hours must be completed at the graduate level.

- Practicum must be supervised by an appropriately certified individual, at a level appropriate to the student's development, but not less than 25% of the student's client contact time.

- Practicum must include experience with clients across the life-span and from culturally different backgrounds, with various types and severities of communication disorders.

- Supervised clinical experiences must include:

  - Evaluation

    - Screening and prevention

    - Case history and report writing

    - Selection and administration of tests, behavioral observation, and other nonstandardized procedures

    - Adaptation of evaluation procedures to meet client needs

    - Interpretation and synthesis of information for diagnosis and recommendations

    - Completion of administration and reporting functions

    - Client referral

  - Intervention

    - Development of intervention plans with measurable, appropriate goals by collaborating with families

    - Implementation of intervention plans

    - Selection of appropriate materials and instrumentation

    - Measurement of performance and progress

    - Completion of administration and reporting functions

    - Identification and referral of clients

  - Interaction

    - Communication effectively, recognizing needs, values, and cultural background of clients and other individuals

    - Collaborate with other professionals

    - Provide counseling regarding communication and swallowing disorders

    - Adhere to the Code of Ethics

STANDARD V: ASSESSMENT

- The candidate must successfully complete formative (ongoing) and summative (final) assessment of the knowledge and skills in Standards II and IV.

STANDARD VI: CLINICAL FELLOWSHIP YEAR

- The candidate must complete a year (36 weeks) of full-time supervised professional employment in clinical service delivery or clinical research.

STANDARD VII: MAINTAINING CERTIFICATION

- As of January 1, 2005, speech-language pathologists must accumulate 3 continuing education credits (30 contact hours) from approved providers every 3 years.

CHAPTER 2

Ethical and Professional Practices

PAUL W. CASCELLA

Case Example 1

Michelle is a speech-language pathologist (SLP) at a local rehabilitation center in a busy urban New England community. Because of ongoing expansion by the rehabilitation agency over the past five years, the speech-language pathology department has employed speech therapy assistants to help manage the clinical caseload. As a supervisor, Michelle has found that these assistants are dedicated and able to implement treatment plans and procedures that she has taught them. Of late, Michelle has found that her own job has spread her thin across agency committees, task forces, and the new satellite birth-to-three program across town. As a result, she finds that she is less often able to directly supervise the speech assistants and she relies on telephone and e-mail consultation to review client data sheets and case notes. After talking with Nicole, one of her especially talented speech assistants, Michelle has allowed Nicole to modify a treatment plan for three adults with aphasia even though Michelle has not directly seen these patients in the past 4 weeks.

Case Example 2

Tom is an audiologist who works at a local teaching hospital which contracts with four skilled nursing facilities. In this contract, residents participate in audiological evaluations and follow-up, usually the first and third Tuesdays of every month. On any of these days, Tom may see up to 20 people from any or all of the four nursing facilities. On one particularly busy day, Tom has a list of residents who are scheduled for appointments, but he loses track of which patients kept their appointments, which residents cancelled, and who was added at the last minute. At the end of the day, Tom sits down to write his casenotes on the residents. Unfortunately, because the day was so busy, Tom cannot be sure of which residents were seen and which ones had cancelled. When he goes to complete billing, he accidentally bills for services for two residents who were not actually seen that day.

Case Example 3

Adam is a preschool SLP who works for a local public school. Whenever a new student is seen for a speech-language evaluation, Adam collects case history information, including medical information about the child. During a recent evaluation, Adam learned that Jasmine, a 3-year-old girl with specific language impairment was born prematurely and had prenatal exposure to alcohol and cocaine. Adam is also an assistant coach for the high school baseball team in the same public school district. That afternoon, he mentions Jasmine's name to one of the other coaches and comments on her prenatal exposure to substances.

INTRODUCTION

As a beginning clinician in speech-language pathology or audiology, you may confront ethical situations not unlike the ones described for Michelle, Tom, and Adam. Each of us has our own personal standards and perceptions of ethical behavior. When thinking about the term **ethics,** it is common to consider the moral and/or civil codes of conduct for a particular person, situation, community, religious group, organization, or society. These codes evolve from a philosophy of human interaction which values behaviors that are personally or collectively regarded as good, honest, proper, and respectable. Each of us has a set of **personal ethics** that have been formed from our upbringing, acculturation, life experiences, personal choices, and education. As children, our parents were likely to stress that certain behaviors were right or wrong. Some of us were taught the Golden Rule (i.e., "Do unto others..."), to treat older people with respect, to tell the truth, to play fairly in sports competitions, and to never cheat on exams. As adults, we consciously choose our own individual ethics and values. These guide us to interact with our families and friends in what we personally consider the right way to behave and our sense of duty, responsibility, and obligation. Personal ethics are important because they enable us to make choices about our own behavior. Personal ethics differ from person to person, and not everyone with similar ethical tenets applies them in the same way. Therefore, many professions abide by a set of **professional ethics** that establish right and wrong actions in serving clients in the workplace. Professional ethics publicly state the common core values and collective obligation shared by persons in a particular discipline. Though each of us brings our personal ethics to clinical practice, the American Speech-Language-Hearing Association (ASHA) and the American Academy of Audiology (AAA) have codified a set of standards for ethical behavior. Each organization has its own **Code of Ethics** that includes tangible expectations that define acceptable conduct and conscientious judgment. As members of the communication disorders discipline, each of us is expected to accept these tenets and apply them to clinical settings. A professional code of ethics enables us to look toward a common set of core values when confronted with ethical dilemmas in the workplace. Table 2.1 gives a list of reasons for a professional code of ethics.

This chapter introduces you to the ethical standards that are the foundation of clinical practice in speech-language pathology and audiology. Ethical principles are presented and case situations that may raise ethical dilemmas are described. As you read the examples of ethical dilemmas, take a moment to pause and

Table 2.1. Reasons for a professional code of ethics

1. Consumer protection and client welfare are safeguarded.
2. The professional reputation of the discipline is maintained.
3. Professional behavior is regulated.
4. Objective guidance is available for ethical dilemmas and deliberation.
5. Practitioners can rely on an external code in addition to their own values.
6. Clients have an objective standard against which to evaluate their clinician's actions.

consider your personal response. The ASHA Code of Ethics is reprinted in its entirety in the appendix at the end of this chapter and you are encouraged to access the AAA Code of Ethics via the webpage http://www.audiology.org. An overview of the two Codes of Ethics follows.

SYNOPSES OF THE AMERICAN SPEECH-LANGUAGE-HEARING ASSOCIATION (ASHA) AND THE AMERICAN ACADEMY OF AUDIOLOGY (AAA) CODES OF ETHICS

The ASHA Code of Ethics

The ASHA Code of Ethics (ASHA, 2003) applies to people who are already credentialed (i.e., the Certificate of Clinical Competence—Speech-Language Pathology [CCC-SLP]; the Certificate of Clinical Competence—Audiology [CCC-A]), candidates in process of earning those credentials (i.e., students, Clinical Fellowship Year [CFY] participants), and members of the organization. The ASHA Code of Ethics consists of three parts: the Preamble, Principles of Ethics, and Rules of Ethics. The Preamble introduces the philosophy of ethical service delivery and the overall content, principles, and structure of the Code. Principles of Ethics are divided into four parts, each of which provides a broad statement about ethical conduct. Principles of Ethics I and II relate to the delivery of services to clients. Principle of Ethics III outlines standards related to interaction with the public, and Principle of Ethics IV outlines standards and responsibilities to the profession. Within each Principle of Ethics there are Rules of Ethics which are statements that articulate acceptable and restricted actions pertaining to each principle. In matters where ethical violations may occur, ASHA has a Board of Ethics that handles the adjudication of alleged violations (ASHA, 2003).

The AAA Code of Ethics

The AAA Code of Ethics (AAA, 2003) applies to current and potential members of this organization. The AAA Code of Ethics consists of two parts: Statements of Principles and Rules and Procedures for Management of Alleged Violations. Statements of Principles and Rules highlight specific actions deemed ethically acceptable to audiology practice. Procedures for the Management of Alleged Violations outline the due process format when violations are suspected, as well as the penalties that can be assigned. This section also outlines record keeping, confidentiality, and public disclosure.

ETHICAL PRINCIPLES IN PROFESSIONAL PRACTICE

To begin our discussion of ethics, we start by considering some of the common core principles shared by AAA and ASHA.

The Principle of Safeguarding Client Welfare

At the core of ethical practice is a guarantee that clinicians will act to ensure the dignity, protection, and autonomy of client rights. Let us look at some concrete examples of how clinicians can guarantee client welfare.

Beneficence and Nonmaleficence   **Beneficence** means that professionals promote the interests and welfare of others while **nonmaleficence** means that professionals deliberately avoid inflicting potential or actual harm (e.g., emotional harm, physical harm) on clients. These principles compel professionals to monitor their own behavior as well as that of caregivers who interact with clients. For example, we are expected to report situations in which we perceive that children, adults, or elders may be victims of physical, emotional, and/or sexual abuse, as well as neglect by their caregivers.

Nondiscrimination   How would you feel at parent-teacher night when you learn that Timothy, a 7-year-old boy who stutters, has two mothers for parents? Or, how would you react when another child's parent asks, "Have you accepted Jesus as your personal savior?" How might you feel when you are assigned to work with a class of preschoolers, one of whom is being raised by her grandparents because her mother is incarcerated? Or, maybe one of your hospital outpatient clients is a transgendered woman who wants speech therapy so that her voice sounds more like a woman's. These may be difficult situations for you based on your own personal values; still, every client's right to quality services is guaranteed because clinicians must practice **nondiscrimination.** This means that clinicians do not exclude clients from their professional practice for reasons other than the person's potential to benefit from our services. Ethical practice is compromised when a clinician discriminates by making a clinical decision based on a client's race, gender, ethnicity, religion, age, national origin, sexual orientation, or disability status.

Referral   Another example of securing a client's welfare is the use of **referral.** This occurs when an SLP or audiologist feels that a client presents a communication disorder beyond the clinician's level of expertise. Professional referrals safeguard a client's right to appropriate clinical services. Let us take our example of the transgendered client. A referral would be appropriate if a clinician has no experience in gender-appropriate voice treatment approaches and thus would be unable to provide that person with competent voice services. In contrast, when we receive a referral, we are expected to exercise independent judgment about the content, frequency, and duration of services that may be recommended. In other words, outside influences should not interfere with evaluation and treatment decisions. For example, an audiologist may receive a physician referral to fit a client with a hearing aid because the physician noted that client had some difficulty hearing case history questions during a physical exam. Before proceeding with a hearing aid, the audiologist should first complete an independent hearing evaluation to assess client need and/or potential to benefit from such equipment. For either type of referral (i.e., *by* the clinician or *to* the clinician), we are prohibited from receiving a commission or gift that could influence our professional practice and decision making.

Informed Consent   **Informed consent** means that clients are told about their speech-language or hearing condition and are informed about the relative strengths, weaknesses, and risks (i.e., side effects) associated with a recommended plan of action or inaction. For people who are unable to authorize legal consent (i.e., children, people with an intellectual disability), this must be obtained from family members or legal guardians. With informed consent, the clinician enables the client to exercise autonomy during the course of treatment. This principle also guarantees that clients can voluntarily withdraw from a treatment protocol at any point during its course. For example, think about how you would react to a middle school child who decides that he no longer wants stuttering therapy even though his speech continues to include blocks, prolongations, and repetitions? How might you attempt to guarantee his welfare if he voluntarily withdraws from treatment?

Confidentiality   In daily practice, we often hear clinical and personal information about clients (i.e., health status, medical history, educational background, cognitive status, financial status, family structure, etc.). Sometimes, it may be very tempting to share this information with people not affiliated with the client's treatment protocol. The principle of **confidentiality** means that professionals share privileged information only with people directly responsible for client management and/or care and only for purposes related to the client's welfare. As professionals, we are bound to neither use privileged information for gossip within a work setting nor to repeat any confidential information outside of the clinical environment. This requires some self-control on the clinician's part, as it is too easy to slip into talking about clients in the teacher's lounge or hospital elevator when others, who should not be privy to the information discussed, may be within earshot. In addition, a federal law (the Health Insurance Portability and Accountability Act of 1996 [HIPAA], PL 104-191) mandates that clients have rights and protections regarding how and to whom their health information is shared. This information includes medical records and conversations between clients and health care providers. Client confidentiality may become an ethical dilemma when precedents override the client's right to confidentiality in law or other compelling circumstances. This might arise, for example, if you are working with an adult with aphasia who expresses in therapy that he wants to kill himself. It might come up too, if a mother confides to you that her child's stepfather has repeatedly hit the child. Should these statements compel you to breach your client's right to confidentiality?

Prognosis and Cures   Implicit in ethical practice is that professionals must not imply or guarantee cures. Instead, clinicians are expected to make a reasonable **prognosis,** or a statement that describes the likelihood that a benefit will be gained from treatment. If a person is not likely to benefit from initial or ongoing treatment, intervention should not be recommended or continued. In practice, this means that we do not recommend treatment for every person who has a speech-language or hearing disorder. Instead we exercise professional judgment about the likelihood that treatment will yield a client benefit. For example, how would you handle a situation in which family members insist on speech therapy services for a person with advanced dementia residing in a nursing facility?

Infection Control   Clinicians are expected to safeguard their clients and themselves from infectious diseases by maintaining **infection control** and prevention procedures. Hygienic precautions usually include hand washing and the use of barriers (e.g., gloves, masks). In addition, clinicians are expected to disinfect equipment and know the proper procedures for the disposal of bodily fluids (e.g., saliva, blood). All clinicians are expected to practice universal precautions, even if they do not work in a medical setting. In other words, universal precautions apply to preschools and schools, child care settings, home health, university clinics, birth-to-3 programs, group homes, and private practices. For example, it would not be remarkable for you to handle bodily fluids if you are working with an infant-toddler early intervention group. Table 2.2 shows a list of common infection control procedures.

The Principle of Competence

Another core ethical principle for audiologists and SLPs is **competent practice.** This occurs when a clinician provides effective diagnostic procedures, accurate prognosis, and appropriate therapy strategies for the particular disorder, as well as an ongoing analysis of client outcomes. Both ASHA and AAA have several practice guidelines that enable clinicians to evaluate their own professional competence. For example, ASHA has preferred practice documents for specific populations, including assessment and intervention for infants and toddlers, swallowing, preschool speech-language and communication, assessment and intervention, and speech-language screenings for children and adults (ASHA, 2004c). Clinicians can refer to these documents for guidance about competent practice.

Ethical practice obligates that each of us clearly understand our own strengths and limitations and that we practice only in those areas in which we regard ourselves as competent. For example, how can you address the communication

Table 2.2.   Infection control procedures

Hand washing	You must vigorously lather and rub your hands, wrists, and forearms with warm water and liquid antibacterial soap before and after each clinical session.
Disposable gloves	You must wear disposable gloves when you have contact with clients' bodily fluids or substances (e.g., saliva, blood, cerumen, vomit).
Contaminated items	Consumable items (e.g., gloves, tongue depressors) that contacted with clients' bodily fluids or substances must be disposed of into a plastic bag and tied securely. Nonconsumable items (e.g., eartips, specula) must be decontaminated.
Decontamination/disinfecting	Disinfectant must be thoroughly applied to all non-consumable items, clinical materials, and clinical furniture. A solution of one-tenth bleach and nine-tenths water is recommended.
Illness	Clinical sessions should be rescheduled when either the clinician or the client has an infectious illness or condition.
Vaccinations	Clinicians should seriously consider vaccination for hepatitis B, rubella, and the mumps. Clinicians are also encouraged to have a yearly tuberculosis test.

needs of a child with autism spectrum disorder if you have no previous experience working with this condition? Or, what if you find yourself in a situation in which you have been laid off from your hospital adult neurogenics position and find that the only local job openings are in home-based birth-to-3 services? Is it ethical to provide services when you do not have prior experience in a particular clinical setting? Many audiologists and SLPs become specialists for a particular population, disorder and/or service delivery model. **Specialization** occurs with in-depth experience, advanced knowledge, and training beyond the initial credential. Whether a specialist or a generalist, each of us is expected to be lifelong learners who maintain clinical competency through continuing education. **Continuing education** enables clinicians to update their skills by keeping current of the latest trends and advances in their discipline. This can be achieved by reading textbooks and journal articles, attending workshops, taking a course at a local university, shadowing professional colleagues, and participating in research activities.

Ethical clinicians judge their own fitness for providing services and withdraw from practice if their own professional conduct is influenced by substance abuse or related health conditions. Similarly, it is expected that clinicians will monitor the ethical compliance of other SLPs and audiologists. Ethical compliance relies on clinicians who keep up to date on contemporary issues that influence clinical practice. Table 2.3 provides examples of several issues that uniquely challenge us to balance our ethics and competency.

The Principle of Acting without a Conflict of Interest

A **conflict of interest** occurs when an SLP or audiologist accepts personal or financial gifts from clients or manufacturers that compromise professional judgment because there are strings and/or expectations attached. When a conflict of interest arises, clinicians can lose their sense of objectivity and their decision making becomes clouded. Examples of potential conflicts of interest include self-dealing (utilizing commercial enterprises in which you have a financial stake) and self-referral (referring patients between two work settings, both of which employ the same clinician). A conflict of interest might also occur when a clinician draws

Table 2.3. Contemporary issues that may influence ethical competence

Competition	Clinicians must balance ethics with competition for employment and the market share (i.e., competitive bidding, marketing, advertising).
Service eligibility	Clinicians must balance client specific data (i.e., prognosis) with federal and state education and health care regulations to decide who is likely to benefit from clinical services and how services should be provided.
Discharge	Clinicians must be able to carefully balance the ethical issues surrounding client discharge, especially when the clinician's judgment disagrees with the client, organizational policies, and/or funding resources.
Resources	When resources are lacking in public education (e.g., budget, shortage of personnel), clinicians must continue to act competently.
Managed care	Clinicians must balance ongoing changes in medical reimbursement and the cost of health care with the needs presented by clients.
Scope of practice	Clinicians must stay both current on and judicious of the latest technologies within clinical practice.
Paraprofessionals	Clinicians must be able to carefully judge the utilization of speech assistants and aides in service delivery.

cases for private practice from their primary place of employment. This can occur especially when school-based clinicians provide private services to children during the summer recess. In and of itself, this is not a conflict of interest so long as the school administration is aware of these services and clients are fully informed about service options and costs.

The Principle of Acting without Misrepresentation

Case Example 4

Adele is an SLP at a local community hospital whose staff is developing a marketing plan to attract more business. Because there are many community-based speech-language-hearing providers, an advertising strategy that "catches the eye" is being sought. After a morning meeting, it has been decided that more clients will be drawn to this hospital if Adele's auditory processing remediation program is advertised as one of the best in the state. Adele does not feel right about this decision, even though she is confidant that the program is effective. Adele knows that she has not done efficacy research or published her results for professional review.[1]

Later that day, Adele participates in a meeting with hospital administration where it is noted that patient billable hours have decreased with the implementation of a new insurance reimbursement system. At the meeting, Adele is informed that without this reimbursement, the speech pathology staff is likely to lose personnel. Adele also learns that particular diagnoses are guaranteed reimbursement, as are persons for whom the prognosis for improvement is rated as "good." Although it is never directly stated, Adele feels as though she is encouraged to reconsider the diagnostic criteria for particular diagnoses, as well as the factors that relate to prognosis.

How would you respond if you were Adele? Because of her morning meeting, she is concerned that the hospital advertising strategy may be a form of misrepresentation. **Misrepresentation** is a type of dishonesty that occurs when truth is distorted or falsified. In this case, misrepresentation occurs because there is an exaggerated description of Adele's auditory processing program. Even though Adele has observed the benefits of the program, she knows that its efficacy has not been scientifically tested. Another example of misrepresentation can occur if clinicians exaggerate their own personal levels of training, experience, and expertise or that of persons who provide clinical services (i.e., Clinical Fellowship Year [CFY] participants, graduate students, speech assistants, aides). Clients should be specifically informed about the educational level of the person providing services.

Because of her afternoon meeting, Adele continues to be concerned about misrepresentation. Here, she is being asked to ignore competent clinical diagnostic procedures (i.e., criteria, prognosis) to secure insurance reimbursement. In effect, Adele would be misrepresenting the client's status by making a diagnosis and a prognosis solely to maintain the financial solvency of her employer.

Finally, another form of misrepresentation occurs when a clinician unfairly influences client decisions by "stacking the deck" a particular way, such as by

---

[1] From American Speech-Language-Hearing Association (1993). *Ethics: Resources for professional preparation and practice.* Rockville, MD: Author; adapted by permission.

deliberately leading the client to a decision in the clinician's, not the client's, best interest. Ethically, clients are guaranteed access to all of the information necessary for making decisions about their care and rehabilitation. We are not supposed to unfairly mislead a client by omitting information that would otherwise be helpful in client decision-making. For example, for clients with a hearing loss, audiologists should provide information about the variety of hearing aids (e.g., brand, type, cost, size) that might be beneficial to a particular client.

Ethical Practice within Professional Supervision and Instruction

SLPs and audiologists often supervise other people as part of their job description. We may supervise people who are already credentialed (i.e., persons with a Certificate of Clinical Competence [CCC], teaching certification, or state license), CFY participants, student-clinicians, or speech assistants/aides. Clinical supervisors should model ethical behavior, and they are expected to monitor the ethical compliance of the persons they supervise. When an unethical behavior is suspected or observed, the supervisor must take specific action to prevent violation of ethical standards, whether or not the person supervised is credentialed or an ASHA or AAA member.

For CFY participants, it is expected that the supervisor will make a good-faith effort to meet the terms (i.e., expectations, follow-up) outlined in the CFY contract (ASHA, 2004a). For student clinicians, ASHA guidelines require that supervisors hold the appropriate CCC credential, provide an appropriate amount and type of diagnostic and clinical supervision, and provide ongoing written and oral feedback to the student. ASHA also has a practice guideline that outlines the supervision requirements of speech-language pathology assistants (ASHA, 2004b).

Ethical Behavior within Professional Relationships

Clinicians are expected to maintain **professional relationships** with other communication specialists, as well as with personnel from other professions. There are many ways to demonstrate collegial behavior. First, we can work to understand the nature of related disciplines and the particular job functions of our teaching, medical, and allied health colleagues. Second, professional behavior includes a give-and-take open communication style so that all team members have the opportunity to discuss pertinent issues in a client's treatment plan. Third, education and rehabilitation professionals are expected to work in a climate of mutual respect and cooperation by avoiding personal conflict. This is especially true given recent efforts in transdisciplinary service provision, inclusive education, and team teaching models.

THE IMPLEMENTATION OF ETHICAL PRACTICE FOR CLINICIANS

With a foundation in ethical principles, it is important that practicing and future clinicians have an understanding of how to judge their own compliance with ethical practice standards. All clinicians benefit from having a framework in which ethical situations can be discussed and debated. One such approach has been developed by Seymour (1994) and called the **Ethics Calibration Quick Test** (ECQT; see Figure 2.1). Using the ECQT, we are able to analyze the ethical

1. What is the problem/conflict/dilemma?

   Is it a professional violation, a legal violation, or both?

2. What values are in conflict?

   Under these circumstances, what do I value the most?

   Will my feelings interfere with my judgment?

3. What evidence is provided by the parties involved?

   Whose evidence is most convincing?

   Is there a consistency in the facts?

   Have I heard all of the facts?

   What is acceptable practice in this situation?

   Who is most believable?

   Have I considered other viewpoints?

4. What courses of action can I take or recommend?

   Do I need outside consultation?

   Have I considered the social, cultural, and political impact of the consequences?

   Have I considered the short-term and long-term impact of the consequences?

5. In whose best interest is the decision?

   Will the decision be fair to all parties concerned?

   If yes, why? If not, why?

6. How will the decision make me feel about myself today and tomorrow?

Figure 2.1. Using the Ethics Calibration Quick Test, clinicians are able to analyze the ethical propriety of a situation by considering the ethical conflict, the values that are involved, the evidence, the possible plans of action, and the decision-making process. (From *Professional issues in speech-language pathology and audiology, first edition,* by R. Lubinki and C. Frattali [Eds]. ©1994. Reprinted with permission of Delmar, a division of Thomson Learning. Fax: 800-730-2215.)

propriety of a situation by considering the ethical conflict, the values that are involved, the evidence, the possible plans of action, and the decision-making process. After you review the ECQT, return to Case Examples 1, 2, and 3 at the beginning of the chapter and make a judgment about Michelle, Tom, and Adam's ethical compliance. In Case Example 1, you should be concerned about the degree of supervision Michelle provides to the speech assistants and whether she should allow a speech assistant, even a talented one, to modify a treatment program. For Michelle, this situation calls for the hiring of another SLP and a review of ASHA's guidelines about the supervision of speech-language pathology assistants (ASHA, 2004b). In Case Example 2, Tom has billed for services not rendered and has unintentionally committed fraud. Also, because Tom cannot be certain about which clients received which services, his ability to keep accurate records should be questioned. Tom needs to develop a more accurate and reliable system for keeping records. In Case Example 3, Adam needs to be careful about client confidentiality and privileged information. Even though other baseball coaches are employed by the school district, there is no reason for them to be told privileged information about a child. Adam needs to review the school district's policy on educational confidentiality.

Another model for ethical decision-making comes from Chabon and Morris (2004; see Figure 2.2) who proposed a consensus model for ethical decisions. In this model, the clinician is encouraged to evaluate the specific facts and values so as to specifically state the ethical dilemma. Then, the analysis includes the possible courses of action and the degree to which these are consistent with professional standards, social rules, and self-interests.

Ethical Practice Review by AAA and ASHA

In addition to our own evaluation of ethical scenarios, both AAA and ASHA have centralized committees that address ethical situations. The AAA committee is called the **Ethical Practice Board,** and the ASHA committee is called the

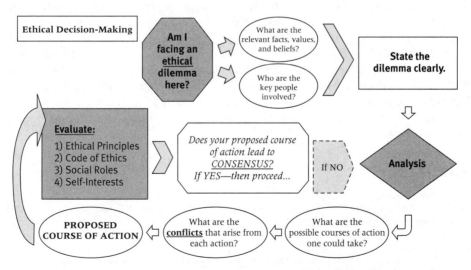

Figure 2.2. A consensus model for ethical decisions. (From Chabon, S.S., & Morris, J.F. [2004, February 17]. A consensus model for making ethical decisions in a less-than-ideal world. *The ASHA Leader,* 17; reprinted by permission.)

Board of Ethics. One role of these groups is to develop position statements that further define particular ethical rules already cited in each code. A second role of these committees is to handle the adjudication process when violations are alleged. Through a due process format, complaints are heard, evidence can be admitted, sanctions or penalties are applied, and appeals are processed. A third role of these committees is to educate ASHA and AAA members about ethics. One way the ASHA committee educates its members is by placing teaching situations in a periodic column in *The ASHA Leader* that discusses case situations that highlight specific ethical actions, for example, the following Case Example. As a final task, try using the ECQT or the consensus model to analyze this case example.

Case Example 5

Ms. Robertson, a 78-year-old, is hospitalized after a hip fracture. A speech-language consultation is requested because her physician is concerned about her cognitive abilities. Scott, a student clinician, conducts the evaluation. He observes mild cognitive deficits, but he also notes that Ms. Robertson coughs immediately after taking sips of water and that she has a wet voice quality for several minutes after drinking. From the medical record, Scott notes that she had pneumonia on admission to the hospital and has been treated for pneumonia at least three times in the past 9 months.

Scott discusses his observations with his supervisor and recommends a swallowing evaluation. His supervisor suggests Ms. Robertson coughs because she is recovering from pneumonia. Furthermore, the supervisor says they were consulted for a cognitive assessment, and thus his observations about her swallowing are inappropriate to include in his report. Scott is concerned about the patient, but unsure of his role as a student and questions how to interpret his own observations.[2]

CONCLUSION

By introducing you to ethical practice, this chapter probably causes you to think about your own personal ethics and the degree to which they are consistent with the professional ethics set by ASHA and AAA. Ethical guidelines will enable you to protect the rights and welfare of your clients. Professional Codes of Ethics provide you with an objective set of standards against which to compare your daily professional actions. By adhering to standards and ethical principles, we are collectively able to promote our clients' welfare, as well as safeguard our own professional reputations and those of the professions of speech-language pathology and audiology.

REFERENCES

American Academy of Audiology. (2003). *Code of ethics*. Houston: Author.
American Speech-Language-Hearing Association (2003). Code of Ethics (revised), *ASHA Supplement, 23*, 13–15.

---

[2] From Blake, A. (1999). When student and supervisor disagree about patient care. *ASHA, 41*(6), 65; reprinted by permission.

American Speech-Language-Hearing Association. (2004a). Clinical fellowship supervisor's responsibilities. *ASHA Supplement, 24*, 36–38.

American Speech-Language-Hearing Association. (2004b). *Guidelines for the training, use, and supervision of speech-language pathology assistants.* Retrieved October 1, 2005, from http://www.asha.org/members/deskref-journals/deskref/default

American Speech-Language-Hearing Association. (2004c). *Preferred practice patterns for the profession of speech-language pathology.* Retrieved October 1, 2005, from http://www.asha.org/members/deskref-journal/deskref/default

American Speech-Language-Hearing Association. (2004d). *Statements of practices and procedures of the Board of Ethics.* Retrieved October 1, 2005, from http://www.asha.org/members/deskref-journals/deskref

Chabon, S.S., & Morris, J.F. (2004, February 17). A consensus model for making ethical decisions in a less-than-ideal world. *The ASHA Leader,* 17.

Health Insurance Portability and Accountability Act (HIPAA) of 1996, PL 104-191, 42 U.S.C. §§ 201 *et seq.*

Lubinki, R., & Frattali, C. (Eds.). (1994). *Professional issues in speech-language pathology and audiology, first edition.* Clifton Park, NY: Thomson Delmar Learning.

STUDY QUESTIONS

1. Why is it important to have ethical standards in professional practice?

2. Give three examples of how a SLP or audiologist can safeguard a client's welfare?

3. Identify two ways in which a clinician can maintain his or her competence.

4. Describe three external factors that influence clinical competence. Why is it important that a clinician understand the influence of these factors?

5. Define and give an example of each of the following terms: *misrepresentation, conflict of interest, non-discrimination, infection control, informed consent,* and *referral.*

6. What is the role of the clinical supervisor in ethical practice?

7. Why is it necessary for ASHA and AAA to have committees that review ethical standards and actions?

8. What revisions might your recommend to the ASHA or AAA Code of Ethics? Why?

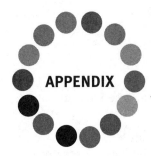

APPENDIX

The ASHA Code of Ethics

Last Revised January 1, 2003

PREAMBLE

The preservation of the highest standards of integrity and ethical principles is vital to the responsible discharge of obligations by speech-language pathologists, audiologists, and speech, language, and hearing scientists. This Code of Ethics sets forth the fundamental principles and rules considered essential to this purpose.

Every individual who is (a) a member of the American Speech-Language-Hearing Association, whether certified or not, (b) a nonmember holding the Certificate of Clinical Competence from the Association, (c) an applicant for membership or certification, or (d) a Clinical Fellow seeking to fulfill standards for certification shall abide by this Code of Ethics.

Any violation of the spirit and purpose of this Code shall be considered unethical. Failure to specify any particular responsibility or practice in this Code of Ethics shall not be construed as denial of the existence of such responsibilities or practices.

The fundamentals of ethical conduct are described by Principles of Ethics and by Rules of Ethics as they relate to the conduct of research and scholarly activities and responsibility to persons served, the public, and speech-language pathologists, audiologists, and speech, language, and hearing scientists.

Principles of Ethics, aspirational and inspirational in nature, form the underlying moral basis for the Code of Ethics. Individuals shall observe these principles as affirmative obligations under all conditions of professional activity. Rules of Ethics are specific statements of minimally acceptable professional conduct or of prohibitions and are applicable to all individuals.

PRINCIPLE OF ETHICS I

Individuals shall honor their responsibility to hold paramount the welfare of persons they serve professionally or participants in research and scholarly activities and shall treat animals involved in research in a humane manner.

From American Speech-Language-Hearing Association. (2003). *Code of ethics (revised)*. Retrieved October 1, 2005, from http://www.asha.org/members/deskref-journals/deskref; reprinted by permission.

Rules of Ethics

A. Individuals shall provide all services competently.

B. Individuals shall use every resource, including referral when appropriate, to ensure that high quality service is provided.

C. Individuals shall not discriminate in the delivery of professional services or the conduct of research and scholarly activities on the basis of race or ethnicity, gender, age, religion, national origin, sexual orientation, or disability.

D. Individuals shall not misrepresent the credentials of assistants, technicians, or support personnel and shall inform those they serve professionally of the name and professional credentials of persons providing services.

E. Individuals who hold the Certificates of Clinical Competence shall not delegate tasks that require the unique skills, knowledge, and judgment that are within the scope of their profession to assistants, technicians, support personnel, students, or any nonprofessionals over whom they have supervisory responsibility. An individual may delegate support services to assistants, technicians, support personnel, students, or any other persons only if those services are adequately supervised by an individual who holds the appropriate Certificate of Clinical Competence.

F. Individuals shall fully inform the persons they serve of the nature and possible effects of services rendered and products dispensed, and they shall inform participants in research about the possible effects of their participation in research conducted.

G. Individuals shall evaluate the effectiveness of services rendered and of products dispensed and shall provide services or dispense products only when benefit can reasonably be expected.

H. Individuals shall not guarantee the results of any treatment or procedure, directly or by implication; however, they may make a reasonable statement of prognosis.

I. Individuals shall not provide clinical services solely by correspondence.

J. Individuals may practice by telecommunication (for example, telehealth/e-health), where not prohibited by law.

K. Individuals shall adequately maintain and appropriately secure records of professional services rendered, research and scholarly activities conducted, and products dispensed and shall allow access to these records only when authorized or when required by law.

L. Individuals shall not reveal, without authorization, any professional or personal information about identified persons served professionally or identified participants involved in research and scholarly activities unless required by law to do so, or unless doing so is necessary to protect the welfare of the person or of the community or otherwise required by law.

M. Individuals shall not charge for services not rendered, nor shall they misrepresent services rendered, products dispensed, or research and scholarly activities conducted.

N. Individuals shall use persons in research or as subjects of teaching demonstrations only with their informed consent.

O. Individuals whose professional services are adversely affected by substance abuse or other health-related conditions shall seek professional assistance and, where appropriate, withdraw from the affected areas of practice.

PRINCIPLE OF ETHICS II

Individuals shall honor their responsibility to achieve and maintain the highest level of professional competence.

Rules of Ethics

A. Individuals shall engage in the provision of clinical services only when they hold the appropriate Certificate of Clinical Competence or when they are in the certification process and are supervised by an individual who holds the appropriate Certificate of Clinical Competence.

B. Individuals shall engage in only those aspects of the professions that are within the scope of their competence, considering their level of education, training, and experience.

C. Individuals shall continue their professional development throughout their careers.

D. Individuals shall delegate the provision of clinical services only to: (1) persons who hold the appropriate Certificate of Clinical Competence; (2) persons in the education or certification process who are appropriately supervised by an individual who holds the appropriate Certificate of Clinical Competence; or (3) assistants, technicians, or support personnel who are adequately supervised by an individual who holds the appropriate Certificate of Clinical Competence.

E. Individuals shall not require or permit their professional staff to provide services or conduct research activities that exceed the staff member's competence, level of education, training, and experience.

F. Individuals shall ensure that all equipment used in the provision of services or to conduct research and scholarly activities is in proper working order and is properly calibrated.

PRINCIPLE OF ETHICS III

Individuals shall honor their responsibility to the public by promoting public understanding of the professions, by supporting the development of services designed to fulfill the unmet needs of the public, and by providing accurate information in all communications involving any aspect of the professions, including dissemination of research findings and scholarly activities.

Rules of Ethics

A. Individuals shall not misrepresent their credentials, competence, education, training, experience, or scholarly or research contributions.

B.   Individuals shall not participate in professional activities that constitute a conflict of interest.

C.   Individuals shall refer those served professionally solely on the basis of the interest of those being referred and not on any personal financial interest.

D.   Individuals shall not misrepresent diagnostic information, research, services rendered, or products dispensed; neither shall they engage in any scheme to defraud in connection with obtaining payment or reimbursement for such services or products.

E.   Individuals' statements to the public shall provide accurate information about the nature and management of communication disorders about the professions, about professional services, and about research and scholarly activities.

F.   Individuals' statements to the public—advertising, announcing, and marketing their professional services, reporting research results, and promoting products—shall adhere to prevailing professional standards and shall not contain misrepresentations.

PRINCIPLE OF ETHICS IV

Individuals shall honor their responsibilities to the professions and their relationships with colleagues, students, and members of allied professions. Individuals shall uphold the dignity and autonomy of the professions, maintain harmonious interprofessional and intraprofessional relationships, and accept the professions' self-imposed standards.

Rules of Ethics

A.   Individuals shall prohibit anyone under their supervision from engaging in any practice that violates the Code of Ethics.

B.   Individuals shall not engage in dishonesty, fraud, deceit, misrepresentation, sexual harrassment, or any other form of conduct that adversely reflects on the professions or on the individual's fitness to serve persons professionally.

C.   Individuals shall not engage in sexual activities with clients or students over whom they exercise professional authority.

D.   Individuals shall assign credit only to those who have contributed to a publication, presentation, or product. Credit shall be assigned in proportion to the contribution and only with the contributor's consent.

E.   Individuals shall reference the source when using other persons' ideas, research, presentations, or products in written, oral, or any other media presentation or summary.

F.   Individuals' statements to colleagues about professional services, research results, and products shall adhere to prevailing professional standards and shall contain no misrepresentations.

G.   Individuals shall not provide professional services without exercising independent professional judgment, regardless of referral source or prescription.

H. Individuals shall not discriminate in their relationships with colleagues, students, and members of allied professions on the basis of race or ethnicity, gender, age, religion, national origin, sexual orientation, or disability.

I. Individuals who have reason to believe that the Code of Ethics has been violated shall inform the Board of Ethics.

J. Individuals shall comply fully with the policies of the Board of Ethics in its consideration and adjudication of complaints of violations of the Code of Ethics.

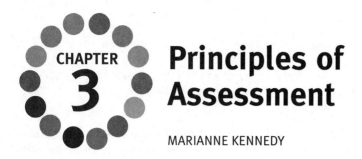

CHAPTER 3

Principles of Assessment

MARIANNE KENNEDY

Case Example 1

Darrell is 4 years, 6 months old, but his speech is more like that of a much younger child. His parents report that he is very difficult to understand and they feel that he is becoming frustrated when he cannot make himself clear. They want him to improve his speech before he begins kindergarten next year.

Case Example 2

Jonah is a 7-year-old and has a severe bilateral sensorineural hearing loss. He uses behind-the-ear hearing aids at home and an auditory trainer at school. His school district has referred him for reevaluation of his hearing, speech, and language and to determine whether his amplification equipment continues to be appropriate for him.

Case Example 3

Anna is a seventh-grade student with significant learning disabilities. She received speech and language therapy when she was younger but was dismissed from services in third grade. Although she receives special education assistance with reading and math, her current teacher believes that she needs more help and wonders whether language therapy would be beneficial at this time.

Case Example 4

Marlene is a 50-year-old woman who has had significant difficulty with communication since her stroke 8 months ago. She received speech and language therapy only for a short time, and her family would like her to pursue more therapy now. They believe that she could continue to make improvements in her ability to communicate if she has the appropriate help.

Case Example 5

Richard, 62 years old, recently underwent a total laryngectomy. He would like to learn to use esophageal speech.

Case Example 6

Thomas is a 27-year-old with a history of severe stuttering. He feels that his speech disorder is interfering with his ability to advance in his career.

The six individuals described previously all appear to have a communication disorder, but they have little else in common. You have been asked to evaluate and make recommendations for these individuals. How will you provide an appropriate assessment for each of these potential clients given the large differences in their problems and the varied assessment protocols that will be necessary to complete the task competently? These examples are provided not to overwhelm the beginning clinician, but to illustrate the breadth of the field of communication disorders. As different as the clients described previously may seem, they are but a sample of the variety of ages, functional levels, and types of disorders to which you will be exposed during training and later in practice. How is it possible to competently assess such a range of problems?

Despite the fact that the needs of these clients are indeed diverse, as are the assessment instruments you will use, there are some general principles that apply. This chapter introduces you to these general principles that guide the process of assessing any communication disorder and provides examples of assessment tools for a variety of communication disorders.

When you hear the word assessment, you may think of testing, but the two terms are not really the same. Testing is only one part of assessment. **Assessment** is the process of collecting and interpreting relevant data for clinical decision-making. The process includes a series of problem-solving activities to assist in making decisions that will result in effective management and intervention for clients with communication disorders. In this chapter, the terms **diagnostic, evaluation,** and assessment are used interchangeably to denote the problem-solving and descriptive process.

Various approaches to assessment in communication disorders have been described in the literature. One approach, derived from the medical model, makes a distinction between **appraisal** and **diagnosis** (e.g., Darley, 1991; Peterson & Marquardt, 1994). Appraisal is seen as the collection of both quantitative and qualitative data about the client. Diagnosis involves interpretation of these data in order to decide whether a problem exists and then differentiating the problem from other similar problems (i.e., **differential diagnosis**). In a medical model, emphasis is also put on identification of possible causes (i.e., **etiology**) and maintaining factors. Another approach is what Miller (1978) and Paul (2001) described as a **descriptive-developmental model** of assessment. In this orientation, the two phases are less distinct. Emphasis is placed on description of the client's present communication behaviors rather than on causal factors or categorization of the disorder. Tomblin (2000) also described a **systems model** of assessment. This model stresses the importance of the family and the cultural context in which the client must function. In this model, there is much emphasis on including the client's significant others in the assessment process to get information about the dynamics of the communication problem. There is a great deal of overlap among the various approaches, and there is no one correct model. For example, use of the descriptive-developmental model certainly does not preclude family involvement or consideration of the client's cultural background.

It is more a question of relative emphasis. The specific model (or combination of models) to be used will depend on the philosophical orientation of the clinician, the setting, and the type of communication problem demonstrated by the client. For example, clinicians who work in medical settings may be more likely than other clinicians to perform assessments that fit the appraisal and diagnosis model. Clinicians who work primarily in educational settings may find the descriptive-developmental approach more useful.

No matter which setting you work in, you will be involved with professionals from other disciplines. Teaming and collaboration among professionals is recognized as the best practice for meeting the needs of clients with a variety of disabilities. Various models of teaming are used in the assessment process, including **multidisciplinary, interdisciplinary,** and **transdisciplinary.** Regardless of the model used, remember that the client and the family are partners in the assessment process; that is, they are critical team members.

Before we can proceed further, several concepts that are important to the diagnostic process must be discussed. The World Health Organization (WHO) has developed a framework for considering health and disability through the International Classification of Functioning, Disability and Health (ICF; WHO, 2001). In ICF, disability and functioning are viewed as outcomes of interactions between health conditions (disorders, diseases, injuries) and contextual factors. Contextual factors include environmental factors (e.g., architectural barriers, social attitudes) as well as personal factors (e.g., age, education, profession). These factors and their interaction influence how the individual experiences a disability. In this framework, functioning is identified at three levels: at the level of the body or body part, at the level of the whole person, and at the level of the whole person in a social context. Disability involves a dysfunction at one or more of these same three levels: **impairments** are problems in body function or structure (such as **aphasia** following a stroke); **activity limitations** are difficulties experienced by an individual in executing one or more activities (such as difficulty producing speech); and **participation restrictions** are problems an individual may experience in involvement in life situations (such as the inability to converse with family). Although it may seem that we should be able to infer activity limitations and participation restrictions from a known impairment, this is not always the case. This can be illustrated in the case example of Richard, the man who underwent a total laryngectomy. Consider two different scenarios: first, that Richard is a computer programmer by profession, and second, that Richard is a trial attorney by profession. Although Richard's obvious activity limitation (inability to communicate by using speech), which is secondary to the impairment (laryngectomy resulting in a structural change to the body), is the same in both cases, the degree of participation restriction relative to his career may be quite different. In the first scenario, Richard may very well be able to continue his career with minor adaptations and compensations. Resuming his career in the second scenario might be more difficult and would most likely require major adaptation and compensation. Knowledge of the impairment is important in describing prognosis and determining an optimal intervention strategy. In Richard's case we know that, barring other medical problems, his status should be stable, and we make prognostic statements and intervention recommendations based on that knowledge. In other cases, with individuals who have neurological impairments known to be degenerative, it is equally important to be familiar with the associated symptoms in order to make appropriate prognostic statements and intervention recommendations. Thus, these issues of disability and functioning must be considered in a comprehensive assessment.

As you develop your clinical skills, keep in mind that assessment, like all types of clinical decision-making, should be undertaken with an evidence-based orientation. The American Speech-Language-Hearing Association (ASHA) has affirmed the importance of **evidence-based practice (EBP),** in which speech-language pathologists (SLPs) and audiologists use current high quality research-based evidence in concert with clinician expertise and client preferences and values to make decisions (ASHA, 2005) (see Chapter 7 for a more in-depth discussion.). By applying EBP criteria, you will be able to choose maximally inform-ative and cost-effective assessment protocols, form valid interpretations from the results, and make meaningful recommendations for treatment.

PURPOSES OF ASSESSMENT

Assessments are completed for various purposes. Understanding the purpose or goal of the assessment is important because it will affect the types of instruments and protocols chosen. The most common reasons for assessment described in this chapter are based on the works of Miller (1978, 1983) and Paul (2001).

Screening

Screening involves the collection of data to decide whether there is a strong likelihood that an individual does or does not have a problem that will require more in-depth assessment. Screening has its roots in medical practices used to identify those who are at risk for a particular disease or disorder (Salvia & Ysseldyke, 1998). Rather than yielding scores, screening results are generally described as *pass* or *fail* based on a predetermined **cut-off score.** A fail will typ-ically result in a referral for more intensive follow-up assessment. You may be familiar with some common uses of screening. Most school districts screen children before they enter kindergarten in a number of areas including speech, language, readiness skills, hearing, and vision. Children who fail one or more of these screenings are referred for further evaluation. Another example is universal newborn hearing screening, now required by 38 states. Examples of frequently used screening procedures in communication disorders are provided in Table 3.1. As Paul (2001) pointed out, it is not always necessary to use a test published as a screening instrument. Any standardized test that samples the relevant areas efficiently and meets certain psychometric criteria can be used.

Screening is also an important component of comprehensive communication assessments. In addition to addressing the presenting concerns, it is important to screen other aspects of speech, language, and communication as well as selected collateral areas. You will see how screening procedures are included into the assessment of Darrell, the 4-year-old whose speech sounds immature. Most likely, you will decide to assess articulation and language skills in depth using several different instruments, both formal and informal. You will also need to screen other areas, however, such as fluency, voice, hearing, and the oral mech-anism in order to determine the possibility that a problem in these areas is also contributing to the concerns that Darrell's parents have described. In addition, you may need to get information about related areas such as play and cognitive skills.

Table 3.1. Examples of screening instruments used in speech, language, and communication assessment

Test	Area	Ages*	Comments
Adolescent Language Screening Test (ALST; Morgan & Guilford, 1984)	Language: Pragmatics, receptive and expressive vocabulary, concepts, sentence formulation, morphology, phonology	11-0 to 17-0 years	Yields pass-fail cut-off score.
Bedside Evaluation Screening Test, Second Edition (BEST-2; West, Sands, & Ross-Swain, 1998)	Aphasia: Speaking, comprehension, reading	Adult	Yields severity ratings. Normed on 200 individuals with aphasia.
Boone Voice Program for Children, Second Edition (Boone, 1993)	Voice	School-aged children	Program includes a voice screening protocol which uses clinician rating scale and s/z ratio.
Brief Test of Head Injury (BTHI; Helm-Estabrooks & Hotz, 1991)	Cognitive, linguistic, communicative abilities	14-0 to adult	Yields standard score, percentile, and severity rating. Assesses post coma abilities following head injury.
Clinical Evaluation of Language Fundamentals—4 Screening Test (Semel, Wiig, & Secord, 2004)	Language: Receptive and expressive morphology, syntax, semantics	5-0 to 21-0 years	Yields criterion referenced score.
Early Language Milestones Scale, Second Edition (ELM-2; Coplan, 1993)	Language: Receptive and expressive semantics, syntax; phonology	Birth to 3-0 years	Pass/fail or point scoring method available. Latter yields standard, percentile, or age scores.
Fluharty Preschool Speech and Language Screening Test, Second Edition (Fluharty, 2001)	Language: Vocabulary, articulation, syntax	3-0 to 6-11 years	Yields standard scores and percentiles for subtests and composites.
Kindergarten Language Screening Test, Second Edition (KLST-2; Gauthier & Madison, 1998)	Language: Receptive and expressive semantics, syntax	3-6 to 6-11 years	Yields percentile rank and stanine. Cut-off score based on stanine is recommended.
Oral Speech Mechanism Screening Exam, Third Edition (OSMSE-3; St. Louis & Ruscello, 2000)	Oral motor mechanism	5-0 to 78-0 years	Yields +/- scores. Provides checklist for noting appropriate structure and function.
Quick Screen of Phonology (Bankson & Bernthal, 1990)	Articulation, phonological processes	3-0 to 7-11 years	Yields ranks and standard scores. Cut-off scores for different ages available.
Screening Test for Developmental Apraxia of Speech, Second Edition (STDAS-2; Blakeley, 2000)	Apraxia	4-0 to 12-0 years	Yields criterion-referenced score. Has four subtests.

*Ages are expressed in years and months with a hyphen dividing the two (e.g., 11-0 means 11 years, 0 months old).

These areas will be discussed in more detail later in the chapter. If the examiner suspects any problems in these areas, more in-depth evaluation should follow.

Determining a Diagnosis or Differential Diagnosis

In some cases, it may be important or useful to label the communication problem or to distinguish the disorder from another disorder with similar symptoms (Emerick & Hatten, 1974). Consider Marlene, the woman who had a stroke 8 months ago. In order to recommend an appropriate course of treatment, we need to understand the basis for her communication problems. Does Marlene's communication problem stem from aphasia, **dysarthria, apraxia,** or some form of **dementia?** In many cases, a diagnostic label may be a prerequisite to obtaining funding for services.

Before assigning a diagnostic label, though, it is always important to ascertain whether the communication issues presented are the result of a difference rather than a disorder. In other words, is it possible that the client's communication differs from the norm because the individual's environment and experiences have been different from the norm? For example, if Darrell's family speaks a language other than English at home, then we must consider the possibility that his current language status is related to the different linguistic experiences he has had rather than a language disorder. Assessing the communication skills of individuals who are from culturally and linguistically diverse backgrounds presents special challenges for the clinician (see Chapter 11). If we find that the presenting concern is a disorder, then it will be important to carefully describe his current level of performance in the various language and communication areas.

Determining Eligibility for Services

Intervention services, which are supported by public or third party funding, may have specific guidelines and eligibility requirements that must be met before those sources of funding can be accessed. For example, the Individuals with Disabilities Education Act of 1990 (PL 101-476) and its subsequent reauthorizations, the most recent being the Individuals with Disabilities Education Improvement Act of 2004 (PL 108-446), require local school districts to provide free special education and related services to those children whose problems have a negative impact on their ability to profit from general education. The law stipulates that in order to be eligible for these services, the child must be shown to have a disability. This usually occurs by documenting the disability through an assessment that identifies what the child knows and can do academically, developmentally, and functionally and then comparing the student's present level of performance with the grade and age level expectations. In many school districts, this means that in order to qualify for services, the child must perform below a predetermined level (usually 1.5 to 2 standard deviations below the mean for the child's age) on an assessment. This point is illustrated by Anna's case. As you will recall, she already receives special education services for her learning disability. Following the referral from her teacher, Anna will have to undergo assessment. In order to qualify for additional services from the school's SLP, the assessment results will have to demonstrate that her performance is significantly below average and that her speech and language status negatively influences her education. These conclusions must be based on several different types of assessment data, never solely on the basis of one test.

Establishing a Baseline

Once we have ascertained that a client has a problem and is eligible for services, it is important to describe the individual's current functioning in all areas of communication. This description, which, as you will see later, can include both qualitative and quantitative data, will serve as a **baseline** or reference point for measuring progress during treatment. It is important to describe what the client is able to do as well as what the client cannot do. The baseline information should be a profile of the client's strengths and weaknesses. Furthermore, because the client's behavior in a clinical setting may not represent typical behavior, baseline information should be gathered in various settings and contexts. Consider the cases of Richard and Thomas to illustrate this. Both clients clearly have a communication problem and both already have a diagnosis. For these clients, the purpose of the current assessment is to document and describe their present level of communication functioning. This description not only will serve as a baseline for comparison with subsequent performance, but it will also lay the basis for the next phase of assessment.

Developing Intervention Targets

Once the client's present status has been described, the next step is to identify potential targets or goals for intervention. Many factors are considered to determine goals and intervention priorities, including developmental appropriateness, targets that would have the greatest impact on the individual's communication, and client and family priorities. As part of this process, the assessment may include **stimulability** testing to determine which communication behaviors can be easily modified or elicited through the use of various levels of cueing or prompting. Similarly, the examiner may use some trial teaching or facilitating techniques to gauge the client's responsiveness. This interactive process, which differs from traditional test administration, is referred to as **dynamic assessment** (e.g., Lidz & Elliott, 2000). When developing goals and intervention methods, it is also important to consider how the client's areas of strength can be used to facilitate or compensate for areas of weakness.

Tracking and Documenting Progress

Finally, assessment procedures are used throughout intervention in order to measure progress toward the stated goals and to assess the effectiveness of the intervention itself. Ongoing assessment is necessary so that adjustments can be made as needed in the intervention targets and techniques. It is also important when you are making decisions about when to dismiss a client from therapy. Just as it was important to sample communication behaviors in a variety of settings when determining baseline functioning, it is also important to document progress in a variety of real-life situations. Tracking and documenting progress will be used as part of the clinical process with all of the clients described previously in the case examples during the course of their therapy.

Periodic reevaluation, a somewhat more formal process than the ongoing assessment described previously, is another way to document changes over time. This is one reason why Jonah, the boy who has a severe hearing loss, gets a referral for testing. Tracking his hearing levels is an essential part of ensuring that he gets the most benefit from his hearing aids and auditory trainer.

METHODS OF ASSESSMENT

Assessment instruments generally fall into one of three main groups: **norm-referenced** or standardized tests, **criterion-referenced tests,** and **observational tools.** Each group has advantages and disadvantages that must be considered in light of the questions being asked of the assessment. Table 3.2 summarizes the major types of instruments and their primary uses in assessment.

Norm-Referenced Tests

Norm-referenced tests are standardized instruments that can be used to compare an individual's performance to the performance of others with similar demographic characteristics such as age and gender. This type of test is most useful for determining the existence of a problem and establishing eligibility for services. Norm-referenced instruments have certain statistical properties that allow meaningful comparisons among individuals and allow us to determine if an individual's performance is significantly different from a typical performance on a given trait or skill. Examples of frequently used norm-referenced tests in the field of communication disorders are provided in Table 3.3. In order to use tests appropriately, clinicians must be informed consumers. This includes investigating the relevant properties of tests and using only those tests that meet acceptable psychometric criteria. Although the detailed explanations of psychometric and statistical theories underlying norm-referenced tests are beyond the scope of this chapter, a brief summary of key characteristics follows (McCauley & Swisher, 1984; Salvia & Ysseldyke, 1998; Paul, 2001; Linn & Miller, 2005; Thorndike, 2005).

Reliability **Reliability** refers to the consistency or dependability with which a test measures what it is supposed to be measuring. When we administer a test, we should be able to make some assumptions about the results that we get. First, we want to be sure that an individual's performance is not unduly influenced by some examiner characteristics. In other words, a different examiner

Table 3.2. Types of assessment instruments and their primary use in assessment

Purpose	Type of instrument			
	Norm-referenced	Criterion-referenced	Behavioral observation	Instrumental
Screening	✓	✓		✓
Determine existence of a problem; diagnosis; differential diagnosis	✓			✓
Determine eligibility for services	✓			✓
Establish baseline		✓	✓	✓
Determine intervention goals		✓	✓	✓
Document or track progress		✓	✓	✓

Table 3.3. Sampling of norm-referenced tests used in speech, language, and communication assessments

Test	Area	Ages*	Comments
Arizona Battery for Communication Disorders of Dementia (ABCD; Bayles & Tomoeda, 1993)	Language (dementia): Auditory comprehension; verbal episodic and semantic memory; oral expression; visual spatial skills	15 years to adult	Yields criterion scores that can be converted to 5-point scaled score. Standardized on patients with Alzheimer's disease and Parkinson's disease as well as younger and older individuals without disabilities. Has 14 subtests.
Boston Diagnostic Aphasia Examination, Third Edition (BDAE-3; Goodglass, Kaplan, & Barresi, 2000)	Language (aphasia): Auditory and written language comprehension, oral expression, writing	Adult	Yields percentile ranks based on a sample of persons with aphasia.
Clinical Evaluation of Language Fundamentals-4 (CELF-4; Semel, Wiig, & Secord, 2003)	Language: Receptive and expressive semantics, syntax, morphology; auditory memory	5-0 to 21-0 years	Yields standard, percentile, and age-equivalent scores. Scoring software available (CELF-4 Scoring Assistant). Spanish edition available. Has 4 core subtests and 14 additional subtests.
Communication Activities of Daily Living, Second Edition (CADL-2; Holland, Frattali, & Fromm, 1999)	Language (aphasia/brain damage): Semantics, pragmatics, reading, writing	Adult	Yields percentile and stanine scores. Normed on 175 adults with neurogenic communication disorders.
Comprehensive Assessment of Spoken Language (CASL; Carrow-Woolfolk, 1999)	Language: Comprehension, expression, and retrieval in lexical/semantic, syntactic, pragmatic, and supralinguistic areas	3-0 to 21-0 years	Yields standard, percentile, stanine, and age-equivalent scores. Has 15 subtests.
Diagnostic Evaluation of Language Variation, Norm-Referenced (DELV-NR; Seymour, Roeper, deVilliers, & deVilliers, 2005)	Language: Syntax, pragmatics, semantics, phonology	4-0 to 9-11 years	Yields standard, percentile, and age-equivalent scores. Designed to neutralize the effect of dialects.
Expressive One Word Picture Vocabulary Test (EOWPVT; Brownell, 2000)	Language: Expressive vocabulary	2-0 to 18-11 years	Yields standard, percentile, and age-equivalent scores. Spanish version available.
Expressive Vocabulary Test (Williams, 1997)	Language: Expressive vocabulary, synonyms	2-6 to 90-0 years	Yields standard, percentile, and age-equivalent scores. Computer scoring program available. Co-normed with PPVT-III.
Goldman-Fristoe Test of Articulation, Second Edition (GFTA-2; Goldman & Fristoe, 2000)	Articulation	2-0 to 21-0 years	Yields standard, percentile, and age-equivalent scores. Separate gender norms available.
Khan-Lewis Phonological Analysis, Second Edition (KLPA-2; Khan & Lewis, 2002)	Phonological processes	2-0 to 5-11 years	Yields composite, percentile, and age-equivalent scores. Has a speech simplification rating. Can be used as companion tool to GFTA-2. Scoring software available.
MacArthur Communicative Development Inventories (Fenson, Dale, Reznick, Thal, Bates, Hartung, Pethick, & Reilly, 1993)	Language: Receptive and expressive vocabulary; gestures, syntax, morphology	0-8 to 2-6 years	Yields percentile ranks. Parent report format. Two versions: "Words and Gestures" for ages 8–16 months and "Words and Sentences" for ages 16–30 months. Spanish version available.

*Ages are expressed in years and months with a hyphen dividing the two (e.g., 5-0 means 5 years, 0 months old).

(continued)

Table 3.3. *(continued)*

Test	Area	Ages*	Comments
Peabody Picture Vocabulary Test-III (PPVT-III; Dunn & Dunn, 1997)	Language: Receptive vocabulary	2-6 to 90-0 years	Yields standard, percentile, and age-equivalent scores. Equivalent forms A and B. Computer scoring program available. Spanish version (TVIP) available.
Preschool Language Scale-4 (PLS-4; Zimmerman, Steiner, & Pond, 2002)	Language: Receptive and expressive semantics, syntax, morphology; articulation	Birth to 6-11 years	Yields standard, percentile, and age-equivalent scores. Spanish version available.
Reynell Developmental Language Scales—US Edition (Reynell & Gruber, 1990)	Language: Receptive and expressive semantics, syntax	1-0 to 6-11 years	Yields standard score, percentile score, and developmental level. Adaptation for children with severe oral impairment available. Uses pictures and objects.
Stuttering Severity Instrument for Children & Adults, Third Edition (SSI-3; Riley, 1994)	Fluency	2-10 to adult	Yields criterion scores, percentile ranks, and severity rating. Computer scoring program available.
Test of Adolescent and Adult Language-3 (TOAL-3; Hammill, Brown, Larsen, & Weiderholt, 1994)	Language: Receptive and expressive semantics and syntax, reading, writing, auditory comprehension	12-0 to 24-11 years	Yields standard, percentile, and age-equivalent scores. Computer scoring program available.
Test of Auditory Comprehension of Language, Third Edition (TACL-3; Carrow-Woolfolk, 1999)	Language: Auditory comprehension of semantics, syntax, morphology	3-0 to 9-11 years	Yields standard, percentile, and age-equivalent scores.
Test of Language Development-Primary: Third Edition (TOLD-P:3; Newcomer & Hammill, 1997)	Language: Receptive and expressive semantics, syntax, morphology; phonology, articulation	4-0 to 8-11 years	Yields standard, percentile, and age equivalent scores. Has nine subtests.
Test of Language Development-Intermediate: Third Edition (TOLD-I:3; Hammill & Newcomer, 1997)	Language: Receptive and expressive syntax and semantics	8-0 to 12-11 years	Yields standard, percentile, and age-equivalent scores. Computer scoring program available.
Test of Narrative Language (TNL; Gillam & Pearson, 2004)	Language: Narrative discourse	5-0 to 11-11 years	Yields standard and percentile scores.
Test of Pragmatic Language (TOPL; Phelps-Terasaki & Phelps-Gunn, 1992)	Language: Pragmatics	5-0 to 13-11 years	Yields standard and percentile scores. Can also be used for adult remedial, English as a Second Language, and aphasic populations.
Western Aphasia Battery (WAB; Kertesz, 1982)	Language (aphasia): Auditory comprehension, verbal fluency, naming, information content	Adolescent to adult	Yields aphasia quotient to indicate severity.
Woodcock Language Proficiency Battery, Revised (WLPB-R; Woodcock, 1991)	Language: Auditory comprehension, oral expression, reading, writing	2-0 to 95-0 years	Yields standard, percentile, age-equivalent, and grade-equivalent scores. Separate norms for college students provided. Computer scoring program available. Spanish version available.

*Ages are expressed in years and months with a hyphen dividing the two (e.g., 5-0 means 5 years, 0 months old).

should be able to get the same results, either by administering the test directly or by rescoring a test given by another examiner. This is called **interrater reliability.** Second, if the test is given to an individual on two separate occasions, theoretically, the results should be identical. This property speaks to the stability of the test and is referred to as **test–retest reliability.** Finally, we want to assume that similar test items would yield similar results and that there is agreement among items within different parts of the test. This third type of reliability is demonstrated in several ways. Some tests have two forms that measure the same skills. This is called **equivalent or alternate form reliability.** A commonly used example in speech-language pathology is the Peabody Picture Vocabulary Test-III (PPVT-III) that has Forms A and B (Dunn & Dunn, 1997). This type of reliability can also be demonstrated by correlating one half of the test with the other half; this is referred to as **internal consistency.** The test can be split by comparing the first half of the items to the second half (**split-half reliability**), by comparing the even items to the odd numbered items (**odd-even reliability**), or by using a statistical procedure which compares all possible divisions of a test into two parts (**Cronbach's coefficient alpha**). Reliability data are reported in correlation coefficients and range from .00 (no reliability) to 1.00 (perfect reliability). These coefficients should be clearly presented in the test manual. Salvia and Ysseldyke (1998) recommend a .90 correlation coefficient as a minimum standard for a test to be considered reliable.

Validity   The most important characteristic to take into account when choosing assessment tools is **validity.** This refers to the relevance and appropriateness of the interpretations and uses of the test results. A test does not have validity in the absolute sense; rather test scores are valid for some uses, but not others (e.g., Thorndike, 2005). For example, if Darrell's family does not speak English at home, how can we interpret and use his PPVT-III scores (see Figure 3.1)? Although his score may be an accurate representation of his current understanding of English vocabulary, it may have questionable validity as a measure of his overall receptive vocabulary. We would have to be very cautious about any inferences we made about his vocabulary recognition skills.

Although validity is considered to be a unitary concept, several types of evidence contribute to overall validity. First, a test has **content related validity** when test items represent a relevant and adequate sample of the domain being measured. This kind of validity is usually judged by experts in the field and is based on the following factors: appropriateness of the items included, completeness of the sample, and the manner in which the items assess the content. Second is **criterion-related validity,** the extent to which performance on a test is correlated with performance on another instrument (i.e., criterion measure) believed to measure the same skill or behavior. Criterion-related validity should be presented as a correlation coefficient in the test manual and can be measured in two ways. **Concurrent validity** refers to the relationship between an individual's performance on the test and a criterion measure when they are administered at the same time, whereas **predictive validity** refers to how well the individual's current performance on the test predicts future performance on a criterion measure. Third, **construct validation,** refers to how a test measures the theoretical trait or construct that it is supposed to measure. This is particularly important for characteristics, such as comprehension, that cannot be directly observed or measured. For example, the PPVT was once used as a measure of IQ. Because

Peabody Picture Vocabulary Test–Third Edition
by Lloyd M. Dunn & Leota M. Dunn

PPVT-III

FORM IIIA

Performance Record

Name __Darrell Thompson__ Sex: ☐F ☒M

Home Address __15 Main St.__ Phone(__210__) __451-3701__

City __Southwick__ State __CT__ ZIP __06510__

School __Jackson__ Grade __Preschool__
(or agency) (or education)

Language of the Home ☒Standard English ☐Other _____
(specify: foreign language, or type of English dialect spoken)

Teacher __Ms Phely__ Examiner __MK__
(or counselor)

Date & Age Data

	Year	Month	Day
Date of testing	06	9	29
Date of birth	02	4	3
Chronological age*	4	6	

*Disregard extra days.

Reason for testing __Parents concerned about__
__speech development — hard to understand__

Other information on test taker __Being treated (with__
__antibiotics) for ear infection__

RECORD OF SCORES

Raw Score
(from oval on page 2) __38__

Deviation-type Norms

Standard Score
(Norms Table 1) __83__

Percentile Rank
(Norms Table 2) __13__

Normal Curve Equivalent
(Norms Table 2) __26__

Stanine
(Norms Table 2) __3__

Developmental-type Norms

Age Equivalent
(Norms Table 3) __3-0__

Graphic Display of Deviation-type Norm Scores

Mark the obtained standard score on the appropriate line below. Draw a straight vertical line through it and across the other scales. (See manual for more information.)

Optional confidence intervals also may be plotted. To do so, draw two lines vertically across all the scales, one on either side of the obtained standard score line. For the 68 percent band width, use ± 4 standard score units. (See manual for other options.)

Copyright 1997, Lloyd M. Dunn, Leota M. Dunn and Douglas M. Dunn. It is illegal to reproduce this form for testing. However, permission is granted to reproduce a completed front page to convey an examinee's scores to other qualified personnel. Unless this form is printed in violet and black, it is not an original and is an illegal photocopy.

For additional forms, call or write AGS, 4201 Woodland Road, Circle Pines, MN 55014-1796; toll-free 1-800-328-2560. www.agsnet.com. Ask for Item #12004 (25 per package).

A09876
Printed in the U.S.A.

Figure 3.1. Darrell's Peabody Picture Vocabulary Test-III results. (From Dunn, L.M., & Dunn, L.M. [1997]. *Peabody Picture Vocabulary Test-III* [p. 1]. Circle Pines, MN: AGS Publishing; permission to reprint this sample page granted by publisher.)

the test is designed to measure receptive vocabulary (which is only one aspect of verbal intelligence), it is not surprising that it is not a good measure of overall intelligence. Evidence for construct validity comes from examination of the theory underlying the construct and the ability of the theory to predict performance. If a test does not have strong construct validity, it may not be measuring the underlying characteristic in question. Construct validity is now considered by testing experts to be the most important evidence of validity (see Thorndike, 2005). Again, it is the examiner's responsibility to be clear about which skills or behaviors are being measured, to choose tests with high levels of validity for measuring the desired areas, and to be mindful of potential consequences (both positive and negative) of the interpretation and use of the results.

Standardization Because it is impossible to test everyone in a given population, test developers rely on a subset of the population from whom the characteristics of the population can be estimated. An individual's performance is then compared with this **norming sample.** The characteristics of the norming or standardization sample are very important because all the norm-referenced scores are based on the performance of this group. Adequate norms depend on several factors. First, the norming sample must be representative; that is, it must include a wide range of persons with characteristics similar to those who will take the test. These characteristics include age, gender, race, ethnicity, socioeconomic background, and geographic distribution in the same proportion as in the general population. McCauley and Swisher (1984) emphasized the importance of noting whether people with disabilities or nonnormal language and communication abilities have been included in the standardization sample. Although the exclusion of such people seems to make intuitive sense, it presents problems. For one thing, if all the participants in the standardization sample are considered typical, then even the lowest score in the sample represents a typical performance. This makes it very difficult to interpret scores, especially those at or below the lowest score of the norming sample. A second factor affecting the adequacy of norms is the number of persons included in the sample. There must be adequate cases at each age level tested. Test experts recommend a minimum of 100 people at each age tested (Salvia & Ysseldyke, 1998). The final factor to be considered is the relevance of the norms to the purpose of the test. In most cases, we will be using national norms based on the general population in a particular age range. In some cases, local norms will be more appropriate. For example, some school districts with high percentages of children with limited English proficiency have developed local norms for language assessment. In other cases, we may wish to use norms based on particular groups, such as the Hiskey-Nebraska Test of Learning Aptitude (Hiskey, 1966) that is standardized on people who are deaf or the Communication Activities of Daily Living, second edition test battery (Holland, Frattali, & Fromm, 1999) that is standardized on adults with neurogenic disorders.

Descriptive Statistics In order to correctly interpret test scores, it is important to understand a few basic concepts of descriptive statistics, which is a way to describe or summarize quantitative data. If a test is given to a sufficiently large number of people, the resulting scores should form a **normal distribution.** This is usually depicted as a symmetrical or "bell-shaped" curve as shown in Figure 3.2. The advantage of this distribution is that the number of cases falling between any two points is known; therefore, scores can be interpreted relative to the distribution. We usually assume that the norming sample for a standardized test had a normal distribution. In a normal distribution, most scores will be clustered close to the **mean,** that is, the arithmetic average of the scores. The mean is known as a **measure of central tendency.** As you move away from the mean, there are fewer scores in either direction. You can see this in the bell curve—as you move away from the middle, the area between the curve and the horizontal axis becomes smaller.

Although the mean tells us about the average performance of the group, we need more information to know just how close to the average the individuals in the group scored. Therefore, in addition to knowing the measure of central

52

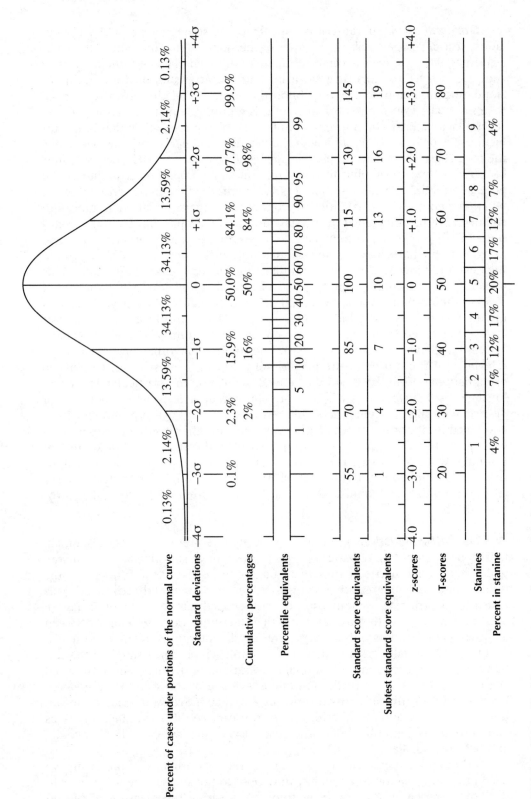

Figure 3.2. Relationship of the normal curve to various types of standard scores.

tendency, we must also know the measure of dispersion or variability. How were the scores of the norming group spread out? The most frequently reported measure of dispersion is the **standard deviation.** Mathematically, this measure is based on another measure of dispersion (variance), but in essence, it represents the average difference of scores from the mean score. In a normal distribution, we expect that approximately 68% of the scores will fall within 1 standard deviation of the mean on either side. Half the scores (34%) will be higher and half will be lower. Approximately 96% of scores will be within 2 standard deviations of the mean. When using a test, it is critical to be aware of the means and standard deviations.

Error   All measurement contains error. Any score that we obtain is only an estimate of the person's true score. Test manuals for norm-referenced tests should provide the examiner with the **standard error of measurement (SEM),** which takes into account the variability that is inherent in human behavior. The SEM is really the standard deviation of error around a person's true score. Because we never really know a person's true score, we use the SEM to determine a **confidence interval** around the person's obtained test score. Figure 3.1 shows how the SEM aids in interpreting test results as it presents results for Darrell on the PPVT-III. You can see the confidence interval around his observed standard score of 83. This means that we can say with 68% confidence that Darrell's true score falls between 79 and 87.

Test Norms and Scores   The raw score obtained on a test has little usefulness in and of itself; it must be interpreted in reference to the test's norms. Test manuals provide tables that allow the examiner to convert raw scores into derived scores. There are two types of derived scores: **developmental scores** and **scores of relative standing.**

1.   The most common kinds of developmental scores are **age equivalents** and **grade equivalents.** Age equivalents are expressed in years and months, usually with a hyphen between the two (e.g., 3-8 means 3 years, 8 months old). Age equivalent means that a person's raw score is the average performance for that age group. Grade equivalents mean that a person's raw score is the average performance for a given grade; they are expressed in grades and tenths of grades, with a decimal point between the two (e.g., 6.2 means sixth grade, second month). Although developmental scores seem easy to understand, they should only be used with great caution. Salvia and Ysseldyke (1998) listed several problems with the use of these derived scores. First, they are easily misinterpreted. Darrell has earned an age-equivalent score of 3-0 (see Figure 3.1). This means that he has answered correctly as many items as the average 3-year-old child, but he may not necessarily have performed as a 3-year-old child would. Let us suppose that another child, James, also received an age equivalent score of 3-0 on the PPVT-III, but James is 7 years old. Most likely, Darrell and James have not performed identically. Furthermore, in the construction of the norms, average age and grade scores may be estimated for groups of individuals that were never actually tested. The average 3-year-old is really a statistical abstraction. Real 3-year-old children represent a range of performance, as you will recall from our

earlier discussion about normal distributions. In fact, the way that equivalent scores are constructed ensures that 50% of any age or grade group will perform below age or grade level. Because developmental scores are not based on equal interval measures (e.g., a 1 year delay in a 3-year-old probably represents a more serious problem than a 1 year delay in a 10-year-old), they cannot be added or subtracted. That means if we retest Darrell next year on the PPVT and he receives an age equivalent score of 3-8, we cannot conclude that he has made 8 months progress. Unfortunately, you will probably see this type of misinterpretation during your career.

2. Scores of relative standing, however, do allow us to make comparisons among individuals of different ages as well as among scores on various tests taken by the same person. There are several types of scores of relative standing and they can be seen in Figure 3.2.

    A. **Percentile ranks** indicate the percentage of people in the norming sample who scored at or below a given raw score. We see in Figure 3.1 that Darrell's PPVT-III raw score converts to the 13th percentile. This means that of 100 children his age who were in the norming sample, 13 of them earned the same or lower raw score than Darrell. Percentile scores are easy to understand and explain to families, but a caution is in order. In looking back at Figure 3.2, note that percentile scores are not equal interval scores. For example, the distance between the 5th and 10th percentiles is larger than the difference between the 45th and 50th percentiles. Therefore, as with developmental scores, you cannot add or subtract them.

    B. **Standard score** is the name for a derived score that has been standardized or transformed so that the mean and standard deviation have predetermined (i.e., standard) values. Standard scores are based on equal interval units so that they can be combined mathematically. Several different standard score distributions are commonly used. The most basic is the **z-score,** which tells us how many standard deviation units a person's score falls from the mean for the particular population. Z-distributions have a mean of 0 and a standard deviation of 1. In Figure 3.2, you can see that a z-score of -1 denotes that an individual's score fell 1 standard deviation below the mean, whereas a z-score of +2 denotes that an individual's score was 2 standard deviations above the mean. **T-scores** are much like z-scores, except that the mean is 50 and the standard deviation is 10. So the z-score of -1 above would convert to a T-score of 40, which shows that the individual scored 1 standard deviation below the mean. Many tests use **scaled scores** (sometimes called deviation IQ scores because they were first used as standard scores for IQ tests) with a mean of 100 and a standard deviation of 15. This means that scores between 85 and 115 are considered to be in the average range, that is, within 1 standard deviation of the mean. Returning to Darrell's PPVT results, you can see that his standard score of 83 places him slightly more than 1 standard deviation below the mean. Tests with subtests frequently use scaled scores with a mean of 10 and a standard deviation of 3. The advantage of T-scores and scaled scores is that you do not have to deal with negative numbers or decimals. Although standard scores may be more difficult to understand and explain to people without some statistical knowledge, they are the best method for deciding whether a client demonstrates a significant deviation from the norm.

Test Administration Procedures   Standardized tests should have clear and sufficiently detailed descriptions of administration procedures so that the clinician can administer the test in the same manner as during test standardization. It is essential that the test be administered exactly as described in the administration manual. Any deviation from the standardized administration can affect the results and must be reported. In such cases, interpretation of the scores must be done with great caution.

Criterion-Referenced Procedures

Rather than measure an individual's performance in comparison to others, **criterion referenced** procedures allow us to measure skills in terms of absolute levels of mastery. These measures do not tell us whether an individual differs significantly from the norm. They are, however, extremely useful in helping to establish baseline functioning, to develop intervention targets, and to document progress. Criterion-referenced procedures include commercially available instruments as well as clinician-constructed procedures. Examples of the former include **developmental scales,** which sample behaviors from specific developmental periods. These scales frequently rely on observational or interview techniques to gather data. Although many of these instruments do yield equivalency score information (usually age scores), they do not meet the strict psychometric criteria for norm-referenced tests. Many commercially available criterion-referenced instruments are standardized in the sense that they have standard procedures for administration and scoring but as mentioned previously, do not provide scores of relative standing. Examples of criterion-referenced procedures frequently used in communication assessments are provided in Table 3.4.

A great advantage of other criterion-referenced procedures is that administration procedures can be modified to suit the needs of the individual client. Tasks can sample **decontextualized** behaviors (i.e., without the support of the context, as in norm-referenced tests) as well as communication behaviors in naturalistic situations. Knowledge about a client's performance in both of these contexts is important to get a complete picture. Many sources are available to help clinicians with developing appropriate tasks. For example, Miller and Paul (1995) discussed the development of criterion-referenced procedures to assess language comprehension in young children. Figure 3.3 is an example of a task for assessing comprehension of prepositions. A variety of procedures are also available for the assessment of speech and language formulation and production. Analyzing samples of a client's speech, language, and communication is an excellent way of gathering information about the individual's current skills in real-life situations (see Chapter 5). Criterion-referenced assessments are scored differently than norm-referenced tests. Remember that these procedures do not yield scores of relative standing but are compared with an absolute standard. Types of scores that you will use include pass/fail, +/-, percentage correct, performance rate, and simple rating scales. For example, the information on page 58 shows procedures and scoring for a frequently used procedure in voice assessment.

Table 3.4. Examples of criterion-referenced tests used in speech, language, and communication assessments

Test	Area	Ages*	Comments
Apraxia Battery for Adults, Second Edition (ABA-2; Dabul, 2000)	Apraxia	9-0 to adult	Yields criterion-referenced score and level of impairment profile. Has six subtests.
Assessment of Phonological Processes, Revised (APP-R; Hodson, 1986)	Phonology	3-0 to 12-0 years	Yields criterion-referenced scores: total number of occurrences, percentage of occurrence. Screening version available.
Burns Brief Inventory of Communication and Cognition (Burns, 1997)	Communication and cognition	18 to 80 years	Yields criterion-referenced scores on three inventories: right hemisphere, left hemisphere, and complex neuropathology. Results can be plotted on a grid.
Contextual Test of Articulation (CTA: Aase, Hovre, Krause, Schelfhout, Smith, & Carpenter, 2000)	Articulation	4-0 to 9-11 years	Yields percentage correct and information about phonetic context of misarticulated sounds. Has six subtests representing most commonly occurring error sounds.
Frenchay Dysarthria Assessment (Enderby, 1983)	Dysarthria	12-0 to adult	Yields criterion-referenced severity rating and profile of strengths and weaknesses. Data on people with dysarthrias as well as individuals without are provided. Has 11 sections.
Minnesota Test for Differential Diagnosis of Aphasia (Schuell, 1973)	Aphasia	Adult	Yields percentage correct and clinical ratings in each area. Results can be used to assist in making a differential diagnosis of different types of aphasia.
Multilevel Informal Language Inventory (Goldsworthy, 1982)	Language: Syntax, semantics, and morphology	4-0 to 12-0 years	Yields a profile that can be used to select intervention targets.
Rossetti Infant-Toddler Language Scale (Rossetti, 1990)	Language and related areas: Interaction-attachment, pragmatics, gesture, play, language comprehension, language expression	Birth to 3-0 years	Yields basal and ceiling levels for each developmental area and global development. Compilation of caregiver reporting, interviews, and child observation.
Voice Assessment Protocol for Children and Adults (VAP) (Pindzola, 1987)	Voice	Children and adults	Yields ratings and descriptions of voice parameters.
Wiig Criterion-Referenced Inventory of Language (Wiig, 1990)	Language: Semantics, pragmatics, syntax, morphology	4-0 to 13-0	Yields raw score and percentage correct. Record forms are available for each area and allow for tracking progress over time.

*Ages are expressed in years and months with a hyphen dividing the two (e.g., 9-0 means 9 years, 0 months old).

Comprehension of Locatives: Search Task

DEVELOPMENTAL LEVEL	30–48 months
LINGUISTIC LEVEL	Lexical
LINGUISTIC STIMULI	Prepositions *in, on, under, behind, in front of*, and *beside*
RESPONSE TYPE	Natural-behavioral compliance
MATERIALS	• Toy mailbox or egg carton for reference object • Six small boxes and six raisins, peanuts, or small candies • A piece of cardboard for use as a screen
PROCEDURE	1. Place the six small boxes in the six locative positions (indicated by the prepositions above) relative to the toy mailbox. 2. Introduce the toy mailbox and the screen to the child. 3. Give the child the following instructions: "Here is a raisin (or peanut or candy). I'm going to hide it and I'll tell you where to find it." 4. Put up the screen between the child and the test items. 5. Hide one raisin (or peanut or candy) under the small box in the mailbox. 6. Remove the screen. 7. Tell the child, "The candy is in the mailbox." 8. Record the child's response on a score sheet. 9. Put the screen up again and repeat the procedure using the next stimulus locative. The stimulus locatives must be presented in the following order: *in, on, under, behind, in front of, beside*. Because the first three locatives are the easiest, they are presented first to ensure some success. Alter the stimulus sentence as appropriate for each locative preposition.
PASSING RESPONSE	The child finds the prize (raisin, peanut, or candy) under the appropriate box. Response is repeated on several trials with different target objects.
RESPONSE STRATEGY	"Probable location" (i.e., child searches for objects where they are usually found)
DEVELOPMENTAL NOTE	Although *in, on,* and *under* are understood by 50%-85% of children at 30 months of age, *in front of* and *beside* are not comprehended by most children until 42 months (Hodun, 1975). Hodun (1975) reports that this search task is easier for children than the placement task.

Figure 3.3. Example of a criterion-referenced task. (From Miller, J., & Paul, R. [1995]. *The clinical assessment of language comprehension* [p. 47]. Baltimore: Paul H. Brookes Publishing Co.; reprinted by permission.)

The s/z ratio is a frequently used task in voice assessment. The ratio shows whether there is a difference in the client's ability to sustain voiced and voiceless expiration. The task is used to help assess respiratory and phonatory efficiency.

PROCEDURE

Ask the client to take a deep breath and say /s/ (or /z/) for as long as possible. You can present a model first. Have the client repeat each phoneme three times. Vary the order of /s/ and /z/. Time each performance with a stopwatch.

SCORING

Use the longest production for each phoneme to compute a ratio as follows:

$$\frac{\text{longest /s/}}{\text{longest /z/}} = \text{s/z ratio}$$

INTERPRETATION

A ratio of 1.0 with normal duration (approximately 10 seconds for children and 20-25 seconds for adults) indicates normal respiration ability and no vocal fold pathology.

A ratio of 1.0 with shortened duration of /s/ and /z/ suggests possible inefficiency of respiration.

A ratio of 1.2 or greater suggests possible vocal fold pathology.

Sources: Boone & McFarlene, 2000; Deem & Miller, 2000.

Curriculum-based assessments (CBAs) are a type of criterion-referenced assessment frequently used in school settings. These assessments are constructed by teachers, SLPs, and other professionals to reflect the content of the curriculum. CBAs can be used effectively to assess curriculum-based language use (Nelson, 1998; Paul, 2001) and may be more sensitive to tracking the progress of students from culturally and linguistically diverse backgrounds than traditional standardized testing (Idol, Nevin, & Paolucci-Whitcomb, 1999).

Clinician-constructed instruments are sometimes referred to as informal assessments. Witt, Elliott, Gresham, and Kramer (1988) pointed out that informal assessment is actually anything but informal. The word *informal* refers to the content rather than the process of the assessment. These techniques, which represent a structured and systematic approach, allow us to examine specific communication behaviors or skills in detail and in a way that is individualized to the client's particular needs. Many clinicians call these techniques probes.

In recent years, several alternative assessment models have evolved, in part as a response to calls for accountability in education and health care and to counter the criticisms of high-stakes standardized testing (Linn & Miller, 2005). Alternative assessments are more likely to take into account contextual and cultural factors that facilitate or impede learning (Losardo & Notari-Syverson, 2001). These models generally have the previously described advantages of criterion-referenced assessments and have much relevance and applicability in the field of communication disorders. You may hear various terms used in reference to these models. For example, **authentic assessment, performance assessment,** and **functional assessment** all emphasize performance on real-life or authentic tasks in naturalistic situations (Baron & Boschee, 1995; Frattali, 1998; Losardo & Notari-Syverson, 2001). Data collected about a client's performance often include various **artifacts** (examples of written work, projects, language samples, etc.) organized into a **portfolio.** Scoring **rubrics** are frequently used to make judgments about the degree to which the performance demonstrates the desired behavior or skill.

Behavioral Observation

The testing methods that we have discussed so far were designed to compare an individual's performance against some standard, whether that standard is the performance of others with similar demographic characteristics or some predetermined criterion. Observational techniques, however, provide a means for describing behavior in a systematic fashion without reference to any predetermined standard. They are useful for measuring the presence or absence of a behavior; the frequency, rate, magnitude, or duration of its occurrence; and the situations in which it is likely to occur. Observations can be made in real time (as they occur) or can be videotaped or audiotaped for later analysis. There are qualitative and quantitative approaches to systematic observation; both have specific, albeit quite different, methodologies associated with them in order to gather meaningful information.

Qualitative systematic observation is primarily descriptive, although it should not be confused with anecdotal records. The latter often precedes quantitative assessment, with the observer watching the individual to get a general impression and recording a description of the behaviors and the contexts in which the behaviors occurred (Salvia & Ysseldyke, 1998). Qualitative methodology involves prolonged observation by highly trained observers with prescribed ways of interpreting results and ensuring reliability and validity (Marshall & Rossman, 1995). **Ethnography,** one type of qualitative methodology, is particularly effective for obtaining information about children and families from different cultural groups (e.g., Crago & Cole, 1991; Hammer, 1998). Another method, **conversation analysis,** has been found to be useful in describing the conversational competence of individuals with aphasia (e.g., Damico, Oelschlaeger, & Simmons-Mackie, 1999).

Dynamic assessments, interactive procedures aimed at providing various levels of support in order to gauge a client's potential for change, are often based on qualitative methodologies (Elliott, 2000; Losardo & Notari-Syverson, 2001). Lidz and Peña (1996) noted three types of information provided by dynamic approaches: a description of how an individual approaches a task, error patterns, and the ability to self-correct; the modifiability of the behavior; and potential directions for effective intervention. Several different dynamic approaches with applicability to communication disorders have been described in the literature, including diagnostic teaching, successive cuing, and mediated learning experiences (Paul, 2001).

When using quantitative approaches to systematic observation, a few guidelines should be kept in mind. First, you must identify the purpose of the observation and be clear about the behaviors that you wish to observe. Define the behaviors and select the contexts in which you will observe. Second, it is important to have a recording system that is appropriate to the behavior you wish to measure. Your recording system can be as simple as a tally sheet you can check every time the behavior of interest is observed. Other recording methods include rankings (e.g., frequently, seldom, never), ratings (e.g., scale of 1–5), and duration (e.g., how many seconds the behavior lasted). An example of a scale for rating speech intelligibility is provided in Table 3.5.

Sometimes it is important to assess affective behaviors, such as attitudes. In many cases, there may be a direct link between a communication disorder and

Table 3.5. Intelligibility rating scale for motor speech disorders

Rating	Dimension	Intelligibility is...

10	Environment[a]
	Content[b]
	Efficiency[c]
		Normal in all environments
		    without restrictions on content
		    without need for repairs

9	Environment
	Content
	Efficiency
		Sometimes[d] reduced under adverse conditions
		    when content is unrestricted
		    but adequate with repairs

8	Environment
	Content
	Efficiency
		Sometimes reduced under ideal conditions
		    when content is unrestricted
		    but adequate with repairs

7	Environment
	Content
	Efficiency
		Sometimes reduced under adverse conditions
		    even when content is restricted
		    but adequate with repairs

6	Environment
	Content
	Efficiency
		Sometimes reduced under ideal conditions
		    when content is unrestricted
		    even when repairs are attempted

5	Environment
	Content
	Efficiency
		Usually[e] reduced under adverse conditions
		    when content is unrestricted
		    even when repairs are attempted

4	Environment
	Content
	Efficiency
		Usually reduced under ideal conditions
		    even when content is restricted
		    but adequate with repairs

3	Environment
	Content
	Efficiency
		Usually reduced under adverse conditions
		    even when content is restricted
		    even when repairs are attempted

2	Environment
	Content
	Efficiency
		Usually reduced under ideal conditions
		    even when content is restricted
		    even when repairs are attempted

1	Speech is not a viable means of communication in any environment, regardless of restrictions in content or attempts at repair

From Duffy, J.R. (2005). *Motor speech disorders: Substrates, differential diagnosis, and management* (2nd ed., p. 97). St. Louis: Elsevier; reprinted by permission.

[a]Environment may be "ideal" (e.g., face-to-face, without visual or auditory deficits in the listener, without competition from noise or visual distractions) or "adverse" (e.g., at a distance, with visual or auditory deficits or distractions).

[b]Content may be "unrestricted" (e.g., all pragmatically appropriate content, new topics, lengthy narratives) or "restricted" (e.g., limited to brief responses to questions or statements that permit some prediction of response content).

[c]Efficiency may be "normal" (e.g., rarely in need of repetition or clarification because of poor speech production) or "repairs" may be necessary (e.g., repetition, restatement, responses to clarifying questions, modified production such as oral spelling, word-by-word confirmation of listener's repetition, spelling).

[d]Intelligibility is reduced in 25% or less of utterances.

[e]Intelligibility is reduced in 50% or more of utterances, but not for all utterances.

Note: Not all combinations of deviant dimensions can be captured by a 10-point scale, and there is an obvious gray area between the meaning of *sometimes* and *usually*. The point on the scale that most closely approximates the clinician's judgment should be used. Many patients will fit into more than one point on the scale. It is appropriate to assign a range rather than a single point in such cases (e.g., 5–6).

a person's feelings and attitudes. For example, in cases of stuttering, feelings and attitudes are considered to be part of the disorder (Guitar, 1998). In other cases, feelings and attitudes may have a direct impact on a person's ability to communicate, as in the effect of stress on a person's voice (e.g., Case, 1996). Thus, information about affective behaviors is helpful in understanding the level of activity, limitations, and participation restrictions that individuals may experience as a result of their disability. Checklists or surveys completed by the client or a family member can be good sources of information about these areas. A number of such surveys are commonly used in communication assessments. An example frequently used in fluency assessments is shown in Figure 3.4. Overall, behavioral observations can be an invaluable source of information in establishing baselines, determining targets for intervention, and gauging progress.

Use of Instrumentation in Communication Assessment

Although instrumentation has always been essential in hearing assessment and certain types of speech assessment, recent advances in technology have resulted in the increased availability and usefulness of instrumentation in the assessment process. Technological tools for assessment include instrumentation for actual testing as well as computer software for scoring and analyzing data. Some examples of technological tools for assessment are the audiometer and **immittance** meter, which are used for behavioral and **electrophysiologic** measures of hearing. It also includes instruments for speech assessment such as the Computerized Speech Lab (www.kayelemetrics.com) for acoustic analysis of speech. Some examples of technology helpful in data scoring and analysis are software programs for scoring tests, such as Clinical Evaluation of Language Fundamentals–4 Scoring Assistant (CELF-4; Semel, Wiig, & Secord, 2003a) and language sample analysis such as Systematic Analysis of Language Transcripts (SALT; Miller & Iglesias, 2003–2005).

AREAS OF ASSESSMENT

In this section, we discuss the areas that you will be covering in an assessment. As illustrated in the beginning of the chapter, assessments may include the evaluation of many different communication disorders. Although the emphasis of the assessment will be on the area of concern, other speech, language, communication, and related areas must also be considered in order to create as complete a picture of the individual's communication profile as possible and to make a differential diagnosis when needed. Many types of speech and language disorders have a high probability of occurring together. For example, articulation disorders are frequently seen in children with language disorders (Bernthal & Bankson, 1998), and children with fluency disorders have a higher than typical rate of associated articulation disorders (Yairi, Ambrose, Paden, & Throneburg, 1996). Motor speech disorders affect not just articulation but all speech systems, resulting in voice and resonance abnormalities (Kent, 1994). Other speech and language disorders have been shown to have high rates of **comorbidity** with other developmental problems. For example, individuals with Down syndrome are at high risk not only for language disorders but also motor speech problems and hearing loss (Miller, Leddy, & Leavitt, 1999). Specific areas to be assessed follow,

Modified Erickson Scale of Communication Attitudes (S-24)

Name: _____ Date: _____ Score: _____

Directions: Mark the "true" column with a check (✓) for each statement that is true or mostly true for you and mark the "false" column with a check (✓) for each statement which is false or not usually true for you.

		TRUE	FALSE
1.	I usually feel that I am making a favorable impression when I talk.	____	____
2.	I find it easy to talk with almost anyone.	____	____
3.	I find it very easy to look at my audience while speaking to a group.	____	____
4.	A person who is my teacher or my boss is hard to talk to.	____	____
5.	Even the idea of giving a talk in public makes me afraid.	____	____
6.	Some words are harder than others for me to say.	____	____
7.	I forget all about myself shortly after I begin a speech.	____	____
8.	I am a good mixer.	____	____
9.	People sometimes seem uncomfortable when I am talking to them.	____	____
10.	I dislike introducing one person to another.	____	____
11.	I often ask questions in group discussions.	____	____
12.	I find it easy to keep control of my voice when speaking.	____	____
13.	I do not mind speaking before a group.	____	____
14.	I do not talk well enough to do the kind of work I'd really like to do.	____	____
15.	My speaking voice is rather pleasant and easy to listen to.	____	____
16.	I am sometimes embarrassed by the way I talk.	____	____
17.	I face most speaking situations with complete confidence.	____	____
18.	There are few people I can talk to easily.	____	____
19.	I talk better than I write.	____	____
20.	I often feel nervous while talking.	____	____
21.	I find it hard to make small talk when I meet new people.	____	____
22.	I feel pretty confident about my speaking ability.	____	____
23.	I wish that I could say things as clearly as others do.	____	____
24.	Even though I knew the right answer, I have often failed to give it because I was afraid to speak out.	____	____

Figure 3.4. Example of a self-report checklist used in stuttering assessment. Score 1 point for each answer that matches the following: 1. False, 2. False, 3. False, 4. True, 5. True, 6. True, 7. False, 8. False, 9. True, 10. True, 11. False, 12. False, 13. False, 14. True, 15. False, 16. True, 17. False, 18. True, 19. False, 20. True, 21. True, 22. False, 23. True, 24. True. For stutterers the mean is 19.22 and the range is 9–24; for non-stutterers the mean is 9.14 and the range is 1–21. (From Andrews, G., & Cutler, J. [1974]. Stuttering therapy: The relation between changes in symptom level and attitudes. *Journal of Speech and Hearing Disorders, 39,* 318–319. ©American Speech-Language-Hearing Association; reprinted with permission.)

and Tables 3.3 and 3.4 show examples of commonly used instruments for assessment of the various areas.

Language

Domains A useful paradigm for language assessment is to consider an individual's performance in the areas of **content, form,** and **use** (Bloom & Lahey, 1978; Lahey, 1988). Effective communicators demonstrate competence in all three areas, and there is interaction among the three areas. Language content, or **semantics,** includes the areas of vocabulary, concepts, and linkages of ideas. Language form includes rules of **syntax, morphology, phonology,** and **prosody.** Language use, or **pragmatics,** includes interactional aspects, such as being able to express a variety of communicative intentions (e.g., requests, protests, comments), using conversational rules (e.g., turn-taking, asking for clarification when necessary, initiating conversation, maintaining a topic), and taking the listener's perspective.

Modalities Each of these domains consists of a receptive and an expressive component. Individuals must both comprehend and be able to produce the elements of content, form, and use in their native language. For older children and adults, language assessment should also include consideration of literacy skills. The following are some specific issues in each major modality of language.

1. *Comprehension:* Because we cannot directly observe comprehension and must rely on various behaviors from which we make inferences about an individual's comprehension, assessment in this area can be challenging, especially in young children and those people whose production skills are impaired. Much has been written in the literature about what constitutes proof of comprehension (e.g., Bates, Bretherton, & Snyder, 1988; Hirsh-Pasek & Golinkoff, 1996). We typically assess comprehension in terms of some motor production, such as pointing to a picture or object or acting out a command or sentence. Consider a young child who does not carry out a command that we give him during an assessment. Is it because he does not understand the words? Is it because he is not compliant? Is it because he does not have the necessary motor skills? It can be difficult to sort out. In such a situation, additional assessment methods such as parent report, dynamic assessment techniques, and observation may be helpful in formulating a hypothesis about the possible reasons for the child's performance.

    One important distinction to make in assessing comprehension is the difference between contextualized (in the presence of routines and nonlinguistic cues) and decontextualized (as in formal testing) tasks. Many authors, including Chapman (1978) and Paul (1990), have noted the differences in performance between the two. Gathering information about both, or in other words, using both standardized and non-standardized procedures, can be helpful in getting a more complete picture of the client's skills. Specific areas to be assessed include receptive vocabulary and concepts, knowledge of syntactic and morphological forms, and comprehension of discourse-level language and social aspects of language use.

2. *Formulation and production:* Although measuring expressive language may appear to be more straightforward than comprehension, expressive language presents its own set of challenges. As Paul (2001) and others have pointed out, the nature of a task may influence the amount and complexity of language that is produced during that task. For example, several studies have noted differences in performance between imitated and spontaneous productions in children (Siegel, Winitz, & Conkey, 1963; Prutting, Gallagher, & Mulac, 1975). Because language is a transactional process, the communication partners influence each other's productions. The types of questions and directions given by the examiner will have an impact on the client's response. Consider the following brief examples:

> Examiner: What color is your car?
> Client: Red.
> Examiner: Tell me about your car.
> Client: It's a red convertible.

It would be a mistake to conclude that the second example represents a more complex response. Both clients were fulfilling their obligations as communication partners by responding contingently. Open-ended questions and requests for information are preferable when trying to elicit multiword utterances.

Assessment of language production and formulation skills include the size and usage of vocabulary, semantic relations in word combinations, usage of grammatical and morphological structures, phonology, pragmatic skills, and prosody. Typical tasks to assess these areas include labeling pictures or objects, describing action in pictures, defining words, filling in the blanks, constructing sentences with a stimulus word, and imitating sentences. Although these types of tasks are useful in testing expressive language skills in a decontextualized manner, more information is needed to describe the person's expressive abilities in actual conversations. For this purpose, language sampling is the most valid and useful method of assessment (see Chapter 5).

Motor Speech

Speech intelligibility is an important factor in communication effectiveness. When intelligibility is affected, the relative contributions of linguistic (i.e., phonologic) and motor (i.e., articulation) skills to the problem must be considered. A variety of perceptual, acoustic, and physiologic instruments are available for assessing motor speech status (Duffy, 2005). Typical perceptual tasks involve naming pictures or objects and reading sentences (for clients who are literate). Again, analysis of spontaneous speech will provide the most valuable information regarding overall intelligibility (see Table 3.5 for an example of an intelligibility rating scale). Examining the oral mechanism and assessing the client's performance in nonspeech tasks are both critical in the investigation of the structure and function of the articulators. Specialized tests are also available to help identify symptoms of dysarthria (weakness or lack of coordination of the speech musculature) or apraxia (motor speech impairment in the absence of weakness or lack of coordination of muscles). See Chapter 4 for an in-depth discussion of speech mechanism assessment.

Voice

Voice assessment includes analysis of various perceptual, acoustic, and physio-logic factors. The assessment should include evaluation of the individual's pitch, loudness, vocal quality, resonance, speaking rate, phonation, and respiration. These areas can be assessed noninstrumentally through perceptual measures, such as criterion-referenced tasks and rating scales, and with a variety of instrumentation, such as the Computerized Speech Lab. **Videostroboscopy,** a way of viewing the anatomy and physiology of the larynx and surrounding structures, has become an invaluable tool in the diagnosis of voice disorders. ASHA (1998) has affirmed the use of this technique to be within the scope of practice for SLPs, but specialized training is required. Teamwork between the SLP and the oto-laryngologist is essential in the assessment process. Whereas the physician makes the medical diagnosis, the SLP makes the diagnosis of a voice disorder. The voice assessment may either precede or follow the medical evaluation, but under no circumstance can therapy be initiated before a complete laryngeal examination by the otolaryngologist is completed (Boone & McFarlane, 2000).

Fluency

Assessment of fluency disorders includes the careful observation and measure-ment of the client's speech behaviors as well as assessment of various aspects of the client's feelings and attitudes about communication and stuttering (Guitar, 1998; Zebrowski, 2000). Speech samples should be obtained in several different situations. This usually includes at least a reading and a conversational sample. Analysis of the samples will include calculating the percentage of syllables and words stuttered and the speech rate, timing the duration of any blocks, and de-scribing the relative percentages of different types of disfluencies (**repetitions, prolongations, blocks**). Physical concomitants such as eye blinks and head nods should be described and rated as to their severity. A variety of surveys and questionnaires are available to assess attitudes and feelings (see Figure 3.4). In the evaluation of a client referred for disfluencies, it is always important to make a differential diagnosis between typical disfluency and stuttering, particularly in young children (Guitar, 1998).

Hearing

The impact of hearing impairment on communication functioning is well docu-mented. Audiologists are the professionals responsible for the evaluation of hear-ing and hearing impairment. The scope of practice of audiology includes the use of a variety of behavioral, electroacoustic, and electrophysiologic methods to assess hearing, balance, and neural system function (ASHA, 1996a) (see Chapter 10).

Early diagnosis of hearing loss is crucial to speech and language development. Testing the hearing of young children, however, can be quite challenging. Based on the child's age and developmental level, behavioral testing techniques would consist of behavioral observation, **visual reinforcement audiometry,** or **play audiometry** techniques. Electrophysiological testing procedures, which measure involuntary responses and therefore do not rely on the child's cooperation, are used to confirm or rule out a hearing loss and to estimate the type and degree of a hearing loss. These procedures include **auditory brain stem evoked response**

audiometry and the measurement of **otoacoustic emissions (OAEs)**. With older children and adults who are able to cooperate in the assessment, audiological evaluation usually consists of **pure tone audiometry, speech audiometry,** and immittance testing.

Because of the critical importance of hearing, all communication assessments should include at least a hearing screening. The scope of practice of speech-language pathology includes pure-tone hearing screening and screening **tympanometry** (ASHA, 1996b). ASHA has developed guidelines for the screening of individuals of all ages (ASHA Audiologic Assessment Panel 1996, 1997). Different techniques and criteria are used for pediatric and adult populations. The following information summarizes criteria for the audiological screening of children ages 5–18, and Figure 3.5 summarizes recommended screening practices for adults. Any client who is unable to participate or who fails the hearing screening must be referred for a full audiological evaluation.

PROCEDURES FOR SCREENING
THE HEARING OF SCHOOL-AGED CHILDREN

Clinical indications

1. Screen school-age children on initial entry to school, annually in kindergarten through third grade, and in seventh and eleventh grades.
2. Screen school-age children as needed, requested, or mandated. In addition, children should be screened upon entrance to special education, in the case of grade repetition, new entry to the school system without evidence of having passed a previous hearing screening, or absence during a previously scheduled screening.
3. The following risk factors suggest the need for a hearing screening in other years:
   A. Parent/care provider, health care provider, teacher, or other school personnel have concerns regarding hearing, speech, language, or learning abilities
   B. Family history of late or delayed onset hereditary hearing loss
   C. Recurrent or persistent otitis media with effusion for at least 3 months
   D. Craniofacial anomalies, including those with morphological abnormalities of the pinna and ear canal
   E. Stigmata or other findings associated with a syndrome known to include sensorineural and/or conductive hearing loss
   F. Head trauma with loss of consciousness
   G. Reported exposure to potentially damaging noise levels or ototoxic drugs
4. School-age children who receive regular audiologic management need not participate in a screening program.

Clinical process

1. These guidelines recommend obtaining informed consent, or, in the case of children, informed parental/legal guardian permission; however, extant state statutes or regulations, or institutional policies, supersede this recommendation.

2. Conduct screening in a manner congruent with appropriate infection control and universal precautions.

3. Conditioned play audiometry (CPA) or conventional audiometry are the procedures of choice.

4. Conduct screening under earphones using 1000, 2000, and 4000 hertz (Hz) tones at 20 decibel hearing level (dB HL)

5. All hearing screening programs should include an educational component designed to provide parents with information, in lay language, on the process of hearing screening, the likelihood of their child having a hearing impairment, and follow-up procedures.

Pass/refer criteria

1. Pass if responses are judged to be clinically reliable at criterion dB level at each frequency in each ear.

2. If a child does not respond at criterion dB level at any frequency in either ear, reinstruct, reposition earphones, and rescreen within the same screening session in which the child fails.

3. Pass children who pass the rescreening.

4. Refer children who fail the rescreening or fail to condition to the screening task.*

*From American Speech-Language-Hearing Association Audiologic Assessment Panel 1996. (1997). *Guidelines for audiologic screening.* Rockville, MD: Author. © American Speech-Language-Hearing Association; reprinted with permission.

Two other areas of assessment fall within the domain of the SLP: **augmentative and alternative communication (AAC)** assessment and swallowing (**dysphagia**) evaluation. Individuals with severely compromised communication skills may benefit from a variety of AAC systems and strategies. These range from low cost, low technology options, such as sign language and pictures, to very expensive, highly sophisticated devices, using computerized screens and synthesized voice output. Because SLPs are knowledgeable about the oral motor and pharyngeal mechanisms, our scope of practice has evolved to include the evaluation and treatment of chewing and swallowing disorders, even in the absence of communication disorders. To competently assess clients in these two areas, additional specialized expertise and instrumentation are required.

Collateral Areas

In getting a complete picture of the client's communication status, it is frequently necessary to gather information about other areas of development or functioning that impact communication. In many settings, you will be working as part of a team, so that team members from other professions will also be evaluating the client simultaneously or will be available for consultation to obtain the relevant data. Some or all of this information may be already available from records or, if you are not working in a team setting, it may be necessary to refer the

---

Hearing Screening (Adults)

Name: _____ Date: _____

Date of birth: _____ Age: _____ Gender: ____ Male ____ Female

Screening unit/examiner: _____ Calibration date: _____

Case history (circle appropriate answers)

Do you think you have a hearing loss?	Yes	No
Have hearing aid(s) ever been recommended for you?	Yes	No
Is your hearing better in one ear?	Yes	No

If yes, which is the better ear? Right   Left

Have you ever had a sudden or rapid progression of hearing loss?	Yes	No

If yes, which ear? Right   Left

Do you have ringing or noises in your ears?	Yes	No

If yes, which ear? Right   Left   Both

Do you consider dizziness to be a problem for you?	Yes	No
Have you had recent drainage from your ear(s)?	Yes	No

If yes, which ear? Right   Left

Do you have pain or discomfort in your ear(s)?	Yes	No

If yes, which ear? Right   Left

Have you received medical consultation for any of the above conditions?	Yes	No

            PASS   **REFER**

Visual/otoscopic inspection

            PASS   **REFER**   Right   Left

Referral for cerumen management _____   Referral for medical evaluation _____

Pure-tone screen (25 decibel [dB] hearing level [HL])   (R = Response, NR = No Response)

Frequency	1000	2000	4000 Hz
Right Ear			
Left Ear			

            PASS   **REFER**

Hearing-disability index

Score: HHIE-S _____   SAC _____   Other _____   Score _____

            PASS   **REFER**

Discharge   ____ Medical examination   ____ Counsel

                ____ Cerumen management   ____ Audiologic evaluation

Comments: _____

_____

Patient signature: _____ Date: _____

Figure 3.5. Protocol for adult hearing screening. (*Key:* Hz = hertz, HHIE-S = hearing handicap inventory for the elderly, SAC = self-assessment of communication.) (From American Speech-Language-Hearing Association Audiologic Assessment Panel 1996. [1997]. *Guidelines for audiologic screening.* Rockville, MD: Author. ©American Speech-Language-Hearing Association; reprinted with permission.)

client to another professional in order to get the required information. Collateral areas include the following:

1. *Cognitive status:* Because cognitive status can have an impact on aspects of language, it helpful to have at least a general sense of the individual's non-verbal cognitive status. Ideally, you will have this information from psycho-logical assessment, but in many instances, this information will not be available. SLPs are not qualified to do IQ testing; however, there are informal screening measures that can help establish whether the client is functioning at or near age level in the nonverbal cognitive area. For children, Paul (2001) suggested play assessments, Piagetian tasks, and drawing as screenings. For adults with suspected cognitive impairments, a combination of informal tasks and a general screening instrument, such as the Mini Mental State exam (Folstein, Folstein, & McHugh, 1975), may be used. In either case, if you have concerns about the client's performance, a referral for cognitive testing should be made.

2. *Literacy:* When testing adults and older children, reading and writing skills should always be considered as part of a comprehensive assessment. In test batteries designed for adults with neurogenic-based language disorders, such as the Western Aphasia Battery (Kertesz, 1982) and the Boston Diagnostic Aphasia Examination, Third Edition (Goodglass, Kaplan, & Barresi, 2000), reading comprehension and written expression subtests are essential com-ponents of the test. In testing older children and adults, a variety of tests, such as the Oral and Written Language Scales (Carrow-Woolfolk, 1995) and the Woodcock Language Proficiency Battery-Revised (Woodcock, 1991), are available to assess reading and writing skills.

3. *Social/emotional/behavioral:* Because communication is an interactive process, it is important to know something about our clients' social environment in order to understand their needs (Paul, 2001). Paul cautioned that commu-nication patterns in families may be an adaptation to the needs of the indi-vidual with a disability rather than a cause of the communication problem. Information about the client's social functioning can be obtained through the interview process, review of records, self-report surveys, and observation of the client. Instruments, such as the Vineland Adaptive Behavior Scales, Second Edition (Sparrow, Balla, & Cicchetti, 2005), can be administered by a trained SLP and can yield important information about the client's status in this domain. Gathering information in this area will also help you in de-termining the degree of activity limitation experienced by the client. Referrals to or consultation with mental health professionals such as social workers, psychologists, or psychiatrists may be necessary.

4. *Motor functioning:* Information about the client's gross and fine motor skills may be very relevant to the communication assessment, particularly in making realistic recommendations. For clients with significant motor problems, knowing about the client's motor status is crucial as proper positioning and use of adaptive equipment are important in getting valid and reliable data during the assessment. Physical and occupational therapists may be part of your team, in which case, they may already be involved in the case or readily accessible to you for consultation. If not, a referral may be in order.

PLANNING FOR ASSESSMENT

In order to obtain the most relevant information in an efficient manner, assessments must be carefully planned. When preparing, it is helpful to organize yourself by asking the following questions:

1. What is the presenting problem or concern? What questions are being asked of the assessment? It is important to know, from the referrer's point of view, how the problem is viewed.

2. What do you already know? This includes obtaining and reviewing pertinent case information such as medical records, school records, previous evaluations, and past therapy reports.

3. What do you want to find out during the assessment? Identify the missing data that you need in order to answer the presenting questions. What communication and collateral areas do you need to assess?

4. How will you find out what you want to know? This includes not only the particular tests you will use but also the contexts in which you want to observe the client and how you will sequence the assessment activities to maximize your productivity and efficiency.

Answering these questions will provide you with a preliminary plan for the assessment session. Remember that you will need to remain flexible enough to make changes in your plan if necessary. Figure 3.6 shows what planning for Darrell's assessment might look like.

Name: Darrell Thompson	**Age:** 4 years, 6 months
Presenting problems or concerns; reasons for the assessment: Speech is difficult to understand. Child seems frustrated when not understood. Speech seems immature.	
What do we know? • Developmental milestones within normal limits (by parent report) • Attends preschool • Youngest of three children; older brother had speech therapy • History of asthma, hay fever, croup, ear infections • Failed audiological evaluation; being treated with antibiotics for ear infection	
What do we need to find out?	**How will we get the information?**
Are speech and language (vocabulary, syntax, morphology, phonology) developmentally appropriate?	Norm-referenced language test (TOLD-P:3); articulation and phonological testing
What percentage of speech is intelligible? What are typical language production skills?	Spontaneous communication sampling
What is status of other speech and communication areas (pragmatics, oral motor, fluency, voice)?	Screening, observation
What are skills in collateral areas (play, readiness, social, motor)?	Observation, informal tasks, parent report
What is stimulability for speech sounds and more advanced language forms?	Informal tasks, imitation

Figure 3.6. Assessment planning worksheet for Darrell. (*Key:* TOLD-P:3 = Test of Language Development—Primary: third edition.)

STEPS IN THE ASSESSMENT PROCESS

The flowchart in Figure 3.7 details the typical sequence and problem solving process involved in communication assessment from the point of referral to the completion of the assessment report. We can summarize the main steps in the diagnostic sequence, keeping in mind that the activities are not always quite as linear as they look. Data gathering, or the preassessment phase as it is sometimes called, is your first major task. This will include getting appropriate releases of information and reviewing relevant records as described previously. In addition to written case history information, you (or another team member) will interview the client and/or family members and possibly consult with other professionals involved in the case. Although many agencies have written case history questionnaires, it is helpful to have a face-to-face discussion with the client and

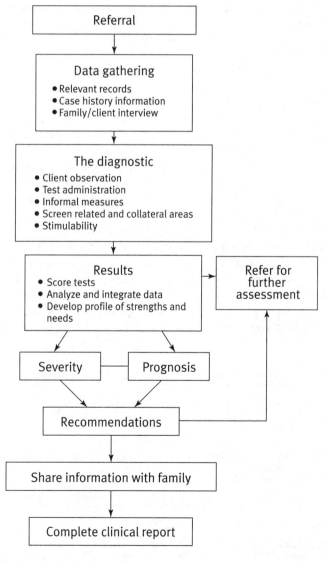

Figure 3.7. Steps in the communication assessment process.

family even if they have filled out a form. This will give you an opportunity to follow up on topics of interest. Interviewing techniques and areas to be covered in a diagnostic interview will be discussed further in Chapter 8. The second major task consists of the administration of the tests, other assessment procedures, and stimulability activities in the communication and collateral areas that you have identified in your assessment plan.

The third major task of the assessment involves the scoring and interpretation of the various pieces of data you have obtained. The information gathered about the client's performance during the assessment must now be integrated with other information gathered during the process. This information is considered in light of other potential issues including the client's particular life circumstances, cultural and linguistic differences, and developmental history.

Once you have analyzed and synthesized the data, you will need to make a statement about the severity of the person's communication problems. Severity is usually described as mild, moderate, severe, or profound. Although these judgments are somewhat subjective, there are some guidelines to follow as shown in Table 3.6. You will also make a statement of prognosis. Prognosis is a prediction about the course and outcome of the communication problem. This is based on all of the information that you have accumulated during the assessment and consideration of the research literature on the specific problem with which you are dealing. Paul (2001) cautioned that, in the case of young children, making short-term prognoses and stating them positively is the best route. In the case of adults with neurogenic impairments, a number of variables including general health, neurologic status, and severity of impairment must be considered in arriving at a prognosis (Brookshire, 2003). Next, you need to state your recommendations. The recommendations must include a statement of whether therapy is indicated. If it is, it is important to include appropriate goals for intervention and specific techniques or strategies that you have observed to be successful with the client during the assessment process.

All of this information must now be shared with the client and family. The feedback should be provided in an empathic, family-friendly, culturally sensitive manner (see Chapter 8). Finally, all of this information has to be put into a clinical report. Diagnostic reports follow a fairly standard format and are discussed in Chapter 8. When preparing your report, keep in mind the intended audience. Foremost, remember that parents and other professionals who may have little knowledge of the field will read your report. To make your report easily understood,

Table 3.6.   Classifications of severity ratings for individuals with mental retardation

Classification	Description
Mild	Some impact on performance but does not preclude participation in age-appropriate activities Able to function independently with minimal assistance
Moderate	Significant degree of impairment that requires accommodations to function in mainstream settings Able to function in a supervised setting
Severe	Extensive support services required to function in typical settings May demonstrate some functional skills with supervision
Profound	Few functional skills Requires maximum assistance with basic activities

Sources: Accardo & Whitman, 2002; World Health Organization, 2004.

you must write it professionally but not use jargon. If the report will be sent to a funding agency, such as an insurance company or school district, it is important to include the information that the agency will use to make decisions regarding funding. An outline for an assessment report can be found in Chapter 8, and a sample report is included in the appendix at the end of this chapter.

CHALLENGES IN ASSESSMENT

During your career, you will be asked to evaluate clients who, for various reasons, may be difficult to assess. Clients may be extremely passive and withdrawn, or they may be overly active, impulsive, and non-compliant. Clients may present with severe physical disabilities, be medically fragile, or easily fatigued. Despite these challenges, no client should be considered untestable. It may be necessary, however, to make adaptations in the environment and in your interactions with the client in order to gather useful information. Paul (2001) pointed out that usually when a client is labeled "untestable," the clinician means that the client was not cooperative or responsive to standardized testing. As we discussed previously, many other types of instruments are available to the clinician. Strategies to elicit information in these less than optimal circumstances include the use of observational data and informal tasks rather than direct testing. Caregivers may be interviewed regarding typical communication behaviors for the client. Giving frequent breaks and providing small snacks may be necessary for the client who is weak or easily fatigued. For clients with behavioral compliance issues, reinforcement, including the use of food reinforcement, may be necessary to complete testing. Multiple sessions and multiple contexts are also helpful in getting representative behavior from such clients. The important thing to remember is that, even for the most difficult client, there are methods and strategies for gathering enough evidence to determine the existence of a problem, determine eligibility for services, and develop some initial goals for intervention.

CONCLUSION

Before ending the discussion on assessment, a final point must be made. No matter how skilled the examiner and how thorough the assessment protocol, it is important to remember that the assessment represents the client's performance in a limited number of situations during a limited time period, and under limited circumstances. The examiner can only observe what the client does, not necessarily what the client is capable of doing. The latter is inferred from the former. A skilled examiner who obtains a representative sample of the client's relevant behaviors and who uses reliable and valid accurately administered, scored, and interpreted assessment instruments will make the most accurate prognoses and appropriate recommendations.

You will discover that assessment and diagnosis are fascinating processes in their own right, but remember that they are only means to an end—the development of effective intervention plans to meet the individual needs of clients. Good assessment forms the beginning of effective intervention, and, conversely, good intervention is characterized by regular assessment of its effectiveness. Communication assessment is an integral component of the chain of events resulting in effective management of communication disorders.

REFERENCES

Aase, D., Hovre, C., Krause, K., Schelfhout, S., Smith, J., & Carpenter, L.J. (2000). *Contextual Test of Articulation*. Eau Claire, WI: Thinking Publications.

Accardo, P.J., & Whitman, B.Y. (Eds.) (2002). *Dictionary of developmental disabilities terminology* (2nd ed.). Baltimore: Paul H. Brookes Publishing Co.

American Speech-Language-Hearing Association. (1996a, Spring). Scope of practice in audiology. *ASHA, 38* (Suppl. 16), 12–15.

American Speech-Language-Hearing Association. (1996b, Spring). Scope of practice in speech-language pathology. *ASHA, 38* (Suppl. 16), 16–20.

American Speech-Language-Hearing Association. (1998). The role of otolaryngologist and speech-language pathologist in the performance and interpretation of strobovideolaryngoscopy. *ASHA, 40* (Suppl. 18), 32.

American Speech-Language-Hearing Association. (2005). *Evidence-based practice in communication disorders [position statement]*. Retrieved June 1, 2006, from http://www.asha.org/members/deskrefjournals/deskref/default

American Speech-Language-Hearing Association Audiologic Assessment Panel 1996. (1997). *Guidelines for audiologic screening*. Rockville, MD: Author.

Andrews, G., & Cutler, J. (1974). Stuttering therapy: The relation between changes in symptom level and attitudes. *Journal of Speech and Hearing Disorders, 39*, 318–319.

Bankson, N.W., & Bernthal, J.E. (1990). *Quick Screen of Phonology*. Itasca, IL: The Riverside Publishing Co.

Baron, M.A., & Boschee, F. (1995). *Authentic assessment: the key to student success*. Lancaster, PA: Technomic.

Bates, E., Bretherton, I., & Snyder, L. (1988). *From first words to grammar: Individual differences and dissociable mechanisms*. New York: Cambridge University Press.

Bayles, K, & Tomoeda, C. (1993). *Arizona Battery for Communication Disorders of Dementia*. Tucson, AZ: Canyonlands.

Bernthal, J.E., & Bankson, N.W. (1998). *Articulation and phonological disorders* (4th ed.). Boston: Allyn & Bacon.

Blakeley, R. (2000). *Screening Test for Developmental Apraxia of Speech* (2nd ed.). Austin, TX: PRO-ED.

Bloom, L., & Lahey, M. (1978). *Language development and language disorders*. Hoboken, NJ: John Wiley & Sons.

Boone, D. (1993). *The Boone Voice Program for Children* (2nd ed.). Austin, TX: PRO-ED.

Boone, D.R., & McFarlene, S.C. (2000). *The voice and voice treatment*. Boston: Allyn & Bacon.

Brookshire, R.H. (2003). *Introduction to neurogenic communication disorders* (6th ed.). St. Louis: Elsevier.

Brownell, R. (Ed.). (2000). *Expressive One Word Picture Vocabulary Test*. Novato, CA: Academic Therapy Publications.

Burns, M.S. (1997). *Burns Brief Inventory of Communication and Cognition*. San Antonio, TX: Harcourt Assessment.

Carrow-Woolfolk, E. (1995). *Oral and Written Language Scales*. Circle Pines, MN: AGS Publishing.

Carrow-Woolfolk, E. (1999a). *Comprehensive Assessment of Spoken Language*. Circle Pines, MN: AGS Publishing.

Carrow-Woolfolk, E. (1999b). *Test of Auditory Comprehension of Language* (3rd ed.). Austin, TX: PRO-ED.

Case, J.L. (1996). *Clinical management of voice disorders*. Austin, TX: PRO-ED.

Chapman, R.S. (1978). Comprehension strategies in children. In J.F. Kavanagh & W. Strange (Eds.), *Speech and language in the laboratory, school, and clinic* (pp. 308–327). Cambridge, MA: The MIT Press.

Coplan, J. (1993). *Early Language Milestones Scale* (2nd ed.). Austin, TX: PRO-ED.

Crago, M.B., & Cole, E. (1991). Using ethnography to bring children's communicative and cultural worlds into focus. In T.M. Gallagher (Ed.), *Pragmatics of language: Clinical practice issues* (pp. 99–131). San Diego: Singular Publishing Group.

Dabul, B. (2000). *Apraxia Battery for Adults* (2nd ed.). Austin, TX: PRO-ED.

Damico, J.S., Oelschlaeger, M., & Simmons-Mackie, N. (1999). Qualitative methods in aphasia research: Conversation analysis. *Aphasiology, 13*, 667–679.

Darley, F.L. (1991). A philosophy of appraisal and diagnosis. In F.L. Darley & D.C. Spriestersbach (Eds.), *Diagnostic methods in speech pathology* (2nd ed., pp. 1–23). Long Grove, IL: Waveland Press.

Deem, J.F., & Miller, L. (2000). *Manual of voice therapy* (2nd ed.). Austin, TX: PRO-ED.

Duffy, J.R. (2005). *Motor speech disorders: Substrates, differential diagnosis, and management* (2nd ed.). St. Louis: Elsevier.

Dunn, L.M., & Dunn, L.M. (1997). *Peabody Picture Vocabulary Test-III*. Circle Pines, MN: AGS Publishing.

Dunn, L.M., Lugo, D.E., Padilla, E.R., & Dunn, L.M. (1986). *Test de Vocabulario en Imagenes Peabody*. Circle Pines, MN: AGS Publishing.

Elliott, J.G. (2000). Dynamic assessment in educational contexts: Purpose and promise. In C.S. Lidz & J.G. Elliott (Eds.), *Dynamic assessment: Prevailing models and applications* (pp. 713–740). New York: Elsevier Science.

Emerick, L.L., & Hatten, J.T. (1974). *Diagnosis and evaluation in speech pathology*. Upper Saddle River: Prentice Hall.

Enderby, P.M. (1983). *Frenchay Dysarthria Assessment*. Austin, TX: PRO-ED.

Fenson, L., Dale, P., Reznick, J., Thal, D., Bates, E., Hartung, J., Pethick, S., & Reilly, J. (1993). *MacArthur Communicative Development Inventories*. San Diego: Singular Publishing Group.

Fluharty, N. (2001). *Fluharty Preschool Speech and Language Screening Test* (2nd ed.). Austin, TX: PRO-ED.

Folstein, M.F., Folstein, S.E., & McHugh, P.R. (1975). "Mini Mental State": A practical method of grading the cognitive state of patients for the clinician. *Journal of Psychiatric Research, 12*, 189-198.

Frattali, C.M. (1998). *Measuring outcomes in speech-language pathology*. New York: Thieme New York.

Gauthier, S., & Madison, C. (1998). *Kindergarten Language Screening Scale* (2nd ed.). Austin, TX: PRO-ED.

Gillam, R.B., & Pearson, N.A. (2004). *Test of Narrative Language*. Austin, TX: PRO-ED.

Goldman, R., & Fristoe, M. (2000). *Goldman-Fristoe Test of Articulation* (2nd ed.). Circle Pines, MN: AGS Publishing.

Goldsworthy, C. (1982). *Multilevel Informal Language Inventory*. Columbus, OH: Charles E. Merrill.

Goodglass, H., Kaplan, E., & Barresi, B. (2001). *Boston Diagnostic Aphasia Examination* (3rd ed.). Philadelphia: Lippincott Williams & Wilkins.

Guitar, B. (1998). *Stuttering: An integrated approach to its nature and treatment* (2nd ed.). Philadelphia: Lippincott Williams & Wilkins.

Hammer, C.S. (1998). Toward a "thick description" of families: Using ethnography to overcome the obstacles to providing family-centered early intervention services. *American Journal of Speech-Language Pathology, 7*, 5–22.

Hammill, D., Brown, V., Larsen, S., & Wiederholt, J. (1994). *Test of Adolescent and Adult Language* (3rd ed.). Austin, TX: PRO-ED.

Hammill, D., & Newcomer, P. (1997). *Test of Language Development-Intermediate* (3rd ed.). Austin, TX: PRO-ED.

Helm-Estabrooks, N., & Hotz, G. (1991). *Brief Test of Head Injury*. Itasca, IL: The Riverside Publishing Co.

Hirsh-Pasek, K., & Golinkoff, R.M. (1996). The intermodal preferential looking paradigm: A window onto emerging language comprehension. In D. McDaniel, C. McKee, & H.S. Cairns (Eds.). *Methods for assessing children's syntax* (pp.105-124). Cambridge, MA: The MIT Press.

Hiskey, M.S. (1966). *Hiskey-Nebraska Test of Learning Aptitude*. Lincoln, NE: Union College Press.

Hodson, B. (1986). *Assessment of Phonological Processes-Revised*. Austin, TX: PRO-ED.

Holland, A., Frattali, C., & Fromm, D. (1999). *Communication Activities in Daily Living* (2nd ed.). Austin, TX: PRO-ED.

Idol, L., Nevin, A., & Paolucci-Whitcomb, P. (1999). *Models of curriculum-based assessment: A blueprint for learning* (3rd ed.). Austin, TX: PRO-ED.

Individuals with Disabilities Education Act of 1990, PL 101-476, 20 U.S.C. §§ 1400 *et seq.*

Individuals with Disabilities Education Improvement Act of 2004, PL 108-446, 20 U.S.C. §§ 1400 *et seq.*

Kent, R.D. (1994). The clinical science of motor speech disorders. In J.A. Till, K.M. Yorkston, & D.R. Beukelman (Eds.), *Motor speech disorders: Advances in assessment and treatment* (pp. 3–18). Baltimore: Paul H. Brookes Publishing Co.

Kertesz, A. (1982). *Western Aphasia Battery.* San Antonio, TX: Harcourt Assessment.

Khan, L., & Lewis, N. (2002). *Khan-Lewis Phonological Analysis* (2nd ed.). Circle Pines, MN: AGS Publishing.

Lahey, M. (1988). *Language disorders and language development.* New York: Macmillan/McGraw-Hill.

Lidz, C.S., & Elliott, J.G. (2000). Introduction. In C.S. Lidz & J.G. Elliott (Eds.), *Dynamic assessment: Prevailing models and applications* (pp. 3–13). New York: Elsevier Science.

Lidz, C.S., & Peña, E.D. (1996). Dynamic assessment: The model, its relevance as a non-biased approach, and its application to Latino American preschool children. *Language, Speech, and Hearing Services in the Schools, 27,* 376–372.

Linn, R.L., & Miller, M.D. (2005). *Measurement and assessment in teaching* (9th ed.). Upper Saddle River, NJ: Pearson Education.

Losardo, A., & Notari-Syverson, A. (2001). *Alternative approaches to assessing young children.* Baltimore: Paul H. Brookes Publishing Co.

Marshall, C., & Rossman, G.B. (1995). *Designing qualitative research* (2nd ed.). Thousand Oaks, CA: Sage Publications.

McCauley, R.J., & Swisher, L. (1984). Psychometric review of language and articulation tests for preschool children. *Journal of Speech and Hearing Disorders, 49,* 34–42.

Miller, J. (1978). Assessing children's language behavior: A developmental process approach. In R.L. Schiefelbusch (Ed.), *Bases of language intervention* (pp. 269–318). Baltimore: University Park Press.

Miller, J. (1983). Identifying children with language disorders and describing language performance. In J. Miller, D. Yoder, & R. Schiefelbusch (Eds.), *Contemporary issues in language intervention* (pp. 61–74). Baltimore: University Park Press.

Miller, J., & Iglesias, A. (2003–2005). *Systematic Analysis of Language Transcripts (SALT), V8.* [Computer software]. Madison: Language Analysis Lab, Waisman Center, University of Wisconsin.

Miller, J.F., Leddy, M., & Leavitt, L.A. (1999). *Improving the communication of people with Down syndrome.* Baltimore: Paul H. Brookes Publishing Co.

Miller, J.F., & Paul, R. (1995). *The clinical assessment of language comprehension.* Baltimore: Paul H. Brookes Publishing Co.

Morgan, D.L., & Guilford, A. (1984). *Adolescent Language Screening Test.* Austin, TX: PRO-ED.

Nelson, N.W. (1998). *Childhood language disorders in context: Infancy through adolescence* (2nd ed.). Boston: Allyn & Bacon.

Newcomer, P., & Hammill, D. (1997). *Test of Language Development: Primary* (3rd ed.). Austin, TX: PRO-ED.

Paul, R. (1990). Comprehension strategies: Interactions between world knowledge and the development of sentence comprehension. *Topics in Language Disorders, 10*(3), 63–75.

Paul, R. (2001). *Language disorders: From infancy through adolescence* (2nd ed.). St. Louis: Elsevier.

Peterson, H.A., & Marquardt, T.P. (1994). *Appraisal and diagnosis of speech and language disorders* (3rd ed.). Upper Saddle River, NJ: Prentice Hall.

Phelps-Terasaki, D., & Phelps-Gunn, T. (1992). *Test of Pragmatic Language.* Austin, TX: PRO-ED.

Pindzola, R. (1987). *Voice Assessment Protocol for Children and Adults.* Austin, TX: PRO-ED.

Prutting, C., Gallagher, T., & Mulac, A. (1975). The expressive portion of the N.S.S.T. compared to a spontaneous language sample. *Journal of Speech and Hearing Disorders, 40,* 40–49.

Reynell, J., & Gruber, C. (1990). *Reynell Developmental Language Scales-U.S. Edition.* Los Angeles: Western Psychological Services.

Riley, G. (1994). *Stuttering Severity Instrument for Children and Adults* (3rd ed.). Austin, TX: PRO-ED.

Rossetti, L. (1990). *Rossetti Infant-Toddler Language Scale.* East Moline, IL: LinguiSystems.

Salvia, J., & Ysseldyke, J.E. (1998). *Assessment in special and remedial education* (7th ed.). Boston: Houghton Mifflin.

Schuell, H. (1973). *Minnesota Test for Differential Diagnosis of Aphasia.* Minneapolis: University of Minnesota Press.

Semel, E., Wiig, E., & Secord, W. (2003a). *CELF-4 Scoring Assistant*. [Computer software]. San Antonio, TX: Harcourt Assessment.

Semel, E., Wiig, E., & Secord, W. (2003b). *Clinical Evaluation of Language Fundamentals–4*. San Antonio, TX: Harcourt Assessment.

Semel, E., Wiig, E., & Secord, W. (2004). *Clinical Evaluation of Language Fundamentals–4 Screening Test*. San Antonio, TX: Harcourt Assessment.

Seymour, H.N., Roeper, T.W., deVilliers, J., & deVilliers, P.A. (2005). *Diagnostic Evaluation of Language Variation—Norm-Referenced*. Austin, TX: Harcourt Assessment.

Siegel, G.M., Winitz, H., & Conkey, H. (1963). The influence of testing instruments on articulation responses of children. *Journal of Speech and Hearing Disorders, 28*, 67–76.

Sparrow, S.S., Balla, D.A., Cicchetti, D.V. (2005). *Vineland Adaptive Behavior Scales* (2nd ed.). Circle Pines, MN: AGS Publishing.

St. Louis, K., & Ruscello, D. (2000). *Oral Speech Mechanism Screening Exam* (3rd ed.). Austin, TX: PRO-ED.

Thorndike, R.M. (2005). *Measurement and evaluation in psychology and education* (7th ed.). Upper Saddle River, NJ: Pearson Education.

Tomblin, J. B. (2000). Perspectives on diagnosis. In J.B. Tomblin & D.C. Spriestersbach (Eds.), *Diagnosis in speech-language pathology* (2nd ed., pp. 2–33). San Diego: Singular Publishing Group.

West, J., Sands, E., & Ross-Swain, D. (1998). *Bedside Evaluation Screening Test* (2nd ed.). Austin, TX: PRO-ED.

Wiig, E.H. (1990). *Wiig Criterion Referenced Inventory of Language*. San Antonio, TX: Harcourt Assessment.

Williams, K. (1997). *Expressive Vocabulary Test*. Circle Pines, MN: AGS Publishing.

Witt, J.C., Elliott, S.N., Gresham, F.M., & Kramer, J.J. (1988). *Assessment of special children*. Glenview, IL: Pearson Scott Foresman.

Woodcock, R. (1991). *Woodcock Language Proficiency Battery-Revised*. Allen, TX: DLM Teaching Resources.

World Health Organization. (2001). *International classification of functioning, disability and health (ICF)*. Geneva: Author.

World Health Organization. (2004). *International statistical classification of diseases and related health problems-10th revision* (2nd ed.). Geneva: Author.

Yairi, E., Ambrose, N., Paden, E.P., & Throneburg, R.N. (1996). Predictive factors of persistence and recovery: Pathways of childhood stuttering. *Journal of Communication Disorders, 29*, 51–77.

Zebrowski, P. (2000). Stuttering. In J.B. Tomblin & D.C. Spriestersbach (Eds.), *Diagnosis in speech-language pathology* (2nd ed., pp. 199–231). San Diego: Singular Publishing Group.

Zimmerman, I., Steiner, V., & Pond, R. (2002). *Preschool Language Scale–4*. San Antonio, TX: Harcourt Assessment.

STUDY QUESTIONS

1. Describe three different models of assessment. How would you decide which model to use?

2. List six purposes of assessment. Give an example of each.

3. Discuss the relative advantages and disadvantages of using norm-referenced tests.

4. List and define five important characteristics of norm-referenced tests.

5. Discuss the relative advantages and disadvantages of using criterion-referenced tests.

6. Discuss the relative advantages and disadvantages of using behavioral observations in assessment.

7. Name and describe the major communication and collateral areas to be covered during a communication assessment.

8. What are some key questions to ask yourself when preparing for an assessment?

9. Describe the main steps in the assessment process.

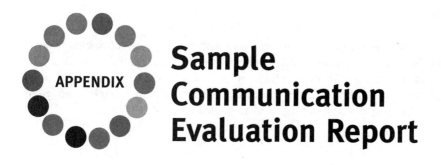

APPENDIX

Sample Communication Evaluation Report

COMMUNICATION EVALUATION

Name: Darrell Thompson
Date of birth: 4/3/02
Dates of evaluation: 9/29/06, 10/6/06

Parents: Margaret and Daniel Thompson
Age: 4 years, 6 months
Home language: English

BACKGROUND

Darrell was referred for a speech and language evaluation by his parents, Margaret and Daniel Thompson. They are concerned that Darrell's speech is very difficult to understand. Mrs. Thompson reports becoming concerned about Darrell's speech approximately 1 year ago when he started nursery school and she noted that the other children were more intelligible than Darrell. Darrell has not had any previous developmental or speech and language evaluations.

An audiological evaluation was recently completed on 9/12/06. Results revealed a mild bilateral conductive hearing loss and restricted eardrum mobility. It was noted that speech discrimination was very good in the right ear, but only fair in the left ear. Recommendations included medical consultation regarding middle ear pathology and a reevaluation in 1 year. It was further recommended that Darrell's middle ear status be monitored. The Thompsons have followed these recommendations and Darrell has just completed a course of antibiotics for an ear infection.

Mrs. Thompson reported that her pregnancy and Darrell's birth history were normal. She does not recall specific ages at which developmental milestones were achieved. Darrell has a history of asthma and hay fever. He has had six episodes of croup and five ear infections since birth. Darrell has no known food allergies and is described by his mother as a good eater who enjoys a variety of food types and textures (e.g., raw vegetables, yogurt, granola bars, peanut butter). Mrs. Thompson described Darrell as a "very neat" eater who uses a fork and a knife.

Darrell lives with his parents and siblings (Jennifer, age 7 and Robert, age 13). Darrell spends much of his free time playing with his sister and a 5-year-old neighbor. Darrell's older brother had a history of speech difficulties and received therapy until third grade.

Darrell currently attends nursery school twice weekly. Darrell seems to love school, and his teachers report that his speech has improved somewhat since last year. He enjoys playing with other children, but he gets easily frustrated if he is not understood. The Thompsons are most interested in helping Darrell to improve his speech before he enters kindergarten next year.

TESTING

Darrell was seen at the clinic for two 1-hour sessions. Mrs. Thompson was present during both sessions. Darrell was initially shy and needed some encouragement to participate in the assessment activities during the first session. During the second session, Darrell was cooperative and actively participated in all tasks.

Results

The following is a summary of tests administered and Darrell's performance:

Test	Standard Score	Percentile Rank
Peabody Picture Vocabulary Test-III (PPVT-III; Form A)	83[a]	13
Expressive One Word Picture Vocabulary Test (EOWPVT)	90[a]	25
Test of Language Development (TOLD-P:3) Composite	80[a]	9
Subtests		
Picture vocabulary	7[b]	16
Relational vocabulary	7[b]	16
Oral vocabulary	7[b]	16
Grammatic understanding	9[b]	37
Sentence imitation	5[b]	5
Grammatic completion	8[b]	25
Supplemental subtests		
Word discrimination	7[b]	16
Phonemic analysis	6[b]	9
Word articulation	5[b]	5
Goldman-Fristoe Test of Articulation (GFTA-2)	71[a]	7
Khan-Lewis Phonological Analysis (KLPA-2)	63	3

Mean length of utterance (MLU): 3.50 (expected mean for age is 5.02; range is 3.96–6.08)

Oral Speech Mechanism Screening: Structures adequate for speech production; difficulty with sequencing movements and speech sounds noted

[a]These tests have a mean of 100 with a standard deviation of 15.
[b]These subtests have a mean of 10 with a standard deviation of 3.

Interpretation

Receptive Language and Comprehension   Darrell's single-word vocabulary recognition skills appear to be in the low average to below average range as demonstrated by his performance on the PPVT and picture vocabulary subtest of the TOLD. He scored in the average range on the grammatic understanding sub-test of the TOLD. This subtest requires comprehension of syntactic differences at the sentence level (e.g., *he* versus *she* versus *they*).

Mrs. Thompson reported that Darrell's comprehension of language appears to be adequate and that he has a good memory for past events. During this eval-uation, Darrell was able to follow two- and three-step directions during play and informal tasks, although he was unable to maintain the correct sequences. For example, given an array of up to 10 small objects, he was able to follow two- to three-step commands involving their manipulation, although out of sequence, approximately 70% of the time (e.g., put the *dog* on the *bed*, put the *baby* on the *chair*, put the *cup* on the *table).*

During informal testing and conversation, it was noted that Darrell had difficulty demonstrating comprehension of some basic concepts such as body parts (e.g., knee, elbow), shapes (e.g. square, triangle), and colors (e.g., yellow, orange). Mrs. Thompson reported that Darrell is usually able to identify colors correctly.

Expressive Language   Darrell scored in the average range on the EOWPVT, a test of expressive naming. Despite this, in his spontaneous speech and during other testing, Darrell demonstrated several instances of word-finding difficulties. He used some immature labels; for example, Darrell called a drum "boom-boom" and a train "choo choo." He also used associative words, for example, calling a Christmas tree "Santa Claus tree." In another instance, he was unable to come up with the label for *scissors.* First he called it a "knife," then "paper." Finally, when given a sentence frame, "You cut paper with _____" he was able to come up with the correct word.

On the relational vocabulary and oral vocabulary subtests of the TOLD, which require the child to tell how two words are related and to define words respectively, Darrell scored in the low average range. He used many gestures to supplement his explanations (e.g., pretending to fly when trying to define *bird*).

Darrell's usage of grammatical forms appears to be somewhat below average to low average for his age, as shown in the results of the grammatic completion subtest of the TOLD and spontaneous language sampling. Darrell's MLU of 3.50 is somewhat below the range typically seen in children of his age (3.96–6.08). Darrell showed evidence of using different sentence types (e.g., statements, ques-tions); however, his usage of grammatical markers such as pronouns and verb tenses was variable. He inconsistently omitted word endings that mark plurals, third person singular, and past tense. These errors may be related to phonological difficulties discussed below. He also substituted immature forms (e.g., "me see horsie in there"). Darrell's spontaneous speech was very difficult to understand; therefore, these results may be a minimal estimate of his actual level of gram-matical knowledge. Darrell had significant difficulty imitating sentences.

Darrell used language for a variety of communicative intentions including requesting, protesting, commenting, and greeting. Several times, he attempted to clarify a message when the examiner said that she did not understand. He frequently turned to his mother for help in getting the examiner to understand him. Darrell was able to maintain a simple conversation about his toys over several turns with the examiner. Mrs. Thompson reported that Darrell is talking much more recently. She commented on the fact that his utterances are more elaborated when he initiates the topic than when he is asked to respond to a direct questions or request. This was also confirmed during the evaluation.

Speech Production and Phonological Skills Darrell demonstrated below average word discrimination, phonemic analysis, and significantly below average word articulation skills (TOLD word discrimination, phonemic analysis, and word articulation subtests, GFTA-2). On the GFTA-2, Darrell correctly produced 47% of the test items that included the consonant sounds of English in initial, medial, and final word positions. His errors were further analyzed using the KLPA-2. Darrell demonstrated difficulties in the following areas: initial voicing (i.e., substituting voiced sounds for voiceless, as in saying "**d**up" for *cup*), syllable reduction (i.e., omitting unstressed syllables in multisyllabic words, as in saying "jamas" for *pajamas*), fronting (i.e., substituting sounds made more forward in the mouth, as in saying "bus" for *bru**sh***), stopping and stridency deletion (i.e., substituting stop sounds for most fricatives, as in saying "diken" for *chicken*), and cluster simplification (i.e., omitting portions of consonant clusters, as in saying "dum" for *drum*).

Darrell's connected speech is very difficult to understand, particularly if the context is not clear. Approximately 50% of Darrell's utterances during this evaluation contained unintelligible elements.

Darrell's pitch, loudness, voice quality, and fluency were judged to be within normal limits for his age and gender.

An oral-mechanism examination revealed Darrell's oral structures to be adequate for speech production. Darrell was able to demonstrate tongue protrusion, tip elevation outside of the mouth, and lateral movements. He had difficulty puffing out his cheeks and biting his lower lip on command. He also had difficulty sequencing oral motor movements (e.g., stick out tongue, blow, then wag tongue from side to side). Darrell had difficulty performing rapid speech movements and sequencing syllables (e.g., "Say *pa* as fast as you can").

SUMMARY AND IMPRESSIONS

Darrell demonstrates a range of speech, language, and communication skills from significantly below average to within the average range for his age. Areas of relative strength include single-word vocabulary recognition, adequate comprehension of grammatical structures, and many appropriate pragmatic skills, including conversational skills when he initiates and controls the topic. Areas of weakness include poor intelligibility of speech, difficulties with oral motor sequencing, usage of immature grammatical forms, and possible word retrieval problems. At this time, Darrell exhibits a mild-moderate expressive language disorder and a moderate phonological disorder. With intensive intervention to address his speech and language problems, Darrell's high level of motivation to communicate and the strong involvement and support of his family are seen as positive indicators for growth.

RECOMMENDATIONS

1. Darrel would benefit from intensive speech and language intervention. Therapy on an individual or small group basis is recommended to address difficulties in speech production and expressive usage of grammar. A phonological process approach to therapy appears warranted for Darrell. Specific activities designed to improve oral motor skills may be helpful as well. Specific long-term goals for therapy might include the following

   - To increase intelligibility of speech

   - To increase age appropriate usage of grammatical forms

2. Periodic monitoring of Darrell's middle ear status as well as audiological re-evaluation in 6 months is warranted given the air-bone gap seen in his audiogram.

3. A developmental/educational evaluation is recommended to assess Darrell's skills in other areas, such as readiness concepts.

4. Darrell would benefit from a preschool group involvement on a more regular and frequent schedule (four to five times per week). This group should contain some peers who could be age-appropriate speech and language models.

_____   _____
Clinician's signature   Date

CHAPTER 4

Assessment of the Speech Mechanism

G. ROBERT BUCKENDORF AND ALLYSON GOODWYN-CRAINE

It is important to assess the speech mechanism in all of your clients, from children through adults. This assessment provides valuable diagnostic information about the role of structural and functional differences in speech production and swallowing. It also offers a baseline measure by which you can evaluate progress. When assessing the speech mechanism, take note of the structure of the client's mouth, which includes lips, tongue, palate, teeth, throat, and jaw, and the symmetry and shape of the client's face. Function is assessed through the client's range of motion, strength, rate of movement, and accuracy of hitting the speech target and through the client's ability to chew and swallow food. It is important to remember that other factors, besides structure and movement of the oral mechanism, also have a bearing on intelligibility and the viability of speech as a mode of communication. Breath support, posture, and general physical condition also impact the client's speech production and ability to eat and drink. Physical structure at times has a direct bearing on speech abilities, such as when a child has a cleft lip and palate or when neuromotor difficulties, such as cerebral palsy, are present. At other times the cause of the speech disorder is linguistically-based and relates to a specific phonological deficit (e.g., final consonant deletion). In these cases, the speech disorder is not likely to be related to structure or function (Ingram, 1997). Still, you need to be sure that there are no significant structural or functional limitations to speech production or swallowing. For this reason, oral-mechanism assessment is an important part of the evaluation.

Norm-based assessments of performance, including rate of tongue and lip movement, can provide initial assessment information as well as data about treatment effectiveness (Fletcher, 1972). It is important to remember, however, that the normal range of function and structure is very broad and that, despite a good deal of variety, most people produce speech that is easily understood. Students and clinicians often assume that, just because a client is missing some teeth or seems to be unable to move his or her tongue as quickly as the norms indicate, any speech problem present is associated with structural or functional deficits. You will see many clients who have marked structural deviations but are

The chapter authors would like to thank Candace J. Gordon for her contributions to the previous edition of this chapter, published as Speech-Mechanism Assessment, by G. Robert Buckendorf and Candace J. Gordon, in Rhea Paul (Ed.), *Introduction to Clinical Methods in Communication Disorders* (2002, pp. 89–109). Baltimore: Paul H. Brookes Publishing Co.

perfectly understandable. You will also see clients whose structure and function appear intact but whose speech is very difficult to understand.

Measures of speech function also allow the clinician to obtain information regarding cranial-nerve function in the adolescent and adult population. The information from this examination could cause the clinician to refer the client to another professional such as a neurologist, **otolaryngologist,** or dentist. For example, Jack, a 68-year-old man was referred for an evaluation by his general practitioner. Jack had complained that his "speech was not as strong as it used to be." During the speech evaluation, Jack's speech was 100% intelligible and his voice volume was within normal limits. It was during the speech-mechanism examination that tongue tremors were noted. This information was communicated to Jack's general practitioner and a referral to a neurologist was recommended. The neurologist who saw Jack diagnosed **Parkinson disease** and was able to prescribe medication that was helpful to his condition. The following outline lists *red flags,* or signs to look for in the examination, and additional testing and considerations for each red flag.

> **Red flag:** Weak phonation, hoarseness, breathiness, and poor pitch/loudness control. These difficulties may be indicative of lower motor neuron damage or vocal fold pathology.
>
> **Test:** In addition to vocal performance, test speech production and swallowing.
>
> **Consider:** Test results may rule out lower motor neuron involvement or vocal fold pathology or indicate referral to an otolaryngologist and/or neurologist.

In another example, Tiffany, a 4-year-old girl, came to the clinic with a parental complaint that her speech was very difficult to understand. During the oral-mechanism examination, Tiffany's oral structure appeared to be within normal limits, but she was extremely hypernasal with no soft-palate movement noted during the functional examination. She also had a significant medical history, including heart surgery at 3 weeks of age. After the examination, she was referred to an otolaryngologist for further evaluation. She was eventually determined to fit the diagnostic profile of velocardiofacial syndrome and was referred to the otolaryngologist for a pharyngeal flap to manage her velopharyngeal incompetence (Shprintzen, 2000). Following surgery, Tiffany still needed extensive articulation treatment to learn new speech behaviors to complement her new structures.

Before Your First Speech-Mechanism Examination

Before you see your first client for a speech-mechanism examination, take the time to observe at least ten typical people during speech production to help you focus on normal tone and structure of the speech mechanism. Complete the speech-mechanism examination on yourself while looking in a mirror to be able to easily identify the structures and using one of the standard forms available for recording the assessment (see Figure 4.1). Complete the examination on at least three colleagues before you try the speech-mechanism examination on a client. The more experience you have assessing normal structure and function, the better you are able to identify problems when they exist.

Oral Mechanism Evaluation Form

Name: _____ Date: _____

1. Lips

   a. Structure

   Touch when teeth are in occlusion: yes _____ no _____

   Upper lip length: normal _____ short _____ long _____
   (describe)

   Evidence of cleft lip or other structural impairment: yes _____ no _____

   b. Function

   Can retract unilaterally

   Left: yes _____ no _____

   Right: yes _____ no _____

   Equal retraction bilaterally: yes _____ no _____

   Number of times can produce /pʌ/ in 5 seconds:

   trial 1 _____ trial 2 _____ trial 3_____

   Does stabilizing the jaw facilitate the activity? yes _____ no _____

   c. Adequacy for speech: 1 _____ 2 _____ 3 _____ 4 _____

2. Teeth

   a. Structure

   Occlusion: normal _____ neutroclusion _____

   distoclusion _____ mesioclusion _____

   Anteroposterior relationship of incisors: normal _____

   Mixed (some in labioversion, some in liguaversion) but all upper and lower teeth contact; all upper incisors lingual to lower incisors but in contact _____ not in contact _____

   Vertical relationship of incisors: normal _____ openbite _____ closebite _____

   Continuity of cutting edge of incisors: normal _____ rotated _____ jumbled _____

   missing teeth _____ supernumerary teeth _____

   If lack of continuity, identify teeth involved and describe nature of deviation.

Figure 4.1. Oral Mechanism evaluation form (From *Diagnosis in speech-language pathology, second edition*, by Tomblin, J.B., Morris, H.L., and Spriestersbach, D.C. © 2000. Reprinted with permission of Delmar, a division of Thomson Learning. Fax: 800-730-2215.)

(continued)

b. Dental appliance or prosthesis: yes _____ (describe)   no _____

c. Adequacy for speech: 1 _____   2 _____   3 _____   4 _____

3. Tongue

a. Structure

Size in relation to dental arches: too large _____   appropriate _____   too small _____

symmetrical _____   asymmetrical _____

b. Function

Can curl tongue up and back: yes _____   no _____

Number of times can touch anterior alveolar ridge with tongue tip without sound in 5 seconds:

trial 1 _____   trial 2 _____   trial 3 _____

above average _____   average _____   below average _____

Number of time can touch the corners of mouth with tongue tip in 5 seconds:

trial 1 _____   trial 2 _____   trial 3 _____

above average _____   average _____   below average _____

Number of times can produce /tʌ/ in 5 seconds:

trial 1 _____   trial 2 _____   trial 3 _____

above average _____   average _____   below average _____

Number of times can produce /kʌ/ in 5 seconds:

trial 1 _____   trial 2 _____   trial 3 _____

above average _____   average _____   below average _____

Restrictiveness of lingual frenum:

not restrictive _____   somewhat restrictive _____   markedly restrictive _____

c. Adequacy for speech: 1 _____   2 _____   3 _____   4 _____

4. Hard palate

a. Structure

Intactness: normal _____   cleft, repaired _____   cleft, unrepaired _____

Figure 4.1.   *(continued)*

Palatal fistula: yes _____ (describe)   no _____

Alveolar cleft: yes _____ (describe)   no _____

Palatal contour:

normal configuration _____ flat contour _____ deep and narrow contour _____

b. Adequacy for speech: 1 _____   2 _____   3 _____   4 _____

5. Palatopharyngeal mechanism

a. Structure

Soft palate

Intactness: normal _____ cleft, repaired _____ cleft, unrepaired _____

symmetrical _____   asymmetrical _____

Length: satisfactory _____   short _____   very short _____

Uvula

normal _____   bifid _____   deviated from midline to right _____

to left _____   absent _____

Oropharynx

Depth: shallow _____ normal _____   deep _____

Width: narrow _____ normal _____   wide _____

b. Function

Soft palate

Movement during prolonged phonation of /ɑ/:

none _____   some _____   marked _____

Movement during short, repeated phonations of /ɑ/:

none _____   some _____   marked _____

Movement during gag reflex:

none _____   some _____   marked _____

If some movement, then amount:

same for both halves _____ more for right half _____ more for left half _____

(continued)

Oropharynx

Mesial movement of lateral pharyngeal walls during phonation of /a/:

none _____   some _____   marked _____

Mesial movement of lateral pharyngeal walls during gag reflex:

none _____   some _____   marked _____

Audible nasal emission while blowing out a match:

yes _____ (describe)   no _____

Inconsistency in nasal emission during speech or blowing tasks:

yes _____ (describe)   no _____

Patient stimulable to oral productions of pressure consonants:

yes _____ (describe)   no _____

Nares construction during speech or blowing tasks:

yes _____ (describe)   no _____

Oral manometer ratio (instrument _____)

trial 1: nostrils open_____   nostrils closed_____   ratio_____

trial 2: nostrils open_____   nostrils closed_____   ratio_____

trial 3: nostrils open_____   nostrils closed_____   ratio_____

c. Adequacy for speech: 1 _____   2 _____   3 _____   4 _____

6. Fauces

a. Structure

Tonsils: normal _____   enlarged _____   atrophied_____   absent _____

Pillars: normal _____   scarred _____   inflamed _____   absent _____

Area of faucial isthmus: above average_____   average_____   below average_____

b. Function

Posterior movement during phonation of /a/: none_____   some_____   marked_____

Mesial movement during phonation of /a/:   none_____   some_____   marked_____

Restriction of velar activity by pillars: none_____   some_____   marked_____

c. Adequacy for speech: 1 _____   2 _____   3 _____   4 _____

Figure 4.1. *(continued)*

Preparation for the Speech-Mechanism Examination

It is important to follow **universal precautions** when performing a speech-mechanism examination. This means that it is necessary to protect yourself and the client from contact with any bodily fluids. You will want to have rubber gloves, a pen flashlight, a tongue depressor, a stopwatch, and facial tissue. In addition, a small dental mirror and gauze pads may be necessary. Before putting the gloves on, clean the table with disinfectant and wash your hands thoroughly with soap. You will need to select an appropriate form to rate your client's performance on the speech-mechanism assessment (see Figure 4.1). Always explain to the client what you will be doing and why you are doing it during the evaluation.

Initial Impressions

The speech-mechanism assessment should begin as soon as you see the client. Generally speaking, the assessment moves from broad to specific. Observe the client's overall motor coordination as he or she walks toward you and reaches out to shake your hand or grab a toy. Note whether there is anything unusual, such as **asymmetry** of facial features. This is also the time when you will want to be aware of the client's breathing. It should be noted if the client has a mouth-open posture and adequate breath support for connected speech. Strong observational skills will allow you to notice asymmetry of oral movement during connected speech and control of saliva when speaking. Be aware of the client's overall voice quality because that could be suggestive of possible speech mechanism problems, such as nasality due to inadequate velopharyngeal closure. Engaging the client in a brief conversation or in play will also allow you to have an idea of overall speech patterns. Some of your most valuable diagnostic information can be noted in functional situations. These initial impressions will guide you in the diagnostic process, directing you to the areas that may require additional attention when completing the speech-mechanism assessment. Remember, too, that accurate results, in any testing situation, are best obtained when you and the client are actively engaged, so try to maintain a light, conversational tone throughout the assessment in order to help the client relax and give the most reliable performance. When working with children, approaching these tasks in an intriguing and playful manner increases the likelihood of compliance.

EXTERIOR FACE

Facial structure is a clue to the presence of certain syndromes (Shprintzen, 2000). In fragile X syndrome in adult males, for example, the face tends to be long and narrow. Low set, rotated ears are characteristic of Noonan syndrome. Facial asymmetry is common in velocardiofacial syndrome. It is important, then, to examine the external face for any indication that some syndrome might be present. Table 4.1 lists syndromes and characteristics that may indicate oral motor concerns. When there is indication of syndromic features, referral to a geneticist is appropriate.

The first step in the formal assessment is the evaluation of the facial symmetry. It is important to watch for any **tremors, spasms,** or **tics,** especially in the

Table 4.1.   Syndromes and characteristics that may result in oral motor concerns

Syndrome	Characteristics that may result in oral motor concerns
Apert syndrome	Premature fusion of cranial sutures, underdevelopment of midface, cleft palate, hyponasality, mouth breathing, forward tongue positioning, articulation concerns
Cornelia de Lange syndrome	Small, dysmorphic nose; thin, downturned upper lip; cleft palate; underdeveloped mandible; severe speech concerns
Cri-du-chat syndrome	Narrow oral cavity
Down syndrome	General hypotonia, flat facial profile, small oral cavity, hard palate abnormalities, malocclusion, tooth grinding, lax ligaments in temporomandibular joint, open-mouth posture, mouth breathing, tongue protrusion, abnormalities of the neuromuscular junctions of the tongue, poor control of oral movements, delayed speech development, dysarthria, motor planning concerns
Ectrodactyly-ectodermal dysplasia-clefting syndrome	Cleft lip and palate, velopharyngeal incompetence, dental abnormalities, underdeveloped maxilla
Fetal alcohol syndrome	Short, upturned nose; underdeveloped maxilla and/or mandible; hypotonia; poor motor coordination; articulation concerns; high incidence of cleft palate
Floating-harbor syndrome	Triangular face, prominent nose, expressive language delay
Fragile X syndrome	Prominent forehead; long, narrow chin; delayed speech and motor development
Goldenhar syndrome	Underdeveloped face and/or head, facial asymmetry, underdeveloped mandible, facial palsy, cleft palate, velar asymmetry and/or paresis, articulation and resonance concerns
Moebius syndrome	Bilateral facial paralysis (involvement of the facial and hypoglossal nerves); tongue lateralization, elevation, depression and protrusion problematic; eating, drinking, and articulatory concerns; high incidence of cleft palate and underdeveloped mandible
Noonan syndrome	Increased distance between eyes; lingual and oral malformations; small, upturned nose; wide mouth; "cupid's bow" lips; micrognathia; narrow upper and lower jaw; high arched hard palate; malocclusion and other dental concerns; articulation concerns
Oro-facial-digital syndrome	Clefting of lip or lip and palate, short labial frenulum, absent central incisors, underdeveloped mandible, micrognathia, tongue malformations, speech impairments
Oto-palatal-digital syndrome	Micrognathia; upper airway obstruction; cleft palate; missing teeth; eating, drinking, and articulation concerns
Pierre-Robin sequence	Underdeveloped mandible, downward placement of tongue, cleft palate, bifid uvula, speech delays, resonance concerns
Prader-Willi syndrome	Hypotonia, speech delays, dysarthria and/or motor planning concerns
Refsum syndrome	Ataxic dysarthria; articulation, voice, rate, and prosody issues
Rett syndrome	Motor planning concerns
Stickler syndrome	Underdeveloped midface; micrognathia; submucosal or overt cleft palate; eating, drinking, articulation, and resonance concerns
Treacher Collins syndrome	Underdeveloped mandible and/or maxilla; submucosal or overt cleft palate short or immobile uvula; malocclusion; underdeveloped teeth; open bite; beak-shaped nose; eating, drinking, and articulation concerns
Turner syndrome	Narrow maxilla and palate, micrognathia
Van der Woude syndrome	Pits or mounds on lower lip; cleft lip or palate; upper lip shaped like "cupid's bow"; velopharyngeal incompetence; eating, drinking, articulation, and resonance concerns
Velocardiofacial syndrome	Hypotonia; long face; prominent nasal bridge; long, tubular nose; narrow palpebral fissures; small mouth; downturned upper lip; cleft lip and/or palate; bifid uvula; eating, drinking, articulation, and resonance concerns; dysarthria; motor planning concerns

Table 4.1. *(continued)*

Syndrome	Characteristics that may result in oral motor concerns
Waardenburg syndrome	Cleft lip or palate, prognathic mandible
Williams syndrome	Short palpebral fissues; depressed nasal bridge; small, upturned nose; long philtrum; prominent lips; open-mouth posture; small, missing, or poorly aligned teeth; eating, drinking, and articulation concerns

From Bahr, D.C. (1991). *Oral motor assessment and treatment: Ages and stages.* Boston: Allyn & Bacon; reprinted by permission.

adult population. Is there any abnormal tension or lack of normal muscle tone in the oral musculature? Is there any drooping on either side of the face at rest or with movement? Second, observe if the client is able to maintain good lip approximation. When at rest, is the jaw held in a position that allows the person to breathe through their nose while maintaining good lip closure? Is there any scarring or evidence of a cleft? Observing overall facial expression, such as symmetrical smiles and elevations of the eyebrow, suggests normal facial innervation while slight drooping on one side of the lips or face could suggest nerve damage. A mask-like appearance with minimal facial expression could be suggestive of Parkinson disease (Duffy, 2005). Table 4.2 provides information from the examination of the external face to assess function of cranial nerves V, VII, X, and XII. Third, look at spacing, shape, and symmetry of the eyes and ears. If there are any facial abnormalities, determine through medical history whether they are acquired (e.g., secondary to injury or disease) or congenital (e.g., cleft palate, related to a syndrome).

> **Red flags:** Lower motor neuron involvement is demonstrated when the client has difficulty raising the eyebrows and presents with asymmetry around the eyes, cheeks, lips, and possibly jaw on one side of the face. Upper motor neuron involvement is demonstrated when the client's asymmetrical movement is limited to the lower face and possibly the lips.
> **Test:** Assess the client's symmetry at rest and with movement in speech and feeding.
> **Consider:** Test results may indicate referral to a neurologist.

Perceptual skills, including tactile sensitivity, give clues as to symmetry, tactile acuity, and localization abilities of the client. An inability to discriminate two points separated by an inch or more may provide clues as to the client's diagnosis and areas that you may need to be aware of in treatment. Assess sensation on the upper and lower lip and cheeks by having your client close his or her eyes and see if he or she can identify a soft touch (e.g., a Q-tip) and hard touch (e.g., tongue depressor). Assess two-point discrimination (e.g., with two tongue

Table 4.2. Summary of physical examination results and patient complaints for cranial nerves V, VII, X, and XII

Cranial Nerve	Function	Technique of examination	Patient complaints	Changes in structure
V—Trigeminal	Motor—masticatory muscles; Sensory—face and mucosal surfaces of the eyes, tongue, and parts of the nasopharyngeal space	Opening the mouth, clenching the teeth for palpation of the masseter and temporalis muscles	Motor—chewing difficulty, drooling, jaw difficult to close; Sensory—decreased sensation in face, cheek, tongue, teeth, or palate	Jaw may hang open
VII—Facial	Muscles of expression	Furrowing the brow, screwing up the eyes, sniffling, whistling, pursing the lips	Drooling, biting the cheek or lip when chewing or speaking, difficulty keeping food in the mouth	Affected side sags at rest; nasolabial fold is often flattened
X—Vagus (recurrent branch only)		Vocal characteristics; laryngoscopic examination		
XII—Hypoglossal	Innervation of tongue muscles	Tongue protrusion	Problem with oral articulation and chewing; difficulty handling saliva; tongue feels "thick"	Atrophy on the weak side
X—Vagus (above the pharyngeal branch)	Motor and sensory —innervation of the muscles of the soft palate, pharynx, and larynx	Gag reflex symmetry; vocal characteristics; laryngoscopic examination	Changes in voice and resonance; nasal regurgitation during swallowing	Soft palate hangs lower on the side of the lesion
X—Vagus (superior branch only)		Vocal characteristics; laryngoscopic examination	Voice changes	

From Yorkston, K., Beukelman, D., Strand, E., & Bell, K. (1999). *Management of motor-speech disorders in children and adults* (pp. 222–224). Austin, TX: PRO-ED; adapted by permission.

Changes in function		Changes in speech	
Unilateral	Bilateral	Unilateral	Bilateral
Jaw deviates to weak side, partly opened jaw may be pushed easily to the weak side by the examiner; decreased contraction on palpation on weak side	Individual may be unable to open or close jaw	None	Imprecise consonants, distorted vowels, slow rate
During lip retraction, face will retract toward the intact side; facial symmetry during movement	Decreased ability to retract, purse, or puff the cheeks	Mild distortion of bilabial and labiodental sounds	Distortion of bilabial and labiodental sounds, slow rate
Affected vocal fold fixed in paramedian position; dysphagia may be present; cough weak; may be airway compromise	Both folds in the paramedian position; airway compromise; inhalatory stridor	Reduced loudness; diplophonia	Reduced loudness
Tongue deviates to weak side; decreased lateral strength may be fasciculations	Atrophy and fasciculations on both sides; protrusion limited but symmetrical	Mild consonant imprecision	Mild to severe consonant imprecision; vowel distortion
Soft palate pulls to the paralyzed side on phonation; gag reflex diminished on weak side	Minimal palatal movement on phonation; nasal regurgitation	Breathiness; decreased loudness and pitch; short phrases; hoarseness; diplophonia; mild hypernasality; nasal emission; mildly weak plosing	Breathiness; aphonia; short phrases; inhalatory strider; moderate hypernasality; nasal emission; weak plosing
Affected vocal fold appears shorter than normal; epiglottis and anterior larynx shifted toward the intact side	Both cords appear short and are bowed; epiglottis will overhang and obscure the anterior portion	Breathy hoarseness; short phrases	Breathy, hoarse voice; decreased loudness and pitch range

blades separated about an inch and asking if the client can tell what he or she feels) and sensitivity to the temperature contrasts of hot and cold (e.g., a spoon held in hot water and placed on the lips about 1 inch apart followed by the same procedure with cold water).

Respiration

Impressions derived from the initial interactive observation provide important information on respiration, as to whether, for example, the client's breathing is easy and smooth or labored. In order to evaluate respiration further, ask your client to take a breath in through the nose and slowly let the air out through the mouth. That task allows you to observe posture, tension, and evenness of exhalation. You should note whether the client appears to run out of air during speech or if speaking occurs on inhalation. Watch and listen for shallow breathing that requires the person to take a breath after only a few words. You should also listen for **stridor** (breath noise on inhalation) or hoarseness and look for neck or chest tension that may indicate poor breathing habits. Have the client place his or her hand on his or her abdomen and then place your hand on top of his or her hand. When the client inhales, observe whether the abdomen pushes out against your hand. If the abdomen goes in instead, he or she may be inhaling by lifting the shoulders or chests instead of using the diaphragm properly. The client may be compensating for some respiratory difficulty and may need further evaluation.

A fun and simple means of testing respiratory adequacy for speech in children is to pour 10 centimeters of water into a glass, insert a regular drinking straw, and ask the child to hold his or her nose and blow water bubbles as long as he or she can. While demonstrating an adequate lip seal around the straw, a child who can blow water bubbles for 5 seconds demonstrates adequate respiratory support to produce speech (Hixon, Hawley, & Wilson, 1982).

Nose

Breathing irregularities can lead to decreased respiratory support for speech and increased fatigue when eating, so it important to assess whether there are any obstructions in the nasal cavity that could affect breath intake. You can ask the client to move his or her head back and assess the nasal area for any abnormalities such as a deviated septum or obstruction of the nasal cavity. This is especially important if you have observed that the client is a mouth breather. Many clients are unable to breathe comfortably through their nose because of allergies or swollen adenoids. This should be noted during the examination and in the case history, and clients should be referred for medical management of these issues. Nighttime snoring and chronically red upper gums are additional clues to this condition. If the client is unable to breathe comfortably through the nose, the adoption of an unhealthy mouth-open breathing posture becomes more likely.

Lips

The lips are very important for eating, drinking, facial expression, and speech production. Lip approximation is an integral part of many speech sounds, and lip closure is part of the swallow process. If a person is unable to easily approximate his or her lips or the movement appears effortful, there may be an impact on speech production, managing oral secretions, and nutrition.

> **Red Flag:** The client's lips may look symmetrical when structures are held in a fixed position (such as when smiling) but demonstrate asymmetry with movement.
> **Test:** Observe the client carefully. If you see lip asymmetry with movement, specifically assess the lips from the point of lip weakness to the facial muscle.
> **Consider:** Evidence of unilateral or bilateral facial weakness with movement may need to be assessed as well?

The initial observation allowed you to determine if the lips were symmetrical in a resting posture and during speech. Limited dynamic lip movement can result in anterior bowing and/or retraction of the upper lip. Observing a natural smile is a good way to assess lip retraction. Scars on the upper lip could suggest a repaired cleft lip or an old injury. To assess lip seal, ask the client to fill his or her cheeks with air and hold that air for 10–15 seconds. Did you notice any air leaking from the lips? Are your client's lips sealed at rest? Can the client round, protrude, and retract the lips bilaterally and sustain a rapid series of bilabial sounds? Can the client rapidly open and close the lips several times a second? When the lips move, is the jaw relatively still or does the person compensate for poor lip movement with excessive jaw movement?

> **Red flag:** When the client cannot adequately move the lips, the lip tissue may retract. The upper lip may look tight on the face and may rest above the margins of the central incisor's biting surface. In severe cases the upper lip may rest at the level of the gums. Similarly, a child who has limited upper lip movement may also present with an anterior bowing of the upper lip.
> **Test:** Place your gloved index finger horizontally across the retracted upper lip. Roll your finger downward with moderate pressure and observe the movement of the lip tissue. Watch to see if the lip moves to the bottom of the central incisors.

Ask the client to pucker the lips and then smile three times. When working with a child, have the child say a familiar repetitive phrase such as baby baby or mama mama rapidly several times. Do you notice groping behaviors during these tasks or does the client repeat these lip movements easily and quickly?

Because lip protrusion and rounding are especially important in the production of vowels, it is a good idea to count the number of times the client can pucker and then smile or open and close his or her mouth. Say "o-e," then ask the client to repeat the sound as many times as possible and count the number of complete repetitions of "o-e." During the production of bilabial sounds (/m/, /p/, /b/), you can observe whether the person uses both lips or makes compensatory movements to achieve closure. You can also observe the speed of alternating movements and look for any drooping of the client's mouth. In the

Dworkin-Culatta Oral Mechanism Examination and Treatment System (1996), the client is asked to perform many of these activities as well as repeat the word *puppy* as rapidly as possible for five seconds. Again, these observations help determine whether there are functional impediments that occur in both speech and non-speech situations or whether articulation errors are confined to speech contexts alone.

Jaw

Jaw movement, including opening and closing, as well as freedom of movement and stability of the **tempo-mandibular joint (TMJ),** is important to speech production and chewing. If freedom of movement is impaired, rate of movement is slowed, or the client has habituated a clenched-jaw posture or poor jaw stability, speech production may be affected.

The jaw performs rapid, gradated movement many times a second during speech, and limited movement secondary to injury or neurological disorder can have a significant effect on speech intelligibility. Does the client have adequate movement of the jaw or present with more of a clenched-jaw posture? This is also a good time to look for anterior or lateral shifting or jutting of the jaw and to listen for any TMJ noise, such as grinding or popping sounds during wide-mouth opening. Some clients may not be able to open their mouths fully because of TMJ problems and a referral to a dentist or oral surgeon may be in order. Jaw lateralization is important for chewing and provides information about cranial nerve function, so you want to observe whether the client can move the jaw in a rotary fashion when chewing. Look at the orientation of the upper and lower jaw at rest. Do they meet symmetrically?

Red Flag: The client's excessive jaw movement during the /p/ or *puppy* task may be a compensation for decreased functional lip movement.
Test: Retest movement with the client's jaw stabilized. Place your thumbs on the boney structure just below the chin, positioning your palms parallel and below the jaw line with your fingertips resting at the jaw base just below the ears. Ask the client to repeat the /p/ task again.

Red Flag: The client's jaw deviates from midline, which may be indicative of lower motor neuron damage or TMJ dysfunction.
Test: Assess the client's ability to function the jaw in speech and chewing.
Consider: Referral to neurologist may be necessary when poor jaw movement control is noted. Referral to dentist may be necessary when the jaw dysfunction appears mechanical.

INTRAORAL EXAMINATION

Looking inside the client's mouth gives you a view of the structures and functions of the articulators. This is necessary in order to determine if there is any obstruction or inadequacy that might contribute to a speech or feeding problem. In preparation for the **intraoral** (within the mouth) examination, you will need to glove and review the characteristics of tissue indicating structural abnormalities in Table 4.3 (Hodge, 1998). Also, you will want to be familiar with terminology, such as tremors, tics, and spasms to describe any involuntary movements you may observe. When working with children, you may want to help them become accustomed to the procedure by letting them look in your mouth first, letting them hold the flash light or tongue depressor, or letting them perform the assessment on a doll or stuffed animal. You can increase children's willingness to open their mouths by telling them fun and interesting phrases such as "Let's see what you had for lunch," or "Are there are any elephants (or dinosaurs or popcorn) in there?" Maintaining a playful tone may help to relieve the natural anxiety children often feel about this procedure.

It is important to note the color of the oral cavity because, according to Shipley and McAfee (1992), a gray color might be a result of **paresis** (weakness), while a translucent color could be a result of a cleft. If dark spots are noted, they should be highlighted in the evaluation write-up and brought to the attention of the referring physician. When evaluating the size and shape of the oral cavity, remember that there is a great deal of normal variation. Still, anything that seems out of the ordinary should be noted. As we have said, it is important to get a good deal of practice in this assessment so that you become familiar with the normal range of variation in mouths and faces.

Palate

The hard and soft palate provides the division between the oral and nasal cavities as well as resonating and directing the voice. The hard palate must be intact

Table 4.3. Characteristics of tissue indicating structural abnormalities

Characteristic	Example
Unusual color	Red (inflammation); blush tint (absence of underlying tissue, as with submucousal cleft; cyanosis)
Rough, fissured, or furrowed texture	Ulceration; atrophy of muscular structure
Unexpected discontinuities in surface or underlying structure (especially at sites of midline union of structures)	Pits or notches in lips, clefts, fistulas, bifid uvula
Absence of structure	Velar musculature inserts anteriorly into hard palate (i.e., no palatal aponeurosis, missing teeth)
Disproportionate size in relation to surrounding structures	Short velum in relation to depth of oropharynx; enlarged palatine tonsils occlude oropharynx
Asymmetry in shape or size of bilateral structures	Unilaterally reduced muscle bulk or wasting on tongue; depressed nasal ala
Misalignment of adjacent or functionally related structures	Mandibular retrusion; dental malocclusion
Unusual contour (elevations or depressions in tissue where not expected)	Peaked hard palate; torus on hard palate
Constrained range of muscular structures	Lingual or labial frenum attached over extended area of structure

From Hodge, M. (1988). Speech mechanism assessment. In D. Yoder & R. Kent (Eds.), *Decision making in speech-language pathology* (p. 106). St. Louis: Mosby; reprinted by permission.

in order for oral sounds to be produced. The soft palate must be able to close off the nasal cavity quickly and repeatedly during running speech and when swallowing. Assessment of these structures is a very important part of the oral-mechanism assessment.

With your flashlight, you will be able to assess the hard and soft palate. Does the hard palate have a normal arch, and healthy looking tissue (uniformly pink, moist, and free from signs of disease) with no growths? Observe the palate for its height and arch. Certainly note if the client has a prosthesis, such as a palatal lift or **obturator.** Are the rugae (the ridges on the alveolar ridge) smooth and rounded, or sharp and angular? In some children, excessively prominent ridges may be associated with an abnormal swallow or indicate habitual mouth breathing.

Look at overall structural intactness. Note whether there are any openings (**fistulas**) through the palate into the nasal cavity. Those openings often occur as a result of cleft palate surgery. They are usually small enough that they do not have any direct effect on speech production, but they may cause difficulties in some clients. Look at the uvula and decide if its shape is uniform and a single, unbroken structure or if it is split (**bifid**). It is possible to have a bifid uvula without any other problems, but it might be suggestive of a submucous cleft and/or of velopharyngeal insufficiency (i.e., the inability of the soft palate to adequately close off the nasal cavity during production of oral sounds). Figure 4.2 provides an illustration of a normal palatal structure for reference. With your gloved hand palpate the hard palate from front to back and side to side. You will be feeling to detect soft indentations or depressions that that might signal a submucous cleft of the palate (i.e., a cleft in the layer of tissue or bone beneath the surface epithelial tissue of the hard palate).

Observe the tonsils. If they are excessively large or almost make contact with each other, a medical referral may be indicated. Sometimes tonsils interfere with movement of the back of the client's tongue, cause problems breathing, or provide additional tissue for the soft palate contact. Usually the tonsils decrease in size as a child matures (see Figure 4.3).

By asking the client to say "ahhh," you will be able to observe soft palate elevation and assess the quality of the phonation. Then have the client try three

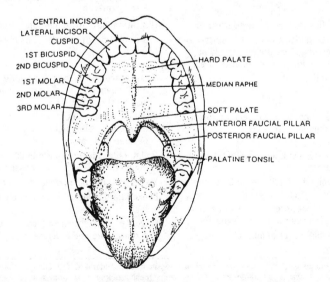

Figure 4.2. Schematic of oral cavity and adjacent structures. (From Meitus, I., & Weinberg, B., *Diagnosis in speech-language pathology* [p. 43]. 1984. Reprinted by permission by Allyn & Bacon.)

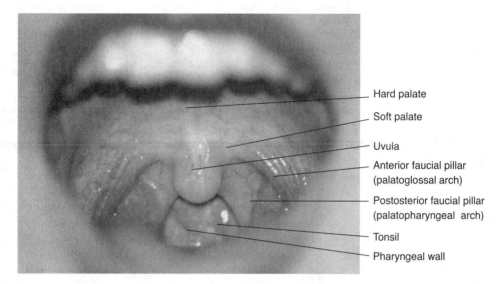

Hard palate
Soft palate
Uvula
Anterior faucial pillar
(palatoglossal arch)
Postosterior faucial pillar
(palatopharyngeal arch)
Tonsil
Pharyngeal wall

Figure 4.3. Photograph of an oral cavity.

quick "ahhhs" in a row. Do you note any weakness on either side of the soft palate? If there is asymmetrical palatal movement, the palate pulls or elevates toward its strongest side. Does the length of the soft palate appear adequate (i.e., long enough to easily reach the posterior pharyngeal wall)? Do the lateral edges of the pharynx move slightly toward midline? Even though adequate soft palate length and elevation do not ensure velopharyngeal closure, a short palate is a risk factor for velopharyngeal insufficiency. Is there any nasal air emission during production of the low-back "ahhh" or the high-front "eee"? **Nasal emission** can be best observed by placing a small dental mirror or small strip of paper under the client's nose. There should be no clouding of the mirror or movement of the paper. Repeat this procedure when the client is asked to produce words containing high-pressure consonants. Again, when a client uses words with no nasal phonemes, there should be no clouding of the mirror or movement of the paper. A test used to assess **hypernasality** in the speech of children with possible velopharyngeal insufficiency is the Iowa Pressure Articulation Test (Morris, Spriestersbach, & Darley, 1961; see Figure 4.4), which provides examples of words containing high-pressure consonants. Children are asked to pronounce a set of words chosen for their sensitivity to problems with nasality. Children who produce nasal emissions or other nasal errors on this test require further evaluation for velopharyngeal problems.

Red Flag: The client has velopharyngeal insufficiency.
Consider: Velopharyngeal insufficiency can occur for many reasons: 1) structural inadequacy (of the boney structure of the hard palate and/or the tissue structure of the soft palate) or 2) cranial nerve damage secondary to neurological insult resulting in uncoordinated or poorly timed movement associated with muscle weakness (dysarthric features) or motor sequencing (apraxic features). Test results may indicate the need to refer the client to an otolaryngologist, craniofacial team, or neurologist.

Iowa Pressure Articulation Test

Name: _____ Date of birth: _____ Age: _____

Date of test: _____ Score: _____

Number correct: _____ Percentage correct: _____

tongue	_____	sheep	_____	fork	_____
kiss	_____	dishes	_____	planting	_____
pocket	_____	fish	_____	clown	_____
duck	_____	jar	_____	glass	_____
girl	_____	bread	_____	block	_____
wagon	_____	tree	_____	wolf	_____
dog	_____	dress	_____	smoke	_____
telephone	_____	crayons	_____	snake	_____
knife	_____	grass	_____	spider	_____
soap	_____	paper	_____	possum	_____
bicycle	_____	cracker	_____	stairs	_____
mouse	_____	tiger	_____	sky	_____
scissors	_____	washer	_____	books	_____

Figure 4.4. Iowa Pressure Articulation Test. (From Morris, H., Spriesterbach, D., & Darley, F. [1961]. An articulation test for assessing competency of velopharyngeal closure. *Journal of Speech and Hearing Research, 4,* 48. © 1961 American Speech-Language-Hearing Association; reprinted by permission).

Oral mechanism assessment also involves evaluating the client's **gag reflex.** Absence of a gag reflex may be indicative of cranial nerve damage. The presence of a hypersensitive reflex has an impact on types and consistency of foods tolerated and also provides the clinician with information about tongue position during swallows and, in a few cases, speech. On occasion in clinical practice you will see children who alter speech patterns in response to gag hypersensitivity. For example, Emma, a 3-year-old child with a particularly sensitive anterior gag demonstrated strong backing tendencies until her clinician could help her regulate these sensations as she learned new feeding and anterior speech patterns. The sensitivity and trigger points of the gag reflex can be assessed informally by asking the caregiver to describe the area in the mouth that elicits a gag during toothbrushing. Many children have anterior gags when stimulated on the lateral margins or tip of their tongue or in the anterior buccal areas. Asking your client to open his or her mouth wide while you gently stimulate the soft palate or the base of the faucial pillars with a tongue blade can complete a formal assessment of the gag reflex. When the gag occurred, did both sides of the soft palate elevate? This procedure may not be appropriate for all clients (particularly children) and needs to be done with care.

> **Red Flag:** The client's absence of a gag reflex may be indicative of cranial nerve damage. The presence of a hypersensitive reflex has an impact on the types and consistency of foods that the client can tolerate, the tongue placement during a swallow, and, on occasion, speech.
>
> **Consider:** Many children have anterior gags when stimulated on the lateral margins, on the tip of the tongue, or in the anterior buccal areas. This may interfere with functional oral skills depending upon the age and clinical presentation of each child. When working with adults, a bilateral gag reflex should be triggered by stimulating the soft palate or the base of the faucial pillars.

Dentition

Although most people compensate quite easily for missing teeth, the overall condition of the client's dentition may affect both speech production and desire to eat or drink. You will want to note the condition of the teeth as well as the gums. Dental caries or impacted food on back molars may be indicative of poor tongue lateralization and an inability to sweep teeth with the tongue.

Dental classification systems provide information regarding relationships between the upper and lower teeth and the maxilla and mandible. You can assess dental alignment by observing the alignment of the first upper molar in relation to the lower by asking the client to bite the teeth together and smile. Note that a client's teeth can occlude (close) in several ways: a Class I condition is a normal occlusion where the dental arches close normally but there may be crooked or misaligned teeth; a Class II condition where the lower molar and jaw is too far back; and a Class III condition where the lower molar and jaw is too far forward in relation to the upper arch (see Figure 4.5) You should also note other dental abnormalities including **crossbites,** when a single tooth or the entire arch of the maxillary teeth overlap the mandibular teeth and **openbites,** when the upper anterior teeth are unable to meet the lower anterior teeth thus resulting in an open space.

> **Red Flag:** The client's abnormal tongue movement patterns, such as a tongue thrust or habitual thumb or finger sucking, can influence orthodontic development. If an overjet or open bite is observed in a child, abnormal tongue movement patterns should be considered as the possible cause.
>
> **Test:** Assess for tongue thrust by observing the client drink from a cup and/or swallowing food. Does he or she stick the tongue out near the lips when swallowing. If there evidence of the tongue pushing against the alveolar ridge or

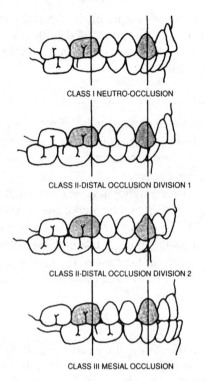

CLASS I NEUTRO-OCCLUSION

CLASS II-DISTAL OCCLUSION DIVISION 1

CLASS II-DISTAL OCCLUSION DIVISION 2

CLASS III MESIAL OCCLUSION

Figure 4.5. Examples of types of occlusions. (From *Head, neck, and dental anatomy, second edition*, by M.J. Short and D.L. Goldstein © 1994. Reprinted with permission of Delmar, a division of Thomson Learning. Fax: 800-730-2215.)

teeth, such as the presence of an open bite? Ask the client or client's guardian if the client sucks on his or her fingers or thumb or uses a pacifier.

If the client has an overjet, measure the space between the client's upper and lower incisors and ask the client to bite the teeth together and smile. Place the tip of a tongue depressor horizontally along the biting surface of the upper central incisors. Gently push the tongue depressor into the mouth until it contacts the lower incisors. With a pencil or ballpoint pen mark the depressor at the point directly in front of the upper incisor. Withdraw the tongue depressor and measure from the tip of the depressor to the mark. If the measurement exceeds 3 millimeters the client has an overjet (Boschart, 1998).

Consider: Further testing for tongue thrust (treatment may be indicated) and possible referral to dentist/orthodontist.

Tongue

The tongue is probably the single most important articulator and critical for moving solids and liquids around in the mouth during chewing and swallowing. Tongue mobility and speed of movement are very important to evaluate. You will want to assess the size, color, symmetry, and mobility of the tongue. Observe the tongue in a resting position on the floor of the mouth to assess the size. A healthy tongue is a velvety-pink muscular organ. According to the Mayo Clinic (http://www.mayoclinic.com/health/geographic-tongue/HQ00747), tongue disorders, such as red and white patches or what appears to be black hair, result from nutritional deficiencies, poor oral hygiene, or the use of some medications. **Atrophy** of one side of the tongue can be seen in clients following damage to the XII cranial nerve. Also, bite marks on the tongue can be noted in clients who have had a stroke due to decreased sensation on the paralyzed side of the tongue. It is important to look for any tremors, spasms, or tics. Ask the client to protrude the tongue and look for any deviation to one side or the other suggesting tongue weakness.

When asymmetrical tongue movement is observed, the tongue pulls toward the weakest side. Some speech-mechanism assessments suggest that the clinician hold the tongue with gauze and lift the tongue to evaluate the floor of the mouth and the **frenum** or **frenulum** (i.e., the thin piece of tissue that connects the underside of the tongue with the floor of the mouth; see Figure 4.6). If you note a thin, white string of tissue, a depression of the tongue tip, and/or the client having difficulty with extending the tongue tip (beyond the lips or up to the alveolar ridge), the frenum may be tethered or shortened.

An oral mechanism assessment includes a variety of nonspeech tasks to assess the client's tongue mobility. These tasks may include moving the tongue from left to right repetitively, tongue elevation to the alveolar ridge, and licking the lips. For young clients, lollipops can be used for the tongue protrusion tasks. The client can be asked to move his or her tongue up, down, and laterally following the lollipop. Attend to the stability of the head and jaw during the movements as some children compensate for poor tongue range or control by moving the head and/or jaw excessively. We have seen several children with a severe speech disorder who were unable to move their tongue independently of their jaw or touch the hard palate or front incisors with their tongue tip.

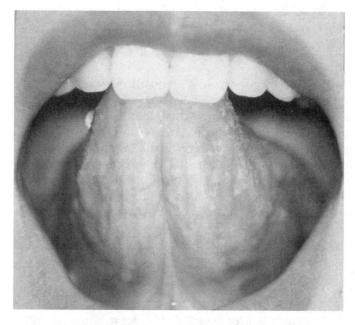

Figure 4.6. Intraoral view of the lingual frenulum.

A few years before visiting our clinic, Kristin, a young woman in her twenties had most of her tongue removed due to cancer. Her oral-mechanism examination revealed that she had only a short, narrow piece of tongue remaining. Based on structure alone, Kristin's prognosis would probably have been "fair to poor" for verbal speech since the tongue is a primary organ for articulation. The oral mechanism examination, however, showed she was able to engage successfully in verbal communication (albeit, with some speech distortions) despite her structural deficiency. This finding impresses, again, the resilience of the speech mechanism and the need for comprehensive structural and functional evaluations when treating clients with speech problems.

Diadochokinesis

One of the classic evaluations of the speech mechanism is the diadochokinetic rate. Slowed rates and imprecise movements are sometimes associated with dysarthria in adults and children following neurological insult.

> **Red Flag:** *Groping* is a term used to describe the client's uncoordinated, halted, or "searching" movement. In adults, groping may be indicative of motor discoordination, poor proprioception, and/or motor planning associated with neurological damage. Interpreting groping behaviors in young children can be a complex task as they are still developing neurologically and will not have the motor control of adults. Mild groping behaviors in children are not necessarily reflective of neurological pathology when the behaviors are not paired with other red flags.
> **Test:** Have the client repeat after you a syllable or word several times and note if the client is able to repeat it accurately.
> **Consider:** Additional testing may be indicated to assess non-verbal and verbal sequencing skills if the client's repeated utterances are varied or the client displays groping behaviors.

Oral-motor sequencing data provide a comparison to normal functioning. The client is timed during the repetition of 20 /pʌ/ productions. The same procedure is completed with /tʌ/ and /kʌ/. The client is then asked to say /pʌtəkə/ 10 times and the length of time required for that production is noted. The norms for this task are listed in Table 4.4 and are used for children from age six through adult. Normed referenced rates for younger children are integrated in the Verbal Motor Production Assessment for Children (VMPAC; Hayden and Square, 1999). Many clinicians use real words in a series, such as *Taco Bell, pat-a-cake*, or *buttercup* that may be more meaningful to children and thus easier for them to say.

> **Red Flag:** If the client's vocal productions are very slow, labored, or erratic, the client may have difficulty sequencing movement (apraxic features) or have poor muscle responsiveness (dysarthric features).
> **Test:** Assess for apraxia and/or dysarthria in order to rule them out.

Table 4.4. Normative data on mean rate of response (MRR) in syllables/second for various syllable patterns

Age (years)	pʌ	tʌ	kʌ	fʌ	lʌ	pʌtə	pʌkə	tʌkə	pʌtəkə
6	4.2	4.1	3.6	3.6	3.8	2.0	1.9	1.9	1.0
7	4.7	4.1	3.8	3.7	3.8	2.0	1.9	1.9	1.0
8	4.8	4.6	4.2	4.1	4.4	2.4	2.1	2.1	1.2
9	5.0	4.9	4.4	4.4	4.4	2.5	2.3	2.3	1.3
10	5.4	5.3	4.6	4.8	4.8	2.7	2.3	2.3	1.4
11	5.6	5.6	5.0	5.0	5.3	3.1	2.6	2.6	1.5
12	5.9	5.7	5.1	5.4	5.4	3.2	2.6	2.7	1.6
14	6.1	6.1	5.4	5.6	5.7	3.6	2.9	2.9	1.8
Adults	6.0–7.0[a]	6.0–7.0[a]	5.5–6.5[a]	6.4[b]	6.5[b]	4.6[c]	—	—	2.5[c]

Data for children are Fletcher's (1972) and Kent, Kent, & Rosenbeck's (1987) time-by-count values converted to count-by-time values; MRR data for adults are shown for comparison. © 1987 American Speech-Language-Hearing Association; reprinted with permission.

[a]Approximate range of means

[b]from Sigurd, 1973.

[c]from Tiffany, 1980.

Chewing and Swallowing

Part of the oral-motor assessment may include information gained as your client eats and drinks. If a history of feeding difficulties, dysphagia, or chronic respiratory issues exists, a more thorough dysphagia evaluation may be indicated. A general feeding screening is an appropriate part of an oral-peripheral examination when swallowing safety is not the problem. You might want to observe the client eating two or three textures of substances (e.g., pudding, crackers, gummy bears) as well as drinking thin liquids from a cup and/or straw. Observation of how the client eats both with a spoon and with finger foods can provide valuable information. For example, note how the client places the food or spoon in his or her mouth. Children who cannot lateralize their tongue to move the food to the molars often place the food on the posterior molars. Children with a tongue thrust often place food at midline then present with food compacted in their palatal arch after swallowing. Clients with poor lip adduction or oral pressure for sucking often turn their spoon upside down as it enters the mouth in order to dump the food into the tongue. During such observations, it is important to note lip and jaw postures as well as the efficiency of the chew itself. Overflow behavior such as upper body tension or tremors should be observed, as should any excessive drooling or coughing.

CONCLUSION

The purpose of the oral-mechanism assessment is to provide diagnostic information as well as ongoing information regarding treatment effectiveness. The coordinated movements of tongue, lips, palate, and jaw are critical for speech production and effective chewing and swallowing. To ensure an accurate prognosis and/or to determine appropriate steps in treatment, clinicians must be aware of normal structure and function and provide referrals to appropriate professionals when necessary. The oral-mechanism evaluation helps to direct you to the appropriate level at which to start treatment.

REFERENCES

Bahr, D.C. (2001). *Oral motor assessment and treatment: Ages and stages.* Boston: Allyn & Bacon.

Boshart, C.A. (1999). *Oral-facial illustrations and reference guide.* Riverside, CA: Speech Dynamics Incorporated.

Duffy, J. (2005). *Motor speech disorders: Substrates, differential diagnosis, and management.* St. Louis: Elsevier.

Dworkin, J., & Culatta, P. (1996). *Dworkin-Culatta oral mechanism examination.* Nicholasville, KY: Edgewood Press.

Fletcher, S. (1972). Time-by-count measurement of diadochokinetic syllable rate. *Journal of Speech and Hearing Research, 15,* 763–770.

Hayden, D., & Swuare, P. (1999). *Verbal Motor Production Assessment for Children.* Austin, TX: Harcourt Assessment.

Hixon, T.J., Hawley, J.L., & Wilson, K.J. (1982). An around-the-house device for the clinical determination of respiratory driving pressure: A note on making the simple even simpler. *Journal of Speech and Hearing Disorders, 47,* 413.

Hodge, M. (1988). Speech mechanism assessment. In D. Yoder & R. Kent (Eds.), *Decision making in speech-language pathology* (p. 106). Toronto, Canada: Decker.

Ingram, D (1997). The categorization of phonological impairment. In B. Hodson & M. Edwards (Eds.), *Perspectives in applied phonology* (pp. 19–38). New York: Aspen Publishers.

Kent, R., Kent, J., & Rosenbeck, J. (1987). Maximum performance test. *Journal of Speech and Hearing Disorders, 52,* 367–387.

Meitus, I., & Weinberg, B. (1984). *Diagnosis in speech-language pathology.* Boston: Allyn & Bacon.

Morris, H., Spriestersbach, D., & Darley, F. (1961). An articulation test for assessing competency of velopharyngeal closure. *Journal of Speech and Hearing Research, 4,* 48.

Shipley, K., & McAfee, J. (1992). *Assessment in speech-language pathology.* San Diego: Singular Publishing Group.

Short, M.J., & Goldstein, D.L. (1994). *Head, Neck, and Dental Anatomy, 2nd edition.* Clifton Park, NY: Thomson Delmar Learning.

Shprintzen, R. (2000). *Syndrome identification for speech-language pathology.* San Diego: Singular Publishing Group.

Sigurd, B. (1973). Maximum rate and minimal duration of repeated syllables. *Language and Speech, 16,* 373–395.

Tiffany, W. (1980). The effects of syllable structure on diadochokinetic and reading rates. *Journal of Speech and Hearing Disorders, 23,* 894–908.

Tomblin, J.B., Morris, H.L., & Spriestersbach, D.C. (2000). *Diagnosis in Speech-Language Pathology, 2nd edition,* Clifton Park, NY: Thomson Delmar Learning.

STUDY QUESTIONS

1. Why do we do a speech-mechanism examination?

2. Why is it important to look at function as well as structure when assessing clients?

3. What are some factors influencing speech intelligibility besides structure and function?

4. What are some important precautions to take before you perform the oral-mechanism examination?

5. When unilateral weakness of the tongue or palate is noted the tongue pulls toward its weakest side, yet the palate pulls or elevates to the strongest side. Explain.

6. Why do we measure diadochokinetic rates?

CHAPTER 5

Communication Sampling Procedures

RHEA PAUL, JOHN TETNOWSKI, AND ELLEN REULER

One of the earliest means of studying children's language was the diary study. Parents who were deeply interested in language development—Charles Darwin among them—kept detailed recordings of their children's early speech productions (Bar-Adon & Leopold, 1971). This method not only yielded both a great deal of quantitative information about what children said at which point in development, but it also introduced the idea of carefully observing, recording, and analyzing natural behavior as a means to understand language use. These early studies were focused on a small number of children, on a small range of questions concerning single-word use and the beginning of two-word combinations, on a narrow age range, on production only, and on typical development only. Nonetheless, the studies set the stage for the development of a broader use of language sampling procedures to address a range of issues in clinical work with people with communication disorders.

There is a simple reason why language sampling became an important part of the assessment of communication problems: It provides a key piece of information about a person's ability to communicate. As you saw in Chapter 3, one of the purposes of assessment is to identify baseline function and target goals for intervention. In order to achieve these purposes, communication sampling is essential. Although standardized tests can tell us whether a person is significantly different from his or her peers, the test cannot tell us how that person uses the communication skills he or she has to interact in real-life situations. It is this ability to interact in day-to-day encounters that we need to address in our interventions. To know what we need to work on, we need to see how the client really communicates—what difficulties he or she has, what strengths he or she shows, and what communicative situations need to be addressed. This is where communication sampling comes in. Communication sampling provides us with our most valid assessment of a client's communicative skill because it examines communication behavior itself, in a naturalistic environment that is closely related to the kinds of settings the client needs to communicate in every day.

A second justification for sampling communication behavior comes from changes made since 2001 in systems for classifying disorders, most notably, the International Classification of Functioning, Disability and Health (ICFDH; World Health Organization 2001). This classification system views disorders from the point of view of their effect on everyday life; that is, whether disorders can result in limitations to aspects of an individual's well-being, beyond the use of speech. For example, a person with a voice disorder may have limitations on career choice because of an inability project the voice sufficiently to be heard by a group of people. This limitation on functioning may affect the person's vocational goals and decisions, if, for example, a teaching career is being considered. In traditional clinical evaluations, this issue may be overlooked because the person might be able to communicate adequately in a clinical setting. Thus, our use of communication sampling contributes to our ability to perform functional assessment. Functional communication assessments add to the understanding of the impact of communication disorders on a person's functioning in a variety of real-world settings. In these days of increased accountability for the costs of our services, we need to be able to demonstrate that our treatments make real, functional differences in our clients' lives. Using communication sampling as a form of functional assessment allows us to meet this requirement.

An important issue in communication sampling is to establish that the sample bears a strong resemblance to the kinds of interactions in which clients really engage. This issue is known as the **representativeness** of the sample. Because we may be seeing clients in a clinical setting with which they are unfamiliar, or in an interaction with an unfamiliar partner (i.e., the clinician, whom the client may not know well yet) who may be from a culturally or linguistically different community, the communication we observe for our sample may not be quite like the client's communication in everyday settings. It is part of our job to ensure that the sample is as representative as possible. We will address some methods for maximizing sample representativeness as we go along, but keep in mind that for every client we see, the issue of the **cultural sensitivity** and relevance of our sampling procedures needs our attention. Cultural sensitivity means realizing that the rules for talking and interacting differ among various communities. To get a valid sample of a client's language, we need to attend to the cultural rules that govern conversation for that person. In some communities, it may not be acceptable for children to talk to strangers; in others it may be rude to ask a question to which the answer is obvious (e.g., "What color is that shirt you are wearing?").

To monitor the representativeness of a speech sample collected from a culturally- or linguistically-different (CLD) client, we will want to learn some details of the cultural conversational practices from interviews with community members. In addition, we may want to observe the client in several conversational situations to select the most representative one to use as the basis for our speech sample analysis. It also is a good idea to check with a family member to ask whether the sample we plan to analyze sounds like the way the client usually talks. With clients for whom English is not the dominant language, we may ask the client to interact with a family member or other fluent speaker of the dominant language. The sample can be collected on audiotape and transcribed by an interpreter, but the interpreter will need to be aware of the clinician's need to have the transcription accurately represent the client's production. If the interpreter *normalizes* the speech (correcting the errors in the transcription), an important source of information about the client's linguistic patterns will be removed. For more information on cultural sensitivity, see Goldstein and Iglesias (Chapter 11), Paul (in press), Roseberry-McKibbin (2002), and Stockman (1996). For now, it is important to remember that language is always embedded in culture and the way people talk differs not only on the basis of their abilities and disabilities, but also on the basis of their own community's conversational rules, which may be different from the clinician's.

Communication sampling can be used with clients of all ages to investigate a broad range of speech, language, and hearing problems. We may use samples of communication to examine the understanding and use of words and sentences (semantics and syntax) in conversations, narratives, and explanations; the appropriateness of communication in context (pragmatics); the sound system and its **intelligibility** (phonology) and **fluency;** the use of **paralinguistics** or prosody in speech; and the quality and **resonance** of the speaking voice. We can divide these kinds of analyses into three broad categories:

1. Nonverbal communication, which includes the range of functions or communicative intentions expressed; the rate or frequency of communication; and the form in which communication is produced, whether with gestures, vocalizations, body movements, and so forth.

2. Language, which includes semantics, syntax, and pragmatics

3. Speech, which includes phonology, prosody, fluency, and voice.

In discussing communication sampling, we look first at sampling procedures for *nonverbal* communication. We then discuss *language* across a range of developmental levels second. Third, we examine sampling for aspects of *speech* production.

Nonverbal Communication

Clients who are at preverbal levels of development, when symbolic language has not yet been acquired, do still communicate, of course. So do clients who have lost previously acquired skills through injury or illness and those whose long-standing level of functioning has precluded symbolic language learning. The issue of collecting a representative sample for clients with nonverbal functioning is particularly difficult. Often, these individuals are hard to engage. If they are very young children, they may be unwilling to interact with an unfamiliar examiner. If they are older, they may be exceedingly passive or withdrawn after years of inability to communicate. If they have lost communicative ability after a stroke or accident, they may be deeply frustrated with the mismatch between the intents they have to express and the means available to them for expression.

The purpose of communicative sampling for nonverbal individuals varies with their developmental level. For young children who are not talking, we may want to determine whether speech or some other form of symbolic communication, such as signs of **American Sign Language (ASL)** (see Figure 5.1) or **Blisssymbols** (see Figure 5.2), would be appropriate, based on the child's current means and rate of communication. We may also use communication sampling in this population to assist in differential diagnosis. For example, we expect children with developmental disorders such as mental retardation, specific language impairment, or hearing impairment to show fairly typical skills in nonverbal communication, even when language in absent. But for children with more pervasive developmental disorders, such as autism spectrum disorders, nonverbal communication is also affected.

For older clients who have developmental delays, we may consider a more sophisticated form of augmentative or alternative communication and need to

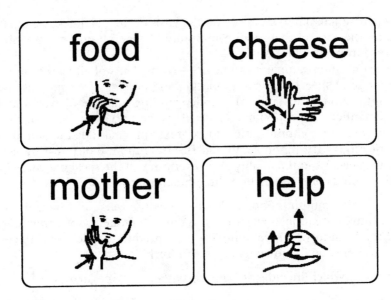

Figure 5.1. Examples of signs from American Sign Language.

determine what kinds of ideas the client is attempting to communicate so that we can match the assistive system to the client's needs. When working with clients who have acquired losses, we may need to determine what kinds of communication skills have been spared so that we can identify the best intervention strategies for making use of the communicative functions the client has. For all these clients, communication sampling is used to answer the following questions:

- What can the client respond to in a linguistic interaction; or, what are functional comprehension skills like?

- What types of communicative intentions can the client express; are a range of intentions available, or is the range very limited?

- How frequently does the client attempt to communicate?

- By what means does the client attempt to get messages across? Does he or she use gestures, gaze, vocalizations, words, or some combination of these?

Collecting the Sample Collecting a representative sample from a nonspeaking client necessitates using a sampling context that is as similar to a typical interaction as possible. For very young clients, this will usually mean a play session with developmentally appropriate toys and a familiar interlocutor, such as a parent. For children with motor impairments, we will need to be especially careful that we provide opportunities for the child to express wants, needs, and intents, because many of these children get used to having everyone around them anticipate their desires and become somewhat passive communicators (Calculator, 1997). Using developmentally appropriate materials in collecting the sample and choosing a context in which communication will be a large part of the activity is important when sampling older clients with severely impaired communication and clients with acquired disorders. This may mean observing the client in a daily living setting and noting various daily behaviors, such as choosing food items from a menu or doing vocational activities that involve interaction. It will

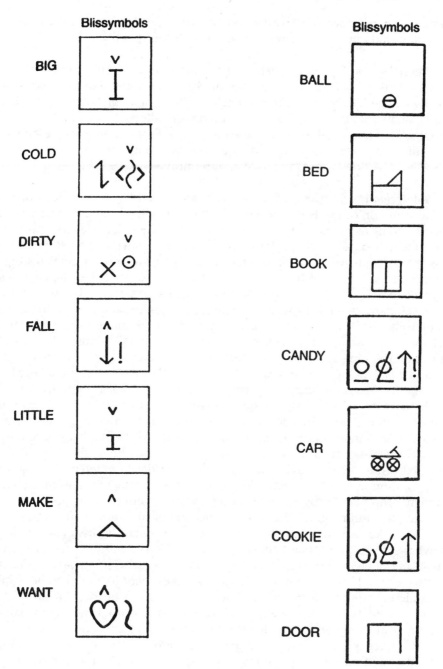

Figure 5.2. Examples of Blissymbols. (Blissymbols used herein copyright Blissymbols Communication International, Toronto, Canada. Exclusive licensee 1982.)

also be important to check in with individuals who know the client well and to ask whether the interaction observed is typical of the client's current communication. The sample we collect should be long enough to exhibit a broad range of communicative behaviors. For active communicators, 15–20 minutes is usually a long enough time period for a reasonable sample. For clients who communicate less frequently, we may need to spend a longer amount of time to collect a sample. Generally, we would want to continue collecting data until we have at least 20 purposeful acts of communication from the client.

Recording the Sample Much of the communicative interaction with non-verbal clients will, of course, take place in visual modalities. For this reason, it is usually a good idea to record the communication sample on videotape so that it can be analyzed at a later time. Videotaping also allows us to watch the interaction several times and to score one aspect of communication during each viewing. This makes it possible to answer all the questions we have posed for the assessment with only one sample of communication.

Analyzing the Sample One issue that we address in our analysis of nonverbal communication is the degree to which the client's behavior suggests an understanding of language. We will want to make some inferences about how the language spoken to the client influences his or her behavior in a natural setting. This information will be an important adjunct to our more formal testing of language comprehension because it will allow us to see whether the client uses what Chapman (1978) has called "comprehension strategies." The use of these strategies allows a client to act as if language comprehension has occurred, even though linguistic knowledge of specific words and grammatical forms may be lacking, as shown when the client is tested in a formal setting. We see these strategies operating in typically developing children, for example, when a mother looks at a ball, points to it and says, "See the ball?" to a 12-month-old. The baby does not have to understand the word *ball* in order to appear to understand; he or she only has to look at what mother points to. This strategic looking gives the impression the child knows the word, even though the child might not be able to identify *ball* in an array of several objects without the mother's gaze cue. If the client does better in these natural interactions than he or she does on standardized testing of language comprehension, we have gathered an important piece of information: The client takes advantage of interactive cues in the environment. This performance would contrast with a client who did poorly on formal receptive testing and did not look much better in natural situations.

Figure 5.3 presents an observation form that might be used to examine a nonverbal client's receptive behaviors in a naturalistic communication sample. The form can be used to record the frequency and context for behaviors that appear to suggest language comprehension. An assessment like this can be helpful for clinicians working with young children who have a hearing impairment in order to assess the degree to which residual hearing is used to support natural communication and also with clients who do not speak for other reasons.

The other questions we posed about nonverbal clients concern the range, frequency, and means of communication expressed. Again, using a videotaped representative communication sample, we can assess how often, in what form, and for what purpose the client communicates. In assessing communication in nonspeakers, it is important to be conservative about attributing intention to the client's actions. We do not want to call every act of the client's an act of communication. In order to count as communicative, a client's action should meet more than one of the following criteria:

1. It should be directed by means of gaze, body orientation, or gesture toward the interlocutor

2. It should have an effect on the interlocutor

Context	Client response		
	Responds appropriately	Responds inappropriately (describe)	Does not respond
Partner gives verbal instruction			
Partner asks question			
Partner offers choice verbally			
Partner suggests joint activity			
Partner remarks on object/event			

Figure 5.3. Assessing comprehension in natural contexts.

3. It should convey a recognizable message that could be translated into words

4. It should be persistent; if the act does not immediately gain its objective, it should be repeated or revised

An observation form like the one in Figure 5.4 can be used to summarize this assessment.

Some more formal procedures have been developed to assess preverbal communication skills. One example is the *Communication and Symbolic Behavior Scales* (Wetherby & Prizant, 2002). This procedure involves a structured play session

Communicative function	Form				
	Gaze	Body movement	Gesture	Vocalization	Word/ approxi- mation
Request object/ action					
Protest					
Comment (joint attention)					
Greeting/social interaction					
Request information					
Give new information					
Acknowledge partner's remark					

Figure 5.4. Assessment of nonverbal communication behaviors.

that can be used to assess behaviors similar to the ones we have been discussing for children at early stages of communicative development.

When assessing nonverbal communication in older clients who have not developed or who have lost speech, we will want to examine the communication that is present, using methods like the ones discussed here. We will also need to investigate the means of communication that can be used or expanded to increase the client's communicative capacity, often using augmentative or alternative modes of communication. Although this assessment is beyond the scope of this chapter, readers will find many useful resources in Beukelman and Mirenda (2005), Fried-Oken (see Chapter 12), and Glennen and DeCoste (1997).

LANGUAGE SAMPLING

We sample client language in order to observe the meanings expressed (semantics), the forms used for expression (syntax), and the appropriateness of communication in a social context (pragmatics). Because language changes and develops over the life span, we use somewhat different methods at each level of development. We discuss language sampling, then, in terms of the broad developmental periods: the preschool level (3–5 years), the school-age level (5–16 years), and the adult level (16 years and older).

Sampling Language in Preschoolers

Children between 3 and 5 years of age are typically in the phase of language development when the basic words and sentence structures of the language are being acquired. Communication sampling in this period often focuses on the syntactic structures and morphological markers that are such significant indicators of growth during this developmental phase, but we can look at other aspects of language as well.

Collecting the Sample   Language samples from preschoolers are usually collected in play interactions. The choice of materials for these play sessions has been shown to make a difference in the kinds of language children produce. For preschoolers, play interactions involving people, activities, materials, and topics that are familiar will elicit the most representative sample (Owens, 2004). The best toys to use represent familiar, domestic objects that easily lend themselves to pretending interactions (this is true with small children of both genders). Toy vehicles or objects that are too exciting or novel tend to elicit more exploratory play and vocalization (e.g., "Vroom! Vroom!") than verbalization (O'Brien & Nagle, 1987).

Even the most appropriate materials will not necessarily get a preschooler to talk, though. Miller (1981) suggested some strategies to help establish rapport and elicit talk from young children. Initially, the clinician is to say nothing except "Hi" for the first few minutes. Later, the clinician may begin parallel play with intermittent comments about ongoing actions (e.g., "You're stacking the blocks; I'll stack mine, too!"). As the play progresses, the clinician can initiate some interactive play, although maintaining a low frequency of talking for the first few minutes. When the child appears comfortable with the clinician, the clinician may begin trying to get some verbal responses from the child.

The clinician's own use of language is critical in obtaining a representative sample. In a study looking at parental questions and topic continuations, Yoder and Davies (1990) found that adult topic continuations elicited the most responses of any length from children. Multiword replies from children were most likely to occur after explicit prompts that continued the child's topic (e.g., Child: "Baby cry" Examiner: "Oh! That's sad! What can we do?"). Questions can be used effectively to break the ice early in the session and to determine interest in a specific topic, but it is unwise to ask many yes-no or **closed questions** (e.g., "What is that?" "Where is the dog?" "Who is this?") because these typically elicit one-word responses. The technique of parallel talk, in which the clinician describes what the child is doing, is often more effective for eliciting language. Clinicians can describe what the child is doing and then lead into an **open-ended question** or comment (e.g., "Tell me about that"). Repetition of a child's utterance, perhaps with a change of inflection, can also be used effectively in increasing child output. (It also helps to repeat a child's utterance when he or she has reduced intelligibility.) Another effective technique is a one-word response followed by silence. An example is *"Really?"* because it shows interest and implies wanting to know more. Playful statements that are obviously false can also be useful in eliciting more elaborated forms (e.g., Examiner: "My doggy is green!" Child: "No it not!").

How long a sample do we need from a preschooler? Most authorities (Miller, 1981; Nelson, 1998) suggest 50–100 utterances. If it is possible to collect two 50 utterance samples in two different settings, this is ideal. For children functioning at the 3–5 year level, a sample of this length can generally be collected from a 15-minute interaction. If language or developmental level is delayed, however, a somewhat longer sample of 20–30 minutes may be needed to get enough speech to analyze.

Recording the Sample   We normally will not need to videotape a communication sample with a preschool-age child. Because we are only interested in the spoken language, audiorecording will usually be sufficient for our purposes. The only exceptions would be for children who are using a visual communication system such as ASL or who are so unintelligible that we will need the non-verbal context to help decide what they are saying. When we plan to analyze a sample from an audiorecording, it is important that the setting be conducive to tape recording. This means that background noise should be at a minimum and that the tape recorder and microphone be carefully chosen and situated in the room. An external, unidirectional microphone is recommended, as are high quality tapes. It is critical that a clinician test the tape recorder and microphone. There is nothing more frustrating than spending 15–20 minutes of time obtaining a language sample only to find that the tape recorder was not working!

Transcribing the Sample   Transcribing a speech sample puts it into a tangible form that we can examine in a variety of ways. It is important to retain in transcription all the errors the child produces so that we can examine these errors for patterns that we will want to address in intervention. Many clinicians are surprised to find that although they understood what a client was saying during the interaction, it is much harder to understand the client when they listen later to the audiotape. For this reason, some clinicians find it helpful to repeat the child's utterances, often with a rising intonation that invites the child to say some more. Others make written notes as they collect the sample to remind them of what was happening.

Another challenging aspect of transcribing the sample is how to separate the child's speech into utterances. This is important because clinicians often calculate the average of particular structures per utterance. Generally, clinicians use syntactic, intonational, contextual, and pausing features to make decisions regarding utterance separation. For preschoolers, Leadholm and Miller (1992) suggested using either a falling or rising intonation contour or a pause of more than two seconds to indicate the end of one utterance and the start of another. Lund and Duchan (1993) also presented rules that can be used at this language phase. These include using intonational, syntactic, and contextual information to make decisions regarding utterance separation.

There are a variety of formats for transcribing language samples. The one suggested by Retherford (2000) appears with a sample transcript in Table 5.1.

Analyzing the Sample   When we look closely at a language sample to discover patterns of error and areas of strength, we cannot truly separate form, meaning, and use. When we do analyses of speech samples, we often artificially divide these aspects of language, but it is wise to remember that in real communication, they are integrated. We examine several analysis procedures for each of these areas of language, but we should remember that, in fact, they all work together to express the clients' intents.

Semantics and Syntax   Analyzing language samples is one of the most time-consuming aspects of our practice. For this reason, it is important to use language sampling judiciously. We should only collect a language sample after we have already established that the client has a deficit in expressive language, as documented by a standardized test (see Chapter 3). Our goal in language sampling is NOT to get a score, but to answer questions about the client's communication and to identify appropriate intervention goals. When completing a language sample analysis, some questions to ask include

- How does the language sample compare to other aspects of the child's language performance, both receptively and expressively?

- Is the child using language structures consistently at one developmental level or stage?

Table 5.1.   Sample transcription format

Adult	Child	Context
1. What have you got there?		Child plays with toy dog and bone.
2. Is it a doggy?	1. Uh-huh.	
3. I have a dog at home.		
4. Tell me about who's at your house.	2. We have kitty.	Child leaves toy and looks up at examiner.
5. Oh, cool!		
6. I like cats.		
7. Tell me about yours.	3. Black. 4. It have white foots.	
8. I'll bet it's pretty!		Child returns to playing with toy dog.

Source: Retherford, 2000.

- Is there variety in the structures the child uses, or does he or she use the same constructions over and over?

- Are there consistent error patterns, or are errors inconsistent and erratic?

Usually when we collect a language sample, in addition to thinking generally about questions like these, we will want to do some formalized analysis to help us understand the sample more fully. There are two basic methods of analyzing language samples: manual methods and computer-assisted procedures.

Manual Methods   There are a variety of paper and pencil methods that have been developed to examine language form during the preschool period. Some examples are given in Table 5.2. Perhaps the most widely used of all language sample analysis procedures is the computation of the mean length of utterance in morphemes (MLU). Roger Brown (1973) first used this measure to index the stages of syntactic development in young children in his pioneering research on child language acquisition. A **morpheme** is a minimal meaningful unit of language. Computing the MLU involves counting the total number of morphemes in the language sample and dividing by the total number of utterances. Brown's rules for counting morphemes and computing MLU are in the following box. A client's MLU can be compared to normative values reported by Leadholm and Miller (1992), Owens (2004), or Paul (in press) to decide if the client's performance represents a significant delay. MLU is also a useful tool to measure a child's growth in the use of syntax. Clinicians who compute an MLU as part of the initial assessment battery have a baseline to which subsequent MLUs can be compared.

RULES FOR COUNTING MORPHEMES AND COMPUTING MEAN LENGTH UTTERANCE

Counting rules

1. Use only completely intelligible utterances.
2. Count morphemes in the first 50 consecutive utterances.
3. Repetitions or false starts within an utterance are assigned morphemes only in the most complete form (e.g., in "My my mom is pretty," count only "My mom is pretty"). If the repetition is for emphasis, count each word (e.g., in "My dad is big BIG," count all words, including the repetition for emphasis).
4. Fillers (e.g., um, well, oh) are not counted. *Hi, no,* and *yeah* are counted.
5. Compound words (e.g., *birthday, somebody*), proper names (e.g., *Mickey Mouse*), and ritualized reduplications (e.g., *choo-choo, night-night*) are counted as one morpheme.
6. Diminutive forms (e.g., *doggie, daddy, toesie*) are counted as one morpheme.
7. Auxiliary verbs are counted as one morpheme, even if they are contracted (e.g., "He is running" = three morphemes; "He's running" = three morphemes).
8. Catenatives (e.g., *gonna, wanna, gotta, hafta*) count as just one morpheme.
9. All inflections (e.g., possessive *'s*, plural *s*, regular past *-ed*) are counted as one morpheme (e.g., shoes = two morphemes; baby's = two morphemes).

10. Negative contractions (e.g., *can't, don't, won't*) are assigned two morphemes only if there is evidence elsewhere in the transcript that the child uses each part of the contraction separately.

Computing mean length utterance

Count the total number of morphemes produced by the speaker.
Divide by the number of utterances counted (usually 50).

Source: Brown, 1973.

Additional analysis of the sample beyond MLU can give more in-depth syntactic and semantic information although still using the framework of Brown's Stages (Miller, 1981). Miller's Assigning of Structural Stage Procedure (ASSP) includes counting the occurrences of the 14 grammatical morphemes originally studied by Brown (1973) and deVilliers and deVilliers (1973) and charting the use of various simple sentence constructions, both of which correspond to Brown's stages. This procedure looks at use of noun and verb phrase elaborations, negations, questions, and complex sentences. Assigning stages to these aspects of language production gives more detailed information about the strengths and weaknesses in the child's use of syntax. It does, though, require a detailed knowledge of the sequence of normal syntactic acquisition. Miller (1981), Retherford (2000), Owens (2004), and Paul (in press) provided information on this sequence that is important for clinicians working in this developmental phase to know.

The ASSP is qualitative in nature and allows us to look at patterns in the child's use of language. Table 5.3 presents a worksheet that might be used to record and summarize information about syntactic development using the ASSP.

Scarborough (1990) presented an extension of Miller's (1981) procedure. The Index of Productive Syntax (IPSyn) includes structures from the ASSP, plus additional forms that Scarborough found to be diagnostic in a child's speech. Use of the IPSyn involves counting the first two correct occurrences of each of these structures to determine whether each is part of the child's repertoire. The IPSyn

Table 5.2. Examples of language sampling procedures

Procedure	Reference
Mean length of utterance (MLU)	Brown, 1973
Language Assessment, Remediation, and Screening Procedure (LARSP)	Crystal, Fletcher, and Garman, 1991
Assigning of Structural Stage Procedure (ASSP)	Miller, 1981
Developmental sentence scoring (DSS)	Lee, 1974
Language Sampling, Analysis, & Training (LSAT)	Tyack and Gottsleben, 1974
Index of Productive Syntax (IPSyn)	Scarborough, 1990

Table 5.3. Sample Assigning of Structural Stage Procedure (ASSP) worksheet

Brown's stage	Grammatical morphemes	Noun phrase	Verb phrase	Negation	Yes–No Qs	Wh-Qs	Complex sentences
I							
II	*-ing* 100%		|||||				
	in 100%						
	plural 100%						
III	*on* 100%	||||| ||||| |||||	||||| |||||	||||| ||	||||	||	
	Possessive 100%						
IV		||||| |||||	||||| |||	|||			|||
V	Copula *be* 33%						
	Regular past 45%						
	Irregular past 50%						
	Regular third person singular 25%						
V+	Auxilliary *be* 33%						
	Irregular third person singular						
V++							

Key: Qs = questions. (*Source:* Miller, 1981.)

provides both norm-referenced and criterion-referenced information that can be useful in selecting treatment goals and in measuring progress in language usage.

Another language sample analysis procedure that has been used widely is Lee's (1974) *Developmental Sentence Analysis* (DSA). This procedure has two components: developmental sentence types (DST) and developmental sentence scoring (DSS). DST is a criterion-referenced analysis for young children whose language is primarily at the one- and two-word phrase level. This procedure analyzes five language categories to determine: 1) which types are frequent in the child's speech, 2) which should be used as a basis for developing longer utterances, and 3) which are infrequent and should be elicited first in one- to two-word utterance form. DSS is more widely used and provides both norm-referenced and criterion-referenced information. It was designed for use with children using subject-verb sentences consistently. This analysis procedure analyzes eight syntactic categories which were selected based on their appearance in the speech of young children and because of the developmental characteristics of their acquisition. DSS scoring can be compared to scores of same-age peers between 2-0 years to 6-6 years. If a child is below the 10th percentile for his or her age, that child is considered to have a language deficit. But, like the ASSP and IPSyn, it is the qualitative information obtained from a DSS analysis that provides the most useful information in understanding an individual child's language usage, determining treatment goals, and measuring progress in intervention.

Computer-Assisted Procedures Computers assist us in much of the work we do today, and they can be used to assist in language sampling as well. There are several computerized forms of language sample analysis available. Miller et al. (1992) described the benefits of computer technology for language sampling in the areas of transcription, analysis, accuracy, and interpretation. The ability to perform multiple analyses on the same transcript is perhaps the biggest advantage in using a computer program. Larson and McKinley (2003) cautioned that it is still up to the clinician to obtain a reliable and representative language sample and to transcribe it accurately.

The widely used Systematic Analysis of Language Transcripts (SALT) was developed by Miller and Chapman (2000) and provides some standard analyses. These include MLU and several kinds of word counts: type–token ratio (TTR), a measure in which the number of different words is divided by the total number of words; number of different words (NDW), a measure of semantic maturity and diversity (Long et al., 2005); and total number of words (TNW), a measure of general language proficiency that reflects talkativeness (Long et al., 2005). Miller and colleagues (1992) showed that both MLU and NDW are sensitive to language development and delay during the preschool and school-age periods. SALT also allows users to design their own analyses. The SALT program provides a reference database (RDB) that incorporates several language groups. This allows a client's performance to be compared to that of children in a culturally relevant reference sample. Some additional computer-assisted forms of language analysis are listed following.

COMPUTER-ASSISTED LANGUAGE ANALYSIS PROCEDURES

Child Language Analysis and Transcription (CLAN, CHAT; McWhinney, 1996): includes programs for doing automatic developmental sentence scoring and index of productive syntax analyses on entered transcripts

Systematic Analysis of Language Transcripts (SALT; Miller & Chapman, 1995, 2000): includes automatic mean length utterance, type-token radio, number of different words, and number of total words analyses

Linquest (Mordecai & Palin, 1982)

Computerized Profiling (Long, Fey, & Channel, 2000): includes programs for doing automatic developmental sentence scoring and index of productive syntax analyses on entered transcripts

---

Pragmatics Pragmatics is defined as the study of how language is used in the context of communication. Evaluating the child's pragmatic skills is a natural extension of evaluating a language sample because they must be assessed in a communicative context. The goal of assessment in this area is to compare a child's pragmatic skills with his or her skills in the areas of syntax, semantics, and phonology to help determine the communicative basis the client has for learning language.

There are several organizing schemes that can be used to evaluate pragmatic skills as observed in the language sample. One that is widely used is Prutting and Kirchner's (1983) *Pragmatic Protocol.* This allows a clinician to look at pragmatic behaviors as they occur within the context of the language sample and make an overall judgment as to whether the behaviors are generally appropriate or inappropriate. An adaptation of this coding scheme appears in Figure 5.5. Owens (2004), Paul (in press), and Roth and Spekman (1984a; 1984b) provided additional guidelines for analyzing communication intentions and discourse organization from a conversational language interaction between the preschool-age child and an adult.

Language Sampling in School-Age Children and Adolescents

In this developmental period, basic sentence structures, vocabulary, and conversational rules have been learned. Analysis focuses on the refinement and elaboration of communication skill.

Collecting the Sample   In collecting a spontaneous speech sample from a school-age child, Evans and Craig (1992) found that the use of an interview format elicited more representative language behaviors than free-play with toys and games. They suggested using the following three open-ended questions to elicit 15-minutes of speech from children in the 7- to 12-year age range:

1.   Tell me about your family.

2.   Tell me about your school.

3.   What do you do when you are not in school?

For students in the school-age period, it may be especially useful to have at least part of the language sample collected during interaction with a peer. Peer conversation tends to contain more complex language than does conversation with adults during this period because children tend to take a relatively passive role in interacting with authority figures and communicate more assertively with those their own age. If a peer interaction can be arranged, information from this portion can be combined with the interview sample for analysis. Suggested topics for a peer conversation would include shared interests, such as sports or entertainment figures, or the explanation of a game or activity by the client.

Recording and Transcribing the Sample   In general, you will continue to use primarily audiorecording for children at this developmental level. The computer-assisted methods of transcription that were discussed in the preschool-age section can be used with school-age children, as well. There are some modifications that are typically used in transcribing speech samples from school-age children, however, which have to do with how utterances are segmented.

Communicative act	Appropriate	Inappropriate	No opportunity to observe
Utterance acts			
A. Verbal/paralinguistic			
1. Voice quality			
2. Vocal intensity			
3. Prosody			
4. Fluency			
B. Nonverbal			
1. Proximity			
2. Posture			
3. Gestures			
4. Gaze			
5. Facial expression			
Expression of meaning			
A. Word use			
1. Specificity			
2. Accuracy			
B. Relations between words			
1. Word order			
2. Given/new information			
C. Register variation			
1. To adults			
2. To peers			
Communicative functions			
A. Speech acts			
1. Remarks relevant to conversation			
2. Uses a broad range of communicative functions*			
B. Topics			
1. Selection			
2. Introduction			
3. Maintenance			
4. Change			
C. Turn-taking			
1. Initiation			
2. Response			
3. Repair/revise			
4. Pause time			
5. Interrupts			
6. Gives feedback			
7. Quantity and conciseness			

Figure 5.5.   A form for recording pragmatic behaviors in communication samples. (Adapted from Prutting, C.A., & Kirchner, D. [1983]. Applied pragmatics. In T.M. Gallagher & C.A. Prutting [Eds.], *Pragmatic assessment and intervention issues in language* [pp. 29–64]. San Diego: College-Hill Press.)

*Some examples of communicative functions are: requests information, follows narrations, provides explanations, gives predictions, pretends, reasons, gives new information, plans conversations, and comments on the conversation.

Hunt (1965) developed a system called **T-unit,** or Terminal unit, segmentation for use with samples of language from school-age children. Hunt observed that school-age children sometimes produced run-on sentences like this:

Well, last weekend I went skiing with my buddies from school and it was gonna be a long trip so I packed a sandwich and a bottle of pop and I put them on my seat on the bus so I would have them for later and I wouldn't get too hungry before we stopped at McDonald's and had some dinner on the way home from the trip but then I got hungry and ate half the sandwich before we got to the mountain.

Hunt reasoned that to count such a long utterance as just one sentence was not really representative of how complex the child's language was. He devised the T-unit to compensate for these run-on sentences. A T-unit is defined as one main clause with all the subordinate clauses and nonclausal phrases attached to it. We would divide the preceding example sentence into T-units as follows:

Well, last weekend I went skiing with my buddies from school

and it was gonna be a long trip

and I packed a sandwich and a bottle of pop

and I put them on my seat on the bus so I would have them for later

and I wouldn't get too hungry before we stopped at McDonald's to have some dinner on the way home from the trip

but then I got hungry and ate half the sandwich before we got to the mountain...

Once the sample is segmented into the T-units, various analyses can be completed, including MLU per T-unit.

Analyzing the Sample At this developmental period, language sample analysis focuses not so much on missing forms but on the degree to which communication is complex and flexible.

Semantics and Syntax There are fewer procedures developed to analyze the expressive language of children in the school-age period. Most clients at this developmental level have mastered the basic syntax, semantics, pragmatics, and phonology of communication. The difficulties they have tend to be in contexts that demand more specific, complex language skills related to literacy and school success. Some of the analyses that we discussed for preschoolers can be used with younger school-age clients. The DSS can be used up to age 7, which usually corresponds to second grade. The SALT reference database contains information on MLU, NDW, and TNW, as well as use of **bound morphemes,** personal pronouns, questions words, negative markers, **conjunctions,** and **modal verbs** (i.e., *can, will, shall, may, could, would, should, must, might*) for children from 3 through 13 years.

Another analysis informative for school-age clients and adapted from analyses used for preschoolers is the client's use of **complex sentences.** Craig and Washington (2002) and Paul (in press) argued that complex sentences are particularly sensitive to development and delay in the school-age period because they reflect the ability to combine ideas within a sentence, an important aspect of literate language. Paul recommends reviewing a transcript for the complex sentences it contains and analyzing the transcript for

- The proportion of complex sentences to total sentences in the sample

- The types of complex sentences used (e.g., infinitive clauses, relative clauses)

- The number and type of conjunctions (e.g., *and, if, because, when, so,*)

This analysis will reveal whether the student is using appropriately complex language and, if not, what aspects of complex language ought to be addressed in the intervention program. A sample worksheet for this analysis appears in Figure 5.6.

Additionally, Paul (in press) and Scott and Stokes (1995) suggested looking at other measures of advanced language use, such as the presence of advanced noun and verb phrase components, adverbs, and morphological features such as prefixes and suffixes. Other aspects of language form that are frequently problematic for students with language disabilities were noted by Miller and colleagues (1992). Clinicians may want to look for the presence of these difficulties in language samples as well:

Utterance formulation difficulties, including false starts, repetitions, and reformulations

Word finding problems as evidenced by single word reformulations and/or circumlocutions

Semantic deficits as evidenced by limited vocabulary and use of general words as opposed to specific names (e.g., *thingy, stuff, whatchamacallit*)

Pragmatics   Larson and McKinley (2003) developed the Adolescent Conversational Analysis, a format that looks at the student's role as both a listener and a speaker. They recommend analyzing a sample with the clinician (i.e., unfamiliar adult) and a peer. As in Prutting and Kirchner's (1983) procedure for younger children, the clinician evaluates the student's conversational behaviors as *appropriate, inappropriate* or *not observed* in a 10-minute sample of conversation with each of several partners, including a peer. As a listener, the client's ability to understand the vocabulary and main ideas of the speaker is evaluated in addition to how he or she responds to non-verbal feedback. As a speaker, the client is evaluated for specific language and paralinguistic features. The client is also evaluated on communication functions and conversational rules, as well as on paralinguistic features such as rate of speech, tone of voice, use of pauses, and fillers. A sample worksheet for this analysis appears in Figure 5.7.

Brinton and Fujiki (2004) found that using probes in interaction increases the efficiency of the sample and can also be effective in identifying various pragmatic behaviors. Some probes that they have found to be effective are

Initiating new topics in the midst of conversation (e.g., "By the way, I went skiing last weekend") to look for responsiveness, maintenance of the new topic, and relevance of the client's response to the comment

Requesting repairs in the context of ongoing conversation (e.g., "What kind of music was it?") to look for responsiveness, adjustment to listener needs, and appropriateness of repair strategies

Inserting sources of communication breakdown (e.g., "Can you get me the scissors?" when no scissors is available) to look for assertiveness, ability to monitor the interaction, and requests for clarification

Student name: A. J. Nevarow   Date of birth: 11/20/94

Teacher: R. Paul   Grade: 6

Clinician: E. Reuler   Date of examination: 10/10/06

School: Ruttles Middle School   Sampling context: Interview

Number of T-units in sample: 50

Number of complex sentences in sample: 22

Percentage of complex sentences in sample: 44%

Complex sentence type	T-unit	Conjunction used
Sentence–conjunction–sentence	5. He plays soccer, and I play baseball. 9. I like ice cream, but I don't want yours.	and but
Simple infinitive	14. I need to go home right after school. 34. He wants to beat me at that game.	
Adverbial clause	16. After I get home, I watch TV. 46. If my mom isn't home, I get a snack.	after if
Propositional clause	27. I wish that I had the new Star Wars DVD.	that
Wh- clause	3. Mom knows where I am. 41. I don't know who that is.	where who
Sentences with three or more verbal phrases	18. I want to go see it, but my mom won't take me. 23. After we go to the circus, we like to stop for ice cream.	but after
Relative clause	25. That's the kind I like. 30. They're the kids that I play ball with.	that that
Infinitive clause with different subject	15. He wants me to go with him. 20. My teacher wants you to teach me.	
Infinitive with wh-	19. I know how to do that. 28. Did you tell me when to stop?	how when
Passive infinitive	7. He doesn't want to get hit by the truck. 10. Do you want to be picked by the teacher?	
Gerund clause	26. Snowboarding is fun. 49. My favorite thing is playing computer games.	

Figure 5.6. Sample worksheet for complex sentence analysis (with example utterances).

Communicative skill	Appropriate	Inappropriate	No opportunity to observe
Listening skills			
1. Understands partner's vocabulary and syntax			
2. Follows conversational topics introduced by others			
3. Indicates understanding or mis-understanding with verbal feedback			
Speaking skills			
A. Linguistic features			
1. Produces a variety of forms			
2. Uses some figurative language, slang			
3. Uses precise vocabulary			
4. Produces few mazes or false starts			
B. Paralinguistic features			
1. Inflection			
2. Pausing			
3. Rate			
4. Fluency			
5. Intelligibility			
C. Communicative functions			
1. Gives information			
2. Requests information			
3. Describes objects and events			
4. Expresses beliefs, intentions, or feelings			
5. Persuades listener to do, believe, or feel			
6. Solves problems with language			
D. Discourse management			
1. Initiates conversation			
2. Chooses topic			
3. Maintains topics			
4. Shifts topics			
5. Repairs/revises when necessary			
6. Yields floor			
7. Interrupts			
E. Conversational rules			
1. Manages quantity (does not talk too much or too little)			
2. Makes sincere comments			
3. Makes relevant comments			
4. Expresses thoughts clearly and concisely			
5. Uses tact, politeness			

Communicative skill	Appropriate	Inappropriate	No opportunity to observe
F. Nonverbal behaviors			
1. Makes gestures and facial expressions			
2. Makes eye contact and holds gaze			
3. Maintains proximity			

Figure 5.7. A worksheet for adolescent conversational analysis. (*Source:* Larsen & McKinley, 2003.)

Narrative and Expository . Larson and McKinley (2003) suggested that for older students, written as well as oral samples of communication should be examined, and **narrative** and **expository** texts should be explored because these more demanding, literate uses of language may reveal weaknesses not seen in ordinary conversation (Scott & Windsor, 2000; Westby, 2005). A variety of methods have become available for analyzing narratives and determining whether clients' narrative skills are age-appropriate. These include Gillam and Pearson (2004); Hughes, McGillivray, and Schmidek (1997); Hedberg and Westby (1993); Larson and McKinley (2003); and Strong (1998). Larson and McKinley (2003) recommended that the clinician obtain two narrative samples, one a reformulation task in which the client retells a story and the other a formulated task in which the client relates a personal experience. If clients' narratives are less mature than would be expected for grade level, intervention can be aimed at advancing both the understanding and production of narrative. Guidance on collecting and analyzing expository and written language samples can be found in Paul (in press), Scott (2005), Scott and Stokes (1995), and Westby (2005).

Language Sampling in Adults with Acquired Disorders

Adults who acquire language disorders through accidents or illness are said to have aphasia. These disorders can affect the ability to retrieve and understand words, to formulate and comprehend sentences and to imitate language. Clinicians may also treat adults with traumatic brain injuries (TBI) that can also lead to cognitive-communication deficits. Clinicians sample language from adults with aphasia and TBIs for the same reasons that they do so for younger clients: to examine the functional use of language in real communicative situations and to supplement standardized evaluation procedures with information from these more naturalistic assessments.

Collecting the Sample Shadden (1998) suggested several contexts for eliciting language samples from adults:

Interactive conversation about a familiar topic

Picture description of a common scene, such as people watching television in a living room; of a well-known picture, such as a Normal Rockwell painting; or of a commonly used clinical stimulus, such as the "cookie theft" picture from the *Boston Diagnostic Aphasia Test* (Goodglass & Kaplan, 1983)

Retelling a story heard verbally

Generating a story from a set of pictures

Listing procedures involved in a well-known event, such as shopping in a grocery store

Shadden, as well as Liles and Coelho (1998) emphasized the importance of collecting samples in more than one of these contexts in order to assess the client's ability to deal with several levels of difficulty in discourse situations. Just as we do when we sample language from children, we want to be sure our sample from an adult validly represents communicative ability. For this reason, sampling in more than one setting is ideal.

Recording and Transcribing the Sample   Most of the recording and transcription conventions used for younger clients are appropriate for transcribing adult language as well. T-unit segmentation is often used in adult samples for the same reasons that it is used in younger populations. Likewise, the same computer-assisted procedures, such as the SALT and CHAT programs, are available to be used to transcribe adult discourse.

Anaylzing the Sample   In analyzing speech from adults with aphasia, we look for disruptions of well-learned language processes and for situations in which frustration occurs due to an inability to find forms for intentions that the adult has in mind.

Semantics and Syntax   According to Shadden (1998), the primary areas of interest in analyzing language form in adult clients include the following

Sentence length

Syntactic complexity, diversity, and completeness

Semantic diversity and accuracy

Use of morphological forms

Because these are many of the same issues we look at in school-age children, we can apply some of the same analysis procedures, including MLU per T-unit, and percent of complex sentences. Shadden (1998) suggested some additional analyses that can be helpful for adults:

Words/clause: total number of words divided by total number of clauses

Clauses/T-unit: total number of clauses (both independent and subordinate) divided by total number of T-units

The percentage of 1-, 2-, and 3+-clause sentences.

All these analyses can be used as baseline measures, against which to monitor progress in increasing syntactic complexity during the course of a therapy program.

As an index of syntactic accuracy and completeness, Shadden (1998) suggested assigning each T-unit in a sample a "+" if it is fully grammatical and a "−" if it contains errors, such as

Verb marking errors

Obligatory word omissions

Additions of extra elements

Incomplete forms

Morphological errors

Pronoun errors

Word order errors

A clinician can then calculate the percentage of syntactically accurate and complete T-units and compare this percentage across discourse tasks or over time in intervention. A similar procedure can be used to assess semantic accuracy and completeness, with "-" scores given for errors such as

Empty or vague word use

Given/new information errors

Neologisms or paraphasias

Inaccurate information

Ambiguous or contentless information

Inappropriate word use

Incompleteness

An additional semantic analysis that is frequently of interest for adult clients concerns the amount, efficiency, conciseness, accuracy, and completeness of the information conveyed. Shadden (1998) suggested that many patients with acquired disorders have specific difficulty with the **informativeness** of their discourse; that is, with conveying the appropriate amount of information and with conveying information of sufficient quality without irrelevancies, redundancies, off-topic interjections, or overly personalized content. Efficiency and conciseness are also problematic for these clients, who may produce discourse that is unfocused and prone to delay, errors, excessive detail, and effortful production. Several approaches have been developed to provide data on these kinds of discourse problems.

Content Unit Analysis or *Correct Information Unit analysis* (Capilouto, Wright, & Wagovich, 2005) involves developing a list of content units for a particular stimulus and comparing a client's response to that stimulus to the list generated by the clinician or a panel of typical controls. The box following this paragraph provides an example of a content unit analysis that might be developed for a picture description task, using a picture created by Nicholas and Brookshire (1993), which appears in Figure 5.8. These units can be derived for a variety of discourse tasks, including procedural descriptions such as "going shopping" or "eating in a restaurant." The number of content units included within a retelling can be tabulated, as well as the number of units that are irrelevant, redundant, or inaccurate. Figure 5.9 presents such an analysis for the Birthday Party picture as it might be produced at two points in time by a client. Capilouto, Wright, and Wagovich (2005) and Nicholas and Brookshire (1995) reported that this analysis allows a clinician to look for increases in quantity of appropriate information and decreases in inappropriate utterances as an index of progress in therapy.

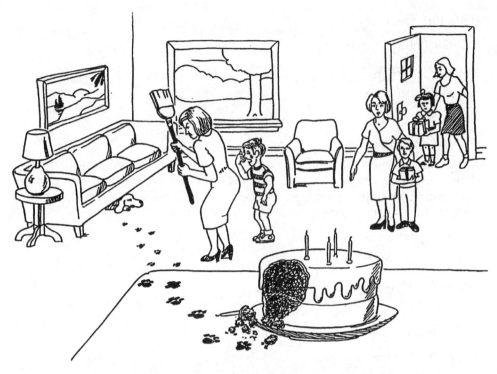

Figure 5.8. Sample picture used in content unit analysis. (From Nicholas, L., & Brookshire, R. [1993]. A system for quantifying the informitiveness and efficiency of the connected speech of adults with aphasia. *Journal of Speech and Hearing Research, 36,* 346. © American Speech-Language-Hearing Association; reprinted by permission.)

CONTENT UNIT ANALYSIS FOR NICHOLAS AND BROOKSHIRE'S (1993) BIRTHDAY PARTY PICTURE IN FIGURE 5.8.

woman	little	women coming	dog
mother[*]	boy	in with children	under couch/sofa
standing (with	crying	to living room	hiding[*]
broom)	sad[*]	mothers[*]	afraid to come
looking (at dog)	standing beside	guests[*]	out[*]
angry[*]	mother[*]	carrying boxes	left footprints
for stealing cake	upset about	birthday gifts[*]	after eating cake[*]
	cake[*]	surprised[*]	ruined party[*]

Sources: Capilouto, Wright, & Wagovich, 2005; Myers, 1979; Nicholas & Brookshire 1993, 1995; Shadden, 1998.
[*]interpretative units.

Informational Content Analysis is used to assess the efficiency of communication. Here, the ratio of meaningful to nonmeaningful units of information can be tracked across several discourse contexts as well as over time. Cheney and Canter (1993) provided data on normal range for this analysis. Figure 5.10 provides a sample worksheet for the information content analysis that can be used

Content units	Time 1	Time 2	Interpretive units	Time 1	Time 2
Woman	X	X	Mother	X	X
Standing with broom	X	X	Angry		X
Looking at dog	X	X	For stealing cake	X	X
Little boy	X	X	Birthday child		
Crying	X	X	Upset		X
Standing beside	X	X	About cake	X	X
Women and children	X	X	Guests and mothers		
Coming into living room	X	X	Surprised		X
With boxes	X	X	With birthday gifts		X
Dog	X	X	Afraid to come out	X	X
Under sofa	X	X	After eating cake		X
Left footprints	X	X	Ruined party		
TOTALS	12/12	12/12		4/12	9/12
Irrelevant/incorrect/ inaccurate units	3	1			

Figure 5.9. Content unit analysis for the Birthday Party picture.

to examine production across several discourse tasks. **Verbosity,** or excessive talking, is often seen in acquired aphasias and can be measured in a variety of ways:

Calculating the number of information units per minute (Yorkston & Beukelman, 1980)

Calculating number of words per story or discourse unit (Gleason et al., 1980)

Calculating the number of content units in the first 50 words in a discourse task (Arbuckle et al., 1989)

Gold and colleagues (1988) suggested distinguishing two kinds of verbosity: off-target verbosity or irrelevant speech, in which clients speak about topics not relevant to the current one; and digressive speech, in which clients remain on topic but say too much about it.

Pragmatic Analysis   As we did for older children, we will want to look at pragmatic aspects of both conversational and narrative samples from adult clients. To analyze conversation, formats that we looked at for younger clients, such as Prutting and Kirchner's (1983) Pragmatic Protocol and Larson and McKinley's (2003) Conversational Analysis, can be used. Halper and colleagues (1996) developed a rating scale specifically for assessing adult communication skills. An adaptation of this form appears in Figure 5.11.

Student name: _____

Teacher: _____

Clinician: _____

School: _____

Date of birth: _____

Grade: _____

Date of examination: _____

Sampling context: _____

| Task/sample date | Meaningful units | | Nonmeaningful units | | | | Efficiency (number of meaningful/nonmeaningful) |
	Essential	Elaborations	Irrelevant	Redundant	Inaccurate	Off-topic	
Cookie theft picture description Date:							
How to make scrambled eggs procedure description Date:							
Story retelling Date:							
Conversation Date:							
Normal range (from Cheney & Canter, 1993)	40%–78%	10%–33%	7%–38%	0%–6%	0%–1%	0%	4%–14%

Figure 5.10. Sample worksheet for information content analysis. (*Source:* Shadden, 1998.)

	1 Markedly abnormal	2 Limited or inconsistent	3 Appropriate most of the time	4 Consistently appropriate
Nonverbal communication				
Intonation				
Facial expression				
Eye contact				
Gestures				
Proxemics				
Verbal communication				
Conversational initiation				
Turn-taking				
Topic maintenance				
Referencing				
Response length				
Repair and revision				
Quantity of information				

Figure 5.11. A Rating Scale for Adult Conversational Skills. (*Source:* Halper, Cherney, Burns, & Mogil, 1996.)

For narrative analysis, too, many of the forms used for older children can likewise be used with adult clients (Coelho & Flewellen, 2003). Assessments including story retelling or story generation, with or without picture supports, have been used. For example, Doyle and colleagues (2000) showed that a wide variety of productive language variables including measures of language form, content, and use can be reliably measured using a story-retelling procedure with adult clients. Hughes and colleagues (1997) outlined a wide variety of narrative assessments designed for school-age clients that can be used effectively with adults as well. One analysis that can be particularly informative for adult narrative samples is the analysis of **cohesive ties,** the structural coherence among parts of a text (Halliday & Hasan, 1976). Liles and Coelho (1998) identified a set of linguistic markers of cohesion that can be examined in stories produced by clients. These markers can be identified within a discourse sample and rated as to whether they are:

Complete: information referred to by the tie is easily found and defined without ambiguity

Example: Alice was hungry. She ate some cake.

Incomplete: information referred to by the tie is not provided in the text

Example: James walked home from school. He saw them at the bus stop.

Cohesive market type	Examples	Cohesive element in client discourse (word)	Found in T-unit number:	Cohesive adequacy		
				Complete	Incomplete	Error
Reference						
Personal	*He, she, mine, it*					
Demonstrative	*This, that, these, those*					
Conjunction						
Causal	*Because, to that end, otherwise*					
Adversative	*Yet, although, instead, but*					
Temporal	*Then, afterward, subsequently*					
Additive	*Likewise, furthermore, incidentally*					
Lexical						
Reiteration •repetition	*I have a <u>house</u> on the beach. It is a tiny <u>house</u>.*					
•synonym	*He's a good <u>boy</u>. One of the finest <u>lads</u>...*					
•superordinate	*You can have the <u>carrot</u>. I don't like <u>vegetables</u>.*					
•general word	*I gave <u>John</u> the money. The <u>doofus</u> lost it.*					
Collocation	*I'll get the <u>doctor</u>. You look <u>sick</u>.*					
Ellipsis						
Nominal	*What do you want to <u>drink</u>? <u>Coke</u>.*					
Verbal	*Who's <u>coming to the store</u>? We <u>are</u>.*					
Clausal	*Has <u>he done it all</u>? He <u>has</u>.*					
Substitution						
Nominal	*I need a <u>coat</u>. Would you get me <u>one</u>?*					
Verbal	*I don't know <u>how to fix this</u>, and I don't think you <u>do</u> either.*					
Clausal	*They <u>won, didn't they</u>? Unfortunately <u>not</u>.*					

Figure 5.12. A worksheet for assessing cohesive adequacy. (*Source:* Liles & Coelho, 1998.)

Table 5.4. Ratings of coherence in narrative

Rating	Global coherence[a]	Local coherence[b]
1	Unrelated	No relation to content of previous utterance
2	Utterance contains more than one clause; one clause relates to the general topic, but the other clause does not	Utterance contains more than one clause; one clause relates to the previous utterance, but the other clause does not
3	Utterance possibly relates to the general topic, but the topic must be inferred; topic is evaluated without substantive information	Utterance relates to the previous utterance, but has a shift in focus or is vague or ambiguous to the point that that relation to the previous utterance must be inferred
4	Utterance contains more than one clause; one clause relates directly to the general topic, but the other clause relates indirectly	Utterance contains more than one clause; one clause relates to directly to the previous utterance, but the other clause may not
5	Utterance provides substantive information that relates to the general topic	The topic of the previous utterance is continued by elaboration, sequencing, examples, or maintaining characters, events, or focus

Source: Coelho & Flewellen, 2003.

[a]The relation of the content or meaning of the utterance to the overall content of the story.

[b]The relation of the content or meaning of the utterance to the previous utterance.

Erroneous: the tie guides a listener to ambiguous information

Example: Tom and Dick were at the video arcade. He had lots of quarters.

Figure 5.12 presents a summary of the cohesive ties identified by Liles and Coelho (1998) in a format that can be used to assess cohesive adequacy in client discourse samples.

A second pragmatic analysis that can be particularly informative for adult narrative samples is the achievement of **coherence.** Coelho and Flewellen (2003) developed a rating system that can be used to examine coherence in stories produced by clients, which is summarized in Table 5.4. LaPointe (2004) and Spreen and Risser (2003) discussed additional communication sampling issues for adult populations with acquired language disorders.

SPEECH SAMPLING

One way in which communication sampling is efficient is that the same sample can be analyzed on a variety of dimensions. Just as we can look at both syntax and pragmatics in the same sample, we can, in addition, look at the same sample in terms of its articulation, intelligibility, fluency, prosody, quality, and resonance. We will look again at the three developmental periods (preschool, school-age, and adult) to see what aspects of speech production can be analyzed through samples of communication.

Preschool Speech Sampling

When sampling speech in the preschool period, we generally have three goals:

Assessing the occurrence of articulation errors and patterns of error

Assessing the contents of the sound inventory

Assessing intelligibility, or the degree to which speech is understandable by listeners

Table 5.5. Examples of procedures for assessing sound errors and patterns

Test	Ages[*]
Assessment of Phonological Processes, Revised (APP-R; Hodson, 2004)	3-0 to 12-0 years
Arizona Articulation Proficiency Scale, Third Edition (Fudala, 2001)	1-6 to 18 years
Bankson-Bernthal Test of Phonology (Bankson & Bernthal, 1990)	3 to 9 years
Contextual Test of Articulation (CTA; Aase, Hovre, Krause, Schelfhout, Smith, & Carpenter, 2000)	4-0 to 9-11 years
Goldman-Fristoe Test of Articulation, Second Edition (GFTA-2; Goldman & Fristoe, 2000)	2-0 to 21-0 years
Khan-Lewis Phonological Analysis, Second Edition (KLPA-2; Khan & Lewis, 2002)	2-0 to 5-11 years
Natural Process Analysis (NPA: Shriberg & Kwiatkowski, 1982)	2 years to adult
Photo Articulation Test, Third Edition (Lippke, Dickey, Selmer, & Soder, 1997)	5 to 10 years

[*]Ages are expressed in years and months with a hyphen dividing the two (e.g., 3-0 means 3 years, 0 months old).

For the purpose of identifying error patterns, there are a variety of published methods that can be used to structure the coding and analysis of phonological errors. Some examples are listed in Table 5.5. To look at the overall number of consonants a child can say, one measure of phonological maturity, the clinician can collect a **phonetic inventory,** a list of all the sounds the client produces in a sample of speech. Shriberg (1993) divided the consonant phonemes of English into three groups, based on their order of acquisition. Figure 5.13 provides a worksheet for recording the appearance of these sounds in a spontaneous language sample in order to assess the range of phonemes in the repertoire, as well as whether the client is following a typical pattern of acquisition. To use the worksheet, the clinician would simply check off each consonant the child produced during a sample of speech.

Intelligibility For young children, the degree to which speech is intelligible is often a concern. Special considerations arise when collecting a sample of speech from unintelligible clients. We cannot analyze speech that we did not understand. For highly unintelligible children, it may be necessary to use a more structured sampling format in order to have a better chance of understanding what the children mean to say. Activities such as having the child make up a story about a set of sequence pictures or tell the story depicted in a picture book may be the best bet for obtaining a sample that can be deciphered and analyzed, although these activities are less ideal than interactive conversation.

Early sounds	/m/	/b/	/j/	/n/	/w/	/d/	/p/	/h/
Middle sounds	/t/	/ŋ/	/k/	/g/	/f/	/v/	/tʃ/	/dʒ/
Late sounds	/ʃ/	/θ/	/s/	/z/	/ð/	/l/	/r/	/ʒ/

Figure 5.13. Worksheet for recording the appearance of developmentally ordered speech sounds. (*Source:* Shriberg, 1993.)

Traditionally, clinicians have used subjective judgments of intelligibility. Probably the most common subjective measure is percentage estimation in which the clinician assigns a percentage of intelligibility to the speech sample based on an "educated guestimate" of the proportion of words understood by the clinician in running speech. There are, however, more objective measurements that lead to quantifiable judgments. One method of assessing intelligibility is to transcribe the sample, using *X*s for any unintelligible words, and compute the percentage of intelligible words per 100-word sample. Another procedure is described by Weiss (1982) in the *Weiss Intelligibility Test.* Using this method, the clinician listens to an interaction between the client and a familiar listener. As the clinician listens, he or she records a dot (.) for each word understood and a slash (/) for each word not understood on a 10 by 10 grid until each cell of the grid is filled in. The percentage of unintelligible words is then computed by dividing the number of slashes by 100. The advantage of this procedure is that it does not require transcription but can be scored during an interaction. Shriberg and Kwiatkowsi (1982) advocated using the percent consonants correct (PCC) as a measure of intelligibility. This measure requires phonemic transcription of a 100-word sample. The clinician transcribes all the consonants the client produced and also transcribes a **gloss,** or the target consonant the client intended to produce. For example, the client may say, "pway" and the clinician may gloss, or interpret, this utterance to mean "play." In this case the clinician would record /pwe/ for the production and /ple/ for the gloss. PCC is derived by counting the number of consonants that agree with their gloss (or are pronounced correctly) and dividing this number by the number of glossed consonants transcribed in the 100-word sample. This number total is the PCC.

School-Age Speech Sampling

Articulation and intelligibility can be issues at the school-age level. When older children present these problems, the same methods of speech sampling can be adapted for this age group as were used for younger children. Another issue that is often problematic for school-age children involves the smoothness or flow of speech, often referred to as fluency.

Fluency   There are two aspects of fluency that we need to think about in sampling communication for school-age children: **stuttering** and **maze** behavior, both of which often affect students with language and learning disorders. We will talk first about sampling for students who stutter and then about other types of **dysfluency.**

Stuttering   The most commonly used means of assessing stuttering through natural speech involves counting stuttering events (i.e., words or syllables) from samples of the client's spontaneous speech and, if age-appropriate, from reading, as well. An example of a commonly used tool for accomplishing this assessment is the Stuttering Severity Instrument-3 (SSI-3; Riley, 1994). The cover sheet is reproduced in Figure 5.14 and illustrates that a client's evaluation is completed through a combination of scores. These scores include: 1) stuttering frequency; 2) stuttering duration, which is measured by the average of the three longest

SSI-3

Stuttering Severity Instrument-3

TEST RECORD AND FREQUENCY COMPUTATION FORM

Name _____

Sex M F Grade _____ Age _____

Date _____ Date of Birth _____

School _____

Examiner _____

Preschool ___ School Age ___ Adult ___ Reader ___ Nonreader ___

READERS TABLE

1. Speaking Task

Percentage	Task Score
1	2
2	3
3	4
4–5	5
6–7	6
8–11	7
12–21	8
22 & up	9

2. Reading Task

Percentage	Task Score
1	2
2	4
3–4	5
5–7	6
8–12	7
13–20	8
21 & up	9

NONREADERS TABLE

3. Speaking Task

Percentage	Task Score
1	4
2	6
3	8
4–5	10
6–7	12
8–11	14
12–21	16
22 & up	18

Frequency Score (use 1 + 2 or 3) ☐

Average length of three longest stuttering events timed to the nearest 1/10th second

		Scale Score
Fleeting	(.5 sec or less)	2
Half-second	(.5– .9 sec)	4
1 full second	(1.0– 1.9 secs)	6
2 seconds	(2.0– 2.9 secs)	8
3 seconds	(3.0– 4.9 secs)	10
5 seconds	(5.0– 9.9 secs)	12
10 seconds	(10.0–29.9 secs)	14
30 seconds	(30.0–59.9 secs)	16
1 minute	(60 secs or more)	18

Duration Score (2 – 18) ☐

Evaluating Scale

0 = none
1 = not noticeable unless looking for it
2 = barely noticeable to casual observer
3 = distracting
4 = very distracting
5 = severe and painful-looking

DISTRACTING SOUNDS	Noisy breathing, whistling, sniffing, blowing, clicking sounds	0 1 2 3 4 5
FACIAL GRIMACES	Jaw jerking, tongue protruding, lip pressing, jaw muscles tense	0 1 2 3 4 5
HEAD MOVEMENTS	Back, forward, turning away, poor eye contact, constant looking around	0 1 2 3 4 5
MOVEMENTS OF THE EXTREMITIES	Arm and hand movement, hands about face, torso movement, leg movements, foot-tapping or swinging	0 1 2 3 4 5

Physical Concomitants Score ☐

Frequency _____ + Duration _____ + Physical Concomitants _____ = ☐

Percentile _____

Severity _____

© 1994 by PRO-ED, Inc.

10 9 8 7 6   96

For additional copies of this form (#6722),
contact PRO-ED, 8700 Shoal Creek Blvd., Austin, TX 78757

Figure 5.14. The Stuttering Severity Instrument-3. (From Riley, G. [1994]. *The Stuttering Severity Instrument-3.* [p.1]. Austin, TX: PRO-ED.; reprinted by permission.)

stuttering events; and 3) physical concomitant behaviors, those behaviors that are associated with stuttering, such as head movements, facial grimaces, and distracting sounds. From these three scores, a total overall score is obtained. The total score is then assigned a percentile and a degree of severity (i.e., very mild, mild, moderate, severe, very severe).

A common critique of many standard stuttering assessments is that they do not evaluate speech in a full range of natural contexts (Conture, 1996; Ingham & Riley, 1998) because stuttering can vary greatly in different situations. Tetnowski (1999) devised a protocol for evaluating stuttering that assesses speech in several settings and at various levels of complexity. This protocol gathers information on percentage of stuttering, length of stuttering events, and physical concomitants, as does the SSI-3; however, it provides clinicians with the opportunity to compare behaviors across several linguistic and non-linguistic contexts. As we discussed for language sampling, clinicians will ideally want to provide as representative a sample as possible, and often this can mean sampling in more than one context.

Maze Behavior   Another type of dysfluency is often referred to as *maze behavior*. These behaviors include the interruption in the smooth flow of speech that is characterized primarily by mazes, speech disruptions that include false starts, repetitions, and revisions. Maze behaviors are often very difficult to differentiate from stuttering, in practice. But because the management implications for these two types of dysfluency are so different (one is treated as a speech disorder, the other as a language disorder), it is especially important to be able to distinguish the two types reliably. A scheme for differentiating stuttering from maze behaviors, developed by Grinager Ambrose and Yairi (1999), appears in Table 5.6.

Dollaghan and Campbell (1992) and Long and colleagues (2005) discussed methods of assessing this kind of dysfluency in spontaneous speech. A description of the kinds of maze behaviors typically seen in the speech of school-age clients with language-learning disorders appears in Table 5.7. Long and colleagues (2005) found that mazes were more common in the narrative genre than in conversation. They suggest that if these maze behaviors occur in more than 25% of the utterances in a conversational sample, the speech can be considered significantly disrupted. Narratives would be considered disrupted if more than 40% of utterances contain mazes.

Voice Quality and Resonance   Children's voice problems typically stem from three main sources:

1. Vocal abuse, or the straining of the voice due to prolonged periods of loud talking, yelling, or attempts to speak at an unnatural pitch

Table 5.6.   Stuttering-like dysfluencies and maze behaviors

Category	Type of dysfluency	Example
Part-word repetition	Stuttering-like dysfluency	"thi-thi-this"
Single-syllable word repetition	Stuttering-like dysfluency	"and-and-and"
Disrhythmic phonations 1. Prolongations 2. Blocks 3. Broken words	1. Stuttering-like dysfluency 2. Stuttering-like dysfluency 3. Stuttering-like dysfluency	1. "coooookie" 2. "#toy" 3. "o#pen"
Interjections	Maze behavior	"um"
Revision/abandoned utterance	Maze behavior	"Mom ate/Mom fixed dinner"
Multisyllable word/phrase repetition	Maze behavior	"because-because" "I want-I want to go"

Source: Grinager Ambrose & Yairi, 1999.
Note: # is a pause in phonation.

Table 5.7. Maze behaviors

Maze behaviors	Description	Example
Pauses		
Filled	Nonword, one-syllable filler vocalization	*um, er*
Silent	Silent intervals of 2 seconds or more	
	More than one silent or filled pause in succession	*He, um, said [pause] I could leave early.*
Repetitions		
Forward	Repetition of an incomplete unit, which is then completed	*He, he said I could leave early.*
Exact	Repetition of a completed unit	*He said I could leave I could leave.*
Backward	Insertion of additional word(s) before the repeated unit, without changing it	*He said I guess he said I could leave.*
Revisions	Modifications to correct errors, add or delete information	*I have two puddies, puppies.* *My older brother my brother hates soccer.*
		My sister, I means my brother, is late.
		I have a sister, two sisters.
Orphans	Linguistic units without obvious relations to other parts of the utterance	*I saved up in all my money.* *And spuh that's her date.*

Source: Dollaghan & Campbell, 1992.

2. Craniofacial anomalies such as a cleft palate or lip, which result in structural differences that affect voice quality and resonance

3. Cerebral palsy, a congenital neurological disorder that may lead to a difficulty in motoric aspects of speech production

Methods of assessment for these kinds of voice problems are similar for children and adults and will be discussed when we look at adult voice problems.

Speech Sampling in Adults

Articulation and Intelligibility Disorders of articulation and intelligibility in adults are most frequently the result of acquired motor speech disorders that affect respiration, phonation, resonance, and articulation. These disorders of speech production are usually classified as dysarthrias and apraxias and are contrasted with acquired language disorders such as aphasia. Aphasia and related disorders affect language understanding and formulation; motor speech disorders, however, affect only the motor production and articulation of the speech signal. Motor speech disorders include the speech patterns associated with Parkinson's disease, multiple sclerosis, amyotrophic lateral sclerosis (ALS), cerebral palsy, tumor, trauma, stroke, as well as other disorders that affect the speech production mechanism.

Dysarthrias are motor speech impairments that are marked by consistent errors, due to a neuromuscular impairment of the speech mechanism. Because the muscles used to control speech also control other functions, dysarthrias affect speech movements as well as non-speech movements such as chewing, smiling, swallowing, and so forth. Apraxias, however, are disturbances of neuromotor programming. Apraxia of speech can exist without any apparent muscle weakness or paralysis, which are the defining characteristics of dysarthria. It should be noted that because dysarthria, apraxia, and aphasia can be a result of damage to the central nervous system, they can, and often do, exist in combination with each other. This can make differential diagnosis quite difficult.

Duffy (1995) outlined principles for assessment of motor speech disorders, which should include complete oral mechanism and standardized motor speech evaluations, in addition to the assessment of intelligibility and the acoustic properties of speech that come out of the analyses of spontaneous speech samples. Many of the same procedures that we discussed for assessing intelligibility in speech samples of children can be applied to those of adults with motor speech disorders. A phonetic transcription of a speech sample could be used to study error patterns produced by the client. PCC or the *Weiss Intelligibility Test* can also be used to determine overall rate of intelligibility in adult speakers. In addition to analysis of spontaneous speech, standard reading passages are often used to gather information on adults with speech disorders. These passages are constructed to contain all the phonemes of English, so that a relatively short sample provides an example of the client's production of each sound in the language. The Rainbow Passage (Fairbanks, 1940) is an example of a reading task often used in this way.

THE RAINBOW PASSAGE

When the sunlight strikes raindrops in the air, they act like a prism and form a rainbow. The rainbow is a division of white light into many beautiful colors. These take the shape of a long round arch, with its path high above, and its two ends apparently beyond the horizon. There is, according to legend, a boiling pot of gold at one end. People look, but no one ever finds it. When a man looks for something beyond his reach, his friends say he is looking for the pot of gold at the end of the rainbow.

Throughout the centuries men have explained the rainbow in various ways. Some have accepted it as a miracle without physical explanation. To the Hebrews it was a token that there would be no more universal floods. The Greeks used to imagine that it was a sign from the gods to foretell war or heavy rain. The Norsemen considered the rainbow as a bridge over which the gods passed from earth to their home in the sky. Other men have tried to explain the phenomenon physically. Aristotle thought that the rainbow was caused by reflections of the sun's rays by the rain. Since then physicists have found that it is not reflection but refraction by the raindrops that causes the rainbow. Many complicated ideas about the rainbow have been formed. The difference in the rainbow depends considerably upon the size of the water drops, and the width of the colored band increases as the size of the drops increases. The actual primary rainbow observed is said to be the effect of superpositioning of a number of bows. If the red of the second bow falls on the green of the first, the result is to give a bow

> with an abnormally wide yellow band, since red and green lights when mixed form yellow. This is a very common type of bow, one showing mainly red and yellow, with little or no green or blue.
>
> From Fairbanks, G. (1940). *Voice and articulation drillbook* (p. 127). New York: Harper & Brothers; reprinted by permission.

Fluency Fluency issues, particularly those related to stuttering, can be problems for adults as well as children. The speech sampling approaches that we talked about for school-age children can be used with adults as well. With adults, reading samples are an especially important part of the sampling procedure and are often contrasted to spontaneous speech.

Prosody Much of the meaning conveyed through language comes not from the words themselves, but from the way they are said: the rate at which we speak, the intonation that we use, the pauses that we insert, the stress that we place on parts of the utterance. All of these paralinguistic cues go into determining the prosody of speech-its rhythm and music. Prosodic function is affected in a variety of communication disorders. Certain kinds of brain damage result in **dysprosody.** Children with autism and some kinds of specific language disorders may show prosodic deficits (Shriberg et al., 2001; Wells & Peppé, 2003). People with impaired hearing often produce abnormal prosody, as do people with apraxia of speech, either developmental or acquired.

Prosody is usually evaluated in spontaneous speech by making a global judgment as to its overall acceptability in conversation. Several of the pragmatic rating scales we looked at earlier include prosody as one element of their checklist. A more formal measure of prosodic production was developed by Shriberg, Kwiatkowski, and Rasmussen (1990). Their *Prosody-Voice Screening Protocol* (PVSP) allows trained raters to assess three independent aspects of prosody (phrasing, rate, and stress)—as well as the pitch, quality, and resonance of the voice—in each utterance in a spontaneous speech sample. The proportion of utterances judged to contain inappropriate prosody in each of these areas can be computed and compared to a database of typical speakers. Shriberg and colleagues have applied this analysis to several types of communication disorders and shown varying patterns of dysprosody across these disabilities.

Voice Quality and Resonance

Vocal Quality Assessment of voice in spontaneous speech relies primarily on the clinician's trained ear. That is, clinicians develop the experience and knowledge to judge when a voice is far enough away from the ideal for age, physique, health status, and gender that a difference or disorder exists. The following dimensions of the voice are usually evaluated using the trained ear:

Fundamental frequency: too high or too low

Loudness: too loud or too soft

Quality: breathy, hoarse, harsh

PERCEPTUAL DESCRIPTIONS OF VOCAL PARAMETERS

Breathiness: the perception of expressive air leakage during voice production due to the vocal folds not completely closing. This can be due to vocal fold paralysis; irregularities along the edge of the vocal fold(s); or mass lesions such as **nodules, polyps,** or **cysts.**

Hoarseness: the perception of breathiness along with the perception of "noise" in phonation. This is caused by irregular vibration of the vocal folds and can be related to mass lesions, inflammation of the vocal folds (laryngitis), or **Reinke's edema.**

Harshness: the perception of excessive tension, tightness, or effort in the voice. This is also associated with hard glottal attacks and overadduction of the vocal folds. Harshness is often associated with many neurological abnormalities or structural abnormalities of the larynx. It can also be noted in learned abnormal behavior patterns or overcompensation for a learned behavior.

Hypernasality: the perception of too much nasality in the voice. It is commonly noted in structural abnormalities like clefting of the palate and with neurological deficits affecting cranial nerves IX, X, and XI.

Hyponasality: the perception of not enough nasality in the voice. This is the perceptual quality that is heard in clients with severe colds or allergies. The voice is marked by a lack of nasal quality in the voice where a nasal quality is normally expected (i.e., /n/, /m/, /g/, and the vowels that surround them). In addition to these descriptive terms, also evaluate clients based upon their appropriate use of pitch and loudness.

Voice specialists also use direct **endoscopic** observation of the larynx, as well as instrumental acoustic and aerodynamic evaluations, to assist in an accurate diagnosis of voice. More information on these formal analyses can be found in Baken (1996); Bless and Bacon (1992); Orlikioff and Bacon (1993); and Till, Yorkson, and Beukelman (1994). Computer-assisted methods are often used to make many of the relevant measurements of the voice without equipment that is invasive to the client. A review of these systems is provided by Bielamowicz, Kreiman, Gerratt, Dauer, and Berke (1996) and Read, Buder, and Kent (1990; 1992). Acoustic analysis tools such as these can provide information related to **fundamental frequency, spectral analysis, formant analysis, signal-to-noise ratio,** and **perturbation** of the speaking voice. Examples of these systems are shown in Figure 5.15.

Resonance An assessment for appropriate nasality, or resonance, is often needed for children with cleft palates, patients who undergo **laryngectomy** surgery, and adults with motor speech disorders (Andrews, 1995; Deem & Miller, 2000; Prater & Swift, 1984). The clinician's trained ear is again the analysis tool used initially to determine the appropriateness of resonance in connected speech. The clinician's determination usually involves a judgment as to whether speech demonstrates

Normal nasality

Hypernasality (overly nasal speech)

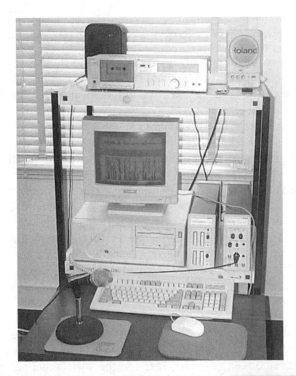

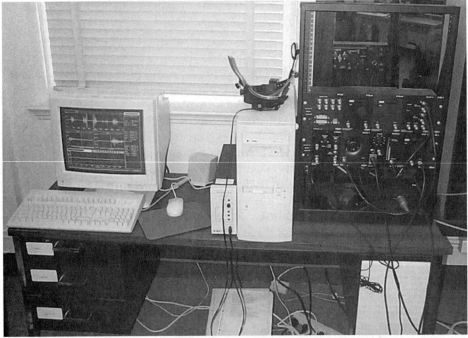

Figure 5.15. Examples of desktop computer speech analysis tools. Top: Kay, Computerized Speech Laboratory. Bottom: Tucker-Davis Technologies, System II with Computerized Speech Research Environment Software.

Hyponasality (denasal speech, such as is produced when a person has "a *code* in the *dose*")

Again, when clinicians detect an abnormal degree of nasality, they will often follow up with more structured tasks, requiring the subject to repeat sentences with high loading of nasal consonants (e.g., "*Mary* has *nine new* stuffed a*nimals*") and those without (e.g., "Ted has a dog with white feet") in order to determine how the client is able to constrain nasality within an utterance. Instrumental evaluations of resonance may also be part of the assessment battery.

Functional measures of voice are also becoming a more standard part of vocal assessments. Tools such as the Voice Handicap Scale (Jacobson et al., 1997) and the Voice Symptom Scale (Dreary, Wilson, Garding, & MacKenzie, 2003) are tools that assess the functional level of communication based on vocal performance. Tools like the Voice Handicap Index (Table 5.8) take a more functional view of a speech disorder.

Table 5.8. Voice Handicap Index (VHI), Henry Ford Hospital

Instructions: These are statements that many people have used to describe their voices and the effects of their voices on their lives. Circle the response that indicates how frequently you have the same experience.

F1.	My voice makes it difficult for people to hear me.
P2.	I run out of air when I talk.
F3.	People have difficulty understanding me in a noisy room.
P4.	The sound of my voice varies throughout the day.
F5.	My family has difficulty hearing me when I call them throughout the house.
F6.	I use the phone less often than I would like.
E7.	I'm tense when talking with others because of my voice.
F8.	I tend to avoid groups of people because of my voice.
E9.	People seem irritated with my voice.
P10.	People ask, "What's wrong with your voice?"
F11.	I speak with friends, neighbors, or relatives less often because of my voice.
F12.	People ask me to repeat myself when speaking face-to-face.
P13.	My voice sounds creaky and dry.
P14.	I feel as though I have to strain to produce voice.
E15.	I find other people don't understand my voice problem.
F16.	My voice difficulties restrict my personal and social life.
P17.	The clarity of my voice is unpredictable.
P18.	I try to change my voice to sound different.
F19.	I feel left out of conversations because of my voice.
P20.	I use a great deal of effort to speak.
P21.	My voice is worse in the evening.
F22.	My voice problem causes me to lose income.
E23.	My voice problem upsets me.
E24.	I am less outgoing because of my voice problem.
E25.	My voice makes me feel handicapped.
P26.	My voice "gives out" on me in the middle of speaking.
E27.	I feel annoyed when people ask me to repeat.
E28.	I feel embarrassed when people ask me to repeat.
E29.	My voice makes me feel incompetent.
E30.	I'm ashamed of my voice problem.

Note: The letter preceding each item number corresponds to the subscale (E = emotional subscale, F = functional subscale, P = physical subscale).

CONCLUSIONS

The sampling of spontaneous communication is an essential part of the assessment of any communication disorder. Only by observing and analyzing clients' real communication in natural settings can we as clinicians understand what they are attempting to get across, where their communication breaks down, and what we can do to improve their communicative effectiveness. Moreover, recent trends in clinical practice require documentation of progress in functional communication to ensure that changes made in therapy have real consequences for clients' ability to participate in real-world settings. Showing changes in communication through the careful assessment of natural language use allows us to demonstrate these changes in levels of functioning. Communication sampling can be accomplished throughout all developmental levels for a wide range of speech and language domains, including syntax, pragmatics, semantics, phonology, and vocal presentation. The sampling and analysis of a client's spontaneous communicative behavior is one of our most fundamental clinical methods and one in which every clinician needs to be competent.

REFERENCES

Aase, D., Hovre, C., Krause, K., Schelfhout, S., Smith, J., & Carpenter, L. (2000). *Contextual Test of Articulation*. Eau Claire, WI: Thinking Publications.

Andrews, M.L. (1995). *Manual of voice treatment*. San Diego: Singular Publishing Group.

Applebee, A. (1978). *The child's concept of a story: Ages 2 to 17*. Chicago: University of Chicago Press.

Arbuckle, T., Gold., D., Frank, I., & Motard, D. (Nov, 1989). *Speech of verbose older adults: How is it different?* Paper presented at the Gerontological Society of America, Minneapolis, MN.

Baken, R. (1996). *Clinical measurement of speech and voice*. San Diego: Singular Publishing Group.

Bankson, N.W., & Bernthal, J.E. (1990). *Bankson-Bernthal Test of Phonology*. San Antonio, TX: Special Press.

Bar-Adon, A., & Leopold, W. (1971). *Child language: A book of readings*. Upper Saddle River, NJ: Prentice Hall.

Beukelman, D.R., & Mirenda, P. (2005). *Augmentative and alternative communication: Supporting children and adults with complex communication needs* (3rd ed.). Baltimore: Paul H. Brookes Publishing Co.

Bielamowicz, S., Kreiman, J., Gerratt, B.R., Dauer, M.S., & Berke, G.S. (1996). Comparison of voice analysis systems for perturbation measurement. *Journal of Speech and Hearing Research, 39,* 126–134.

Bless, D., & Bacon, R. (1992). Introduction: Assessment of voice. *Journal of Voice, 6,* 95–97.

Brinton, B., & Fujiki, M. (2004). *Conversational management with language impaired children: pragmatic assessment and intervention*. San Antonio, TX: PRO-ED.

Brown, R. (1973). *A first language, the early stages*. Cambridge, MA: Harvard University Press.

Brutten, G.J. (1985). *Communication Attitude Test*. Unpublished manuscript, Southern Illinois University, Department of Communication Disorders and Sciences, Carbondale.

Calculator, S. (1997). Fostering early language acquisition and AAC use: Exploring reciprocal influences between children and their environments. *Augmentative and Alternative Communication, 13,* 149–157.

Capilouto, G., Wright, H., & Wagovich, S. (2005). CIU and main event analyses of the structured discourse of older and younger adults. *Journal of Communication Disorders, 38,* 431–444.

Chapman, R. (1978). Comprehension strategies in children. In J.F. Kavanaugh and W. Strange (Eds.), *Speech and language in the laboratory, school, and clinic* (pp. 308–327). Cambridge, MA: The MIT Press.

Cheney, L., & Canter, G. (1993). Informational content in the discourse of patients with probably Alzheimer's disease and patients with right brain damage. *Clinical Aphasiology, 21,* 123–134.

Coelho, C., & Flewellen, L. (2003). Longitudinal assessment of coherence in an adult with fluent aphasia: A follow-up study. *Aphasiology, 17,* 173–182.

Conture, E.G. (1996). Treatment efficacy: Stuttering. *Journal of Speech and Hearing Research, 39,* S18–S26.

Craig, H., & Washington, J. (2002).Oral language expectations for African American preschoolers and kindergartners. *American Journal of Speech-Language Pathology, 11,* 59–70.

Crystal, D., Fletcher, P., & Garman, M. (1991). *The grammatical analysis of language disability: A procedure for assessment and remediation.* San Diego: Singular Publishing Group.

De Nil, L., & Brutten, G. (1990). Speech-associated attitudes. Stuttering, voice disordered, articulation disordered and normal speaking children. *Journal of Fluency Disorders, 15,* 127–134.

Deem, J.F., & Miller, L. (2000). *Manual of voice therapy.* Austin, TX: PRO-ED.

deVilliers, J., & deVilliers, P. (1973). A cross-sectional study of the acquisition of grammatical morphemes. *Journal of Psycholinguistic Research, 2,* 267–278.

Dollaghan, C., & Campbell, T. (1992). A procedure for classifying disruptions in spontaneous language samples. *Topics in Language Disorders, 12,* 56–68.

Doyle, P., McNeil, M., Park, G., Goda, A., Rubenstein, E., Spencer, K., et al. (2000). Linguistic validation of four parallel forms of a story retelling procedure. *Aphasiology, 14,* 537–549.

Dreary, I.J., Wilson, J.A., Garding, P.N., & Mackenzie, K. (2003). VoiSS: A patient derived Voice Symptom Scale. *Journal of Psychometric Research, 54*(5), 483–489.

Duffy, J.R. (1995). *Motor speech disorders: Substrates, differential diagnosis, and management.* St. Louis: Elsevier.

Evans, J., & Craig, H. (1992). Language sample collection and analysis: Interview compared to freeplay assessment contexts. *Journal of Speech and Hearing Research, 35,* 343–353.

Fairbanks, G. (1940). *Voice and articulation drillbook.* New York: Harper & Brothers.

Fudala, J.B. (2001). *Arizona Articulation Proficiency Scale* (3rd ed.). Los Angeles: Western Psychological Services.

Gillam, R., & Pearson, N. (2004). *Test of Narrative Language.* Greenville, SC: SuperDuper Publications.

Gleason, J., Goodglass, H., Obler, L., Green, E., Hyde, M., & Weintraub, S. (1980). Narrative strategies of aphasic and normal-speaking subjects. *Journal of Speech and Hearing Research, 23,* 370–382.

Glennen, S., & DeCoste, D. (1997). *Handbook of augmentative and alternative communication.* San Diego: Singular Publishing Group.

Gold, D., Andres, D., Arbuckle, T., & Schwartzman, A. (1988). Measurement and correlates of verbosity in older people. *Journal of Gerontology, 43,* 27–34.

Goldman, R., & Fristoe, M. (2000). *Goldman-Fristoe Test of Articulation, second edition (GFTA-2).* Circle Pines, MN: AGS Publishing.

Goodglass, H., & Kaplan, E. (1983). *The Boston Diagnostic Aphasia Examination.* Philadelphia: Lea & Febinger.

Grinager Ambrose, N. & Yairi, E. (1999). Normative dysfluency data for early childhood stuttering. *Journal of Speech, Language, and Hearing Research, 42,* 895–909.

Halliday, M., & Hasan, R. (1976). *Cohesion in English.* New York: Longman Publishers.

Halper, A., Cherney, L., Burns, M., & Mogil, S. (1996). *Clinical management of right hemisphere dysfunction* (2nd ed.). New York: Aspen Publishers.

Hedberg , N., & Westby, C. (1993). *Analyzing storytelling skills: Theory to practice.* Tucson, AZ: Communication Skill Builders.

Hodson, B. (2004). *Hodson Assessment of Phonological Patterns* (3rd ed.). Austin, TX: PRO-ED.

Hughes, D., McGillivray, L. & Schmidek, M. (1997). *Guide to narrative language: Procedures for assessment.* Eau Claire, WI: Thinking Publications.

Hunt, K. (1965). *Grammatical structures written at three grade levels (Research Report No. 3).* Urbana, IL: National Council of Teachers of English.

Ingham, J.C., & Riley, G. (1998). Guidelines for documentation of treatment efficacy for young children who stutter. *Journal of Speech, Language and Hearing Research, 41,* 753–770

Ingham, R.J. (1990). On the valid role of reliability in identifying what is stuttering: Comment. *Journal of Speech and Hearing Disorders, 55,* 394–397.

Jacobs, B. (2001). Social validity of changes in informativeness and efficiency of aphasic discourse following linguistic specific treatment (LST). *Brain and Language, 78,* 115–127.

Jacobson, B.H., Johnson, A., Grywalski, C., Silbergleit, A., Jacobson, G., Benninger, M.S., et al. (1997). The Voice Handicap Index (VHI): Development and validation. *American journal of Speech-Language Pathology, 6*(3), 66–70.

Khan, L., & Lewis, N. (2002). *Khan-Lewis Phonological Analysis* (2nd ed.). Circle Pines, MN: AGS Publishing.

Klecan-Aker, J., & Kelty, K. (1990). An investigation of the oral narratives of normal and language-learning disabled children. *Journal of Childhood Communication Disorders, 13,* 207–216.

LaPointe, L.L. (2004). *Aphasia and related neurogenic language disorders.* New York: Thieme New York.

Larson, V., & McKinley, N. (2003). *Communication solutions for older students: Assessment and intervention strategies.* Eau Claire, WI: Thinking Publications.

Leadholm, B., & Miller, J. (1992). *Language sample analysis: The Wisconsin guide.* Madison: Wisconsin Department of Public Instruction.

Lee, L. (1974). *Developmental sentence analysis.* Evanston, IL: Northwestern University Press.

Liles, B., & Coelho, C. (1998). Cohesion analysis. In L. Cherney, B. Shadden, & C. Coelho (Eds.). *Analyzing discourse in communicatively impaired adults* (pp. 65-84). New York: Aspen Publishers.

Lippke, B., Dickey, S., Selmar, J., & Soder, A. (1997). *Photo Articulation Test (PAT-3).* Austin, TX: PRO-ED.

Long, S., Fey, M., & Channell, R. (2000) *Computerized Profiling (CP; Version 9.26)* (Computer software, Windows only). Cleveland, OH: Case Western Reserve University. Available from http://www.computerizedprofiling.org/

Long, S., McKinley, N., Thormann, S., Jones, M., & Nockerts, A. (2005). *Language sample analysis II: The Wisconsin guide.* Madison: Wisconsin Department of Public Instruction.

Lund, N., & Duchan, J. (1993). *Assessing children's language in naturalistic contexts,* (3rd ed.). Upper Saddle River, NJ: Prentice Hall.

McWhinney, B. (1996). The CHILDES system. *American Journal of Speech-Language pathology, 5,* 5–14.

Miller, J. (1981). *Assessing language production in children: Experimental procedures.* Boston: Allyn & Bacon.

Miller, J., & Chapman, R. (2000). *SALT: Systematic analysis of Miller language transcripts* (computer programs to analyze language samples). Madison: Language Analysis Laboratory, Waisman Center, University of Wisconsin-Madison.

Miller, J., Freiberg, C., Rolland, M., & Reeves, M. (1992). Implementing computerized language sample analysis in the public school. *Topics in Language Disorders, 12*(2), 69–82.

Mordecai, D., & Palin, M. (1982). *Lingquest 1 & 2* (computer program). East Moline, IL: Lingquest Software.

Morrison, J., & Shriberg, L. (1992). Articulation testing versus conversational speech sampling. *Journal of Speech and Hearing Research, 35,* 259-273.

Müller, N. (2006), *Multilayered transcription.* San Diego: Plural Publishing.

Myers, P. (1979). Profiles of communications deficits in patients with right cerebral hemisphere damage. In R. Brookshire (Ed.), *Clinical aphasiology: Conference proceedings* (pp. 38–46). Minneapolis, MN: BRK.

Nelson, N. (1998). *Childhood language disorders in context: Infancy through adolescence* (2nd ed.). Columbus, OH: Charles E. Merrill.

Nicholas, L., & Brookshire, R. (1993). A system for quantifying the informativeness and efficiency of the connected speech of adults with aphasia. *Journal of Speech and Hearing Research, 36,* 338–350.

Nicholas, L., & Brookshire, R. (1995). Presence, completeness, and accuracy of main concepts in the connected speech of non-brain-damaged adults and adults with aphasia. *Journal of Speech and Hearing Research, 38,* 145–156.

O'Brien, M., & Nagle, K. (1987). Parents' speech to toddlers: The effect of play context. *Journal of Child Language, 14,* 269–279.

Orlikioff, R., & Bacon, R. (1993). *Clinical speech and voice measurement: Laboratory exercises.* San Diego: Singular Publishing Group.

Owens, R. (2004). *Language disorders* (4th ed.). Boston: Allyn & Bacon.

Paul, R. (in press). *Language disorders from infancy through adolescence: Assessment and intervention* (3rd ed.). St. Louis: Elsevier.

Prater, R.J., & Swift, R.W. (1984). *Manual of Voice Therapy.* Austin, TX: PRO-ED.

Prutting, C.A., & Kirchner, D. (1983). Applied pragmatics. In T.M. Gallagher and C.A. Prutting (Eds.), *Pragmatic assessment and intervention issues in language* (pp. 29–64). San Diego: College-Hill Press.

Read, C., Buder, E.H., & Kent, R.D. (1990). Speech analysis systems: A survey. *Journal of Speech and Hearing Research, 33,* 363–374.

Read, C., Buder, E.H., & Kent, R.D. (1992). Speech analysis systems: An evaluation. *Journal of Speech and Hearing Research, 35,* 314–332.

Retherford, K. (2000). *Guide to analysis of language transcripts* (3rd ed.). Eau Claire, WI: Thinking Publications.

Riley, G. (1994). *Stuttering Severity Instrument-3.* Austin, TX: PRO-ED.

Roseberry-McKibbin, C. (2002). *Multicultural students with special language needs* (2nd ed.). Oceanside, CA: Academic Communication Associates.

Roth, F., & Spekman, N. (1984a). Assessing the pragmatic abilities of children: Part 1. Organizational framework and assessment parameters. *Journal of Speech and Hearing Disorders, 49,* 2–11.

Roth, F., & Spekman, N. (1984b). Assessing the pragmatic abilities of children: Part 2. Guidelines, considerations, and specific evaluation procedures. *Journal of Speech and Hearing Disorders, 49,* 12–17.

Sackett, D.L. (1998). Evidence-based medicine. *SPINE, 23,* 1085-1086.

Scarborough, H. (1990). Index of productive syntax. *Applied Psycholinguistics, 11,* 1–22.

Scott, C. (2005). Learning to write. In H. Catts & A. Kamhi (Eds.), *Language and reading disabilities* (2nd ed., pp. 233–273). Boston: Allyn & Bacon.

Scott, C., & Stokes, S. (1995). Measures of syntax in school-age children and adolescents. *Language, Speech, and Hearing Services in Schools, 26,* 309–317.

Scott, C., & Windsor, J. (2000). General language performance measures in spoken and written narrative and expository discourse of school-age children with language learning disabilities. *Journal of Speech, Language, and Hearing Research, 43,* 324–39.

Shadden, B. (1998). Sentential/surface level analyses. In L. Cherney, B. Shadden, & C. Coelho (Eds.), *Analyzing discourse in communicatively impaired adults.* (pp. 35–64). New York: Aspen Publishers.

Shriberg, L. (1993). Four new speech and prosody-voice measures for genetics research and other studies in developmental phonological disorders. *Journal of Speech and Hearing Research, 36,* 105–140.

Shriberg, L., & Kwiatkowski, J. (1980). *Natural process analysis.* New York: Macmillan/McGraw-Hill.

Shriberg, L., & Kwiatkowski, J. (1982). Phonological disorders III: A procedure for assessing severity of involvement. *Journal of Speech and Hearing Disorders, 47,* 256–270.

Shriberg, L., Kwiatkowski, J., & Rasmussen, N. (1990). *Prosody Voice Screening Protocol.* Tuscon, AZ: Communication Skill Builders.

Shriberg, L., Paul, R., McSweeney, J., Klin, A., Cohen, D., & Volkmar, F. (2001). Speech and prosody characteristics of adolescents and adults with high functioning autism and Asperger syndrome. *Journal of Speech, Language and Hearing Research, 44,* 1097–1115.

Spreen, O., & Risser, A. (2003). *Assessment in aphasia.* New York: Oxford University Press.

Stockman, I. (1996). The promises and pitfalls of language sample analysis as an assessment tool for linguistic minority children. *Language, Speech, and Hearing Services in Schools, 27,* 355–366.

Strong, C., (1998). *Strong Narrative Assessment Procedure.* Eau Claire, WI: Thinking Publications.

Tetnowski, J.A. (1999). *A stuttering profile.* Unpublished manuscript, University of Louisiana at Lafayette.

Tetnowski, J.A., & Franklin, T.C. (2002). The clinical analysis layer of transcription. *Clinical Linguistics and Phonetics, 15*(5), 361–369.

Tetnowski, J.A., & Franklin, T.C. (2006). The clinical analysis level. In N. Müller (Ed.), *Multilayered transcription.* San Diego: Plural Publishing.

Till, J.A., Yorkson, K.M., & Beukelman, D.R. (Eds.). (1994). *Motor speech disorders: Advances in assessment and treatment.* Baltimore: Paul H. Brookes Publishing Co.

Tyack, D., & Gottsleben, R. (1974). *Language sampling, analysis, and training* (Rev. ed.). Palo Alto, CA: Consulting Psychologists Press.

Ulatowska, H., Doyle, A., Freedman-Stern, R., Macaluso-Haynes, S., & North, A. (1983). Production of procedural discourse in aphasia. *Brain and Language, 18,* 306–316.

Weiss, C. (1982). *Weiss Intelligibility Test.* Tigard, OR: CC Publications.

Wells, B., & Peppé, S. (2003). Intonation abilities of children with speech and language impairments. *Journal of Speech, Language, and Hearing Research, 46*(1), 5–20.

Westby, C. (2005). Assessing and facilitating text comprehension problems. In H. Catts & A. Kahmi (Eds.), *Language and reading disabilities* (2nd ed., pp. 157–232). Boston: Allyn & Bacon.

Wetherby, A.M, & Prizant, B.M. (2002). *Communication and Symbolic Behavior Scales: Developmental profile*^{TM} *(CSBS DP*^{TM}*).* Baltimore: Paul H. Brookes Publishing Co.

World Health Organization. (2001). *International classification of functioning, disability and health.* Geneva: Author.

Wright, H., Capilouto, G., Wagovich, S., Cranfill, T., & Davis, J. (2005). Development and reliability of a quantitative measure of adults' narratives. *Aphasiology, 19,* 262–272.

Yoder, P., & Davies, B. (1990). Do parental questions and topic continuations elicit replies from developmentally delayed children: A sequential analysis. *Journal of Speech and Hearing Research, 33,* 563–573.

Yorkston, K., & Beukelman, D. (1980). An analysis of connected speech samples of aphasic and normal speakers. *Journal of Speech and Hearing Disorders, 45,* 27–35.

Yorkston, K., & Beukelman, D. (1981). *Assessment of Intelligibility of Dysarthric Speech.* Tigard, OR: CC Publications.

STUDY QUESTIONS

1. Why is communication sampling an important part of assessment?

2. What are the specific questions an assessment of nonverbal communication attempts to answer?

3. For what kind of samples is videorecording needed? Audiorecording?

4. What sampling contexts are appropriate for preschoolers? School-age children? Adults?

5. What are the advantages and disadvantages of computer-assisted analysis methods? Of manual methods?

6. How are utterances segmented in transcription of preschool language samples? School-age samples? Adult samples?

7. In addition to looking at syntax, what other areas need to be examined in communication samples of adults with acquired disorders?

8. Discuss two methods for assessing speech intelligibility.

9. Discuss the difference between stuttering and maze behavior dysfluencies. Why is this distinction important?

10. What is the Rainbow Passage and for what is it used?

11. How are voice quality, resonance, and prosody typically assessed using communication sampling?

CHAPTER
6

Communication
Intervention

Principles and Procedures

FROMA ROTH AND RHEA PAUL

Perhaps you will recall the six clients we talked about in Chapter 3:

1. Darrell, a preschooler with immature, unintelligible speech, whose parents want him to improve his speech before he begins kindergarten next year

2. Jonah, a 7-year-old with a severe bilateral sensorineural hearing loss. His school district referred him for reevaluation of his hearing, speech, and language and to determine whether his amplification equipment continues to be appropriate for him

3. Anna, a seventh-grade student with significant learning disabilities

4. Marlene, a 50-year-old woman with communication difficulty since her stroke 8 months ago

5. Richard, aged 62, who recently underwent a total laryngectomy and wants to use esophageal speech

6. Thomas, a 27-year-old with a history of severe stuttering, who feels that his speech disorder is interfering with his ability to advance in his career

We talked in some detail about assessment strategies for these and other clients. Once the assessment is completed, though, a clinician is faced with implementing the recommendations made in the assessment. This phase of clinical practice is called intervention. The purpose of intervention is to effect change in communicative behavior in order to maximize an individual's potential to communicate effectively. The way we achieve this purpose varies according to the nature of the disorder, the age and therapy history of the client, the family situation, and the client's learning style and preferences. Whatever the methods of intervention are, though, intervention is designed to teach strategies for improving overall communication, rather than teaching specific behaviors.

Olswang and Bain (1991) discussed three basic purposes that intervention can serve:

1. In some cases, the purpose is to *eliminate the underlying cause* of the disorder. For example, the provision of amplification to a 9-month-old baby with a mild hearing impairment may prevent, or at least minimize, the emergence of developmental speech and language difficulties. For Jonah, audiological reevaluation might determine that his current speech and language difficulties are due to a change in hearing status that requires a change in amplification. In this case, the new intervention program, involving new hearing aids, may eliminate the underlying disorder.

2. In other cases, the purpose may be to teach a client *compensatory strategies* to improve functional communication. This purpose may be appropriate for Marlene, who needs to learn new ways to get her ideas across when her speech is unintelligible due to the motor neuron damage suffered during her stroke. Anna, too, may need to learn compensatory strategies to help her cope in the school setting. And Richard's desire to learn esophageal speech shows that he is eager to find a compensatory mechanism to allow him to communicate vocally despite the loss of his larynx.

3. A third purpose for intervention is to *modify the disorder* by teaching specific speech, language, or pragmatic behaviors that enable an individual to become a more effective communicator. Darrell, for example, may receive instruction on the correct production of his error sounds or sound classes to achieve improved speech production skills and better overall speech intelligibility. Thomas, the client with dysfluency, may not be able to entirely eliminate stuttering moments. If this is the case, he may need to learn to modify his stuttering so that it interferes less with his social communication.

There are a variety of approaches to planning intervention. The common thread among all these, however, is that communication intervention is a dynamic process that proceeds in a systematic progression. Following the diagnosis of a communication disorder, the clinician completes a detailed assessment of current strengths and needs and selects appropriate target behaviors for therapy. Training procedures are then developed and implemented to promote the acquisition of the target behaviors. The intervention process is completed when the client demonstrates mastery of these target behaviors. Periodic monitoring is often performed to ensure the retention and stability of the newly acquired behaviors (Roth & Worthington, 2005).

Essential to the selection of an intervention approach is the degree to which it is evidence-based-that is, supported by the highest quality scientific research in conjunction with the clinical expertise of a speech-language pathologist or audiologist. Using evidence-based practices (EBP) enables clinicians to critically appraise the available body of research as it applies to each client's needs, culture, and value system. Efficacy and effectiveness data are not currently available for all aspects of intervention or for all clinical populations. Still, it is the responsibility of the clinician to work within an EBP framework and approach intervention scientifically by providing specific rationales for intervention procedures and hypotheses about a client's responsiveness to those procedures. Of course, best practices change with evolving research and individual clinical experience, and so, EBP is best viewed as an ongoing, dynamic clinical decision-making process (Dollaghan, 2004). Fey and Justice (Chapter 7) discuss ways clinicians can apply EBP to their daily activities.

When planning intervention, there are three aspects of a program that need to be considered: its products, processes, and contexts (McLean, 1998; Paul, in press). This chapter discusses the products and processes of intervention. The contexts, or the circumstances under which intervention takes place, will be discussed in Chapter 10.

INTERVENTION PRODUCTS

The first step in planning intervention is the identification of the communicative behaviors to be acquired in the program. These are drawn from our assessment data and are usually called **long-term goals.** Long-term goals for a client are the relatively broad changes in communicative behavior to be achieved during a course of therapy. The achievement of these goals will be justification for terminating therapy.

For example, Marlene's stroke left her very limited in speech production, unable to verbalize her wants and needs, and depressed as a result of her frustration. Long-term goals for Marlene could include

1. Increasing amount of intelligible speech

2. Increasing ability to communicate wants and needs

3. Decreasing her frustration by providing alternative means of communication

Once general long-term goals have been identified, clinicians must decide how to help the client to progress toward them. This is accomplished by formulating the steps that will lead the client toward the long-term goal in such a way that progress can be observed and measured. To facilitate this, these steps are stated in a specific form as **behavioral objectives.** There are three components of a behavioral objective:

1. The *do* statement identifies the action the client is to perform. This statement should contain verbs that name observable actions, such as *point, label, repeat, say, match, write, name,* or *ask.* Words to avoid in behavioral objectives are those that talk about processes that cannot be observed directly, such as *understand, know, learn, remember, comprehend,* or *discover.*

2. The *condition* identifies the situation in which the target behavior is to be performed; such as when it will occur, where, in whose presence, and with what materials or cues. Some examples of condition statements include

    Following a clinician's model
    In response to a question
    Given a list of written words
    In response to pictures
    In presence of other therapy group members

3. The *criterion* specifies how well the target must be performed for the objective to be achieved. Typically used criteria include

    90% correct
    8 correct trials out of 10
    Fewer than four errors in three consecutive sessions
    Consistently over a 10-minute period

At this point, you might try writing a behavioral objective for one of Marlene's long-term goals. One example follows, to help you get started.

Do statement	Condition	Criterion
1. Marlene will produce the words *no* and *yes* appropriately	In response to the clinician's questions	With 8 out of 10 intelligible, appropriate responses
2. Marlene will...		

Before beginning a therapy program, the clinician must be sure that the client cannot already perform the target behavior independently. This might seem obvious; but often a diagnosis is made on the basis of standardized tests that include only one item for a particular communication element, and a client may have missed that one item for a variety of reasons. Perhaps Darrell was given an articulation test, and he substituted a /t/ for the final /ʃ/ in the one item that tests final /ʃ/ (e.g., *dish*). Should we include final /ʃ/ as a therapy target? It is possible that Darrell would NOT say /ʃ/ in other final /ʃ/ words and did so in *dish* because he was influenced by the sound /d/ at the beginning of *dish*. This is an example of why potential therapy targets must be pretested before an intervention program is initiated. The **pretest** allows a clinician to establish that the client is not already consistently correct on a target behavior. When clinicians observe that a client is achieving target behaviors in most intervention activities, they administer a **posttest** to determine the client's consistency with target behavior. The pretest and posttest are usually the same; they consist of a set of 10–20 opportunities for the client to produce the target form when presented with minimal cues, prompts, or support from the clinician. The items in the pre- and post-test are different from the items used during instruction. Suppose one behavioral objective for Darrell was as follows:

Do statement	Condition	Criterion
Darrell will produce fricative sounds (/s/, /z/, /ʃ/) in final position	In imitation of the clinician's model with picture cues	With 8 of 10 correct responses

Before beginning intervention, a pretest (such as the example that appears in the following box) would be administered to ensure that a reasonable goal has been set:

Stimulus	Response	Criterion
The client will view a picture card and will be given a prompting statement and question (e.g., "Here's a fish. What is it?").	*"fish"*	With 9 of 10 correct productions of final fricatives

If the client fails to attain the criterion on the pretest, intervention on this target would be provided using the techniques described below. When the client achieves criterion levels of correct production in the intervention situation, a posttest is given to determine whether the objective has been met, using the same stimuli, responses, and criterion that were used in the pretest.

Once long-term and short-term objectives have been established and pretested, it is necessary to determine how to move the client toward achieving these objectives. This process usually involves **task analysis.** In a task analysis, a larger goal is broken down into small steps that can be followed to achieve it. To accomplish this breakdown, a clinician examines the input and output prerequisites necessary for completing the task. Consider Marlene's first long-term goal: increasing the amount of intelligible speech. The requirements of the goal could be analyzed this way:

Sensory: She must hear the speech spoken to her

Motor: She must be able to make oral articulatory movements

Language: She must have some degree of semantic (word meaning) and syntactic (sentence structure) skill

Cognitive: She must have some degree of conceptual and problem-solving ability; she must not be inordinately confused or demented

A clinician would then proceed, by means of informal assessment, to determine whether Marlene has the requisite skills. If not, the clinician might revise the goal or work on developing its prerequisites. If Marlene does have the requisite abilities, however, the clinician would devise a series of steps, or a **task sequence,** through which Marlene will be guided in order to achieve the goal. The whole process, from establishing task prerequisites to sequencing steps to achieve goals, is the task analysis. Figure 6.1 presents a sequence of difficulty for both verbal and nonverbal behaviors that are typically used in communication intervention. A task analysis encourages the clinician to move from the current form of response through of sequence of increasingly complex forms in the course of the intervention program. Table 6.1 gives an example of the sequence of steps a clinician might choose for Marlene to increase her production of intelligible speech. In summary, identifying the products or targets of intervention requires a clinician to

1. Establish long-term goals

2. Identify short-term objectives that build toward the long-term goals

3. Use task analysis to create task sequences through which clients progress toward their goals

Once these steps have been accomplished, the next challenge is to find activities that facilitate this progress. To face this challenge, a clinician has a range of intervention processes.

Table 6.1. Task sequence for Marlene

1. Using sounds she can produce, Marlene will imitate simple words, such as *no, uh-huh, come, stop, hi.*

2. Marlene will produce these words without a direct imitative model (using delayed imitation—for example, "Hi, Marlene; nice to see you").

3. Marlene will practice using the words in scripts designed around daily activities, using picture cues. For example, with a series of pictures, tell Marlene a story about a woman's day, starting with greeting a friend, refusing a cigarette, agreeing with a colleague, and so forth. Marlene will produce the target word at an appropriate point in the story. The clinician will prompt her if necessary.

4. Marlene will practice using these words in conversations with family members, as the clinician coaches her with cues and prompts.

	Nonverbal	Verbal
Simple ↓	Manipulated movement/gesture (clinician moves client's hand to form a gesture)	Immediate imitation (client repeats immediately after clinician)
	Imitated movement/gesture (clinician provides a model and asks client to imitate it)	Delayed imitation (clinician gives verbal model, some intervening speech, then asks client to imitate)
	Elicited movement/gesture (clinician asks client to produce gesture or movement without a direct model)	Partial imitation (clinician produces part of the target; client is asked to produce the whole target)
	Spontaneous movement/gesture (client produces movement/gesture appropriately without model or request for it)	Elicitation with object cue (clinician asks client for verbal response with an object as a cue)
		Elicitation with picture cue (clinician asks client for verbal response with a picture as a cue)
		Elicitation with written cue (clinician asks client for verbal response with a written word as a cue)
		Elicitation with question (clinician asks client for verbal response with a conversational question as a cue)
Complex		Spontaneous response (client produces target appropriately without model or request for it)

Figure 6.1. Task sequence for nonverbal and verbal clinician prompts.

INTERVENTION PROCESSES: THE CONTINUUM OF NATURALNESS

Intervention activities vary in their degree of naturalness. These variations have been described by Fey (1986) as falling along a **"continuum of naturalness."** This continuum represents the degree to which intervention contexts correspond to everyday communication situations and interactions (see Table 6.2). This framework can be adapted for a broad range of communication disorders and ages.

According to Fey (1986), three factors affect naturalness: 1) the intervention activity itself, 2) the physical context in which the activity takes place, and 3) the individuals with whom the client interacts during intervention (see Table 6.3). Clinician-directed (CD) approaches and Client-centered (CC) approaches represent the end points of this continuum.

Table 6.2. Continuum of naturalness for a broad spectrum of communication disorders

Least natural ←	→	Most natural
Clinician directed	Hybrid	Client centered
Drill	Organized activities	Daily activities
Drill play	Milieu teaching	Facilitative play
Modeling	Focused stimulation	Daily routines
	Script therapy	Vocational activities
	Role playing	
	Conversational coaching	
	More naturalistic modifications of clinician directed activities (e.g., structured scripts)	

Source: Fey, 1986.

Clinician-Directed Approaches

In CD approaches, the clinician controls all aspects of the intervention from determining therapy goals, selecting stimulus materials, choosing the type and frequency of reinforcement, determining the order of activities, and identifying the specific target responses to be elicited. Behavioral theorists (e.g., Roth & Worthington, 2005; Skinner, 1957) referred to these antecedent, behavior, and consequence activities using the acronym ABC:

A. Antecedent or stimulus: The clinician provides a model of the desired behavior or a prompt to produce it.

B. Behavior: The client responds by producing a target behavior.

C. Consequence: The clinician provides reinforcement if the client's behavior was produced correctly. If not, the clinician provides feedback or correction or may ignore the incorrect behavior.

Behaviorist theory holds that all behavior occurs following some identifiable antecedent that prompts it and is maintained or discouraged by its consequences. What a clinician needs to do, in this view, is to manage the antecedents and consequences so that they facilitate the production of desired behaviors. To accomplish this management, behaviorists rely heavily on the operant procedures listed in the following box. These approaches are not considered naturalistic because of the degree of clinician control and their lack of adherence to the conventions of genuine reciprocal communication.

Table 6.3. Factors affecting the degree of naturalness of intervention

Activity	Drill	Organized activities	Daily activities
Physical context	Clinic	School/place of work	Home
Social context	Clinician	Teacher/co-worker	Family members

Source: Fey, 1986.

PROCEDURES USED IN OPERANT CONDITIONING

Cue: A verbal or nonverbal signal that tells the client when to produce the response; for example, the clinician taps child on the hand to cue the response to each stimulus.

Delayed imitation: The clinician inserts an intervening statement after the stimulus, but the client still echoes the stimulus; for example, the clinician says, "This is green. It's my favorite color. What color is it?"

Direct (immediate) imitation: The client echoes the clinician immediately after the stimulus is presented; for example, the clinician says, "This is green," and the client says, "Green."

Fading: A systematic withdrawal of reinforcement, either by decreasing the amount of reinforcement or by requiring more instances of the target behavior before reinforcement is given, after a behavior is established.

Prompt: A verbal or nonverbal hint, directive, or minimal guidance that assists the client in producing a behavior; for example, the clinician strokes his or her neck with a finger to remind the client with dysfluency to use easy onset.

Reinforcement: An item or activity that increases the frequency of a correct response; for example, a favorite food, a turn with a toy, or a monetary payment.

Reinforcer: An item or activity that is offered following a behavior to the increase or decrease of a particular behavior. Reinforcers can be

    A. *Primary:* A biological necessity; for example, food or water.

    B. *Secondary:* An item or activity that becomes important because it is linked to a primary reinforcer; for example, a bell that is rung when food is presented.

    C. *Social:* The praise, approval, or attention that is given as a consequence for a behavior; for example, the clinician says, "You said everything clearly! That was a good job."

Reinforcement schedule: The frequency with which reinforcement is given. Schedules can be

    A. *Continuous:* A reinforcement is given for every correct/target behavior.

    B. *Intermittent:* A reinforcement is not given for every correct/target behavior; instead behaviors are rewarded at certain intervals.

Shaping: A reinforcement is provided contingent on successive approximations toward a target behavior; for example, the clinician uses a series of reinforcements on different behavioral steps until the client's behavior at each step is consistent and, eventually, the target behavior is consistent as well.

The most common CD approaches are *drill* and *drill play.* Drill is considered the most highly structured format (Paul, in press; Roth & Worthington, 2005; Shriberg & Kwiatkowski, 1982). The clinician selects the training stimuli; explains the specific target response to the client; presents stimulus items in a predetermined order; and reinforces correct responses tangibly (e.g., with candy or a token), verbally (e.g., "Good job!"), or nonverbally (e.g., the client gets a high-five from the clinician). In drill play, the drill is embedded in a game format so that the client is motivated by the activity itself to produce the target forms as well as by the reinforcement that follows the production. For example, Darrell's clinician might have him play a game in which five paper bags are labeled with target words. He is given a sponge ball to toss into one of the bags (motivating activity), and then he must say the word on the bag. He is only reinforced for correct production. Reinforcement may be tangible or the chance to take another turn at the game.

CD approaches are thought to be most effective during the initial stages of intervention to establish a new target behavior. Once established, transitional activities can be introduced to provide the client with more naturalistic contexts in which to practice and use the new communicative behavior to achieve carry-over or **generalization**—the use of target behaviors outside the therapy situation without support from the clinician.

Client-Centered Approaches

CC approaches emphasize the provision of communication therapy in authentic settings. The assumption underlying these approaches is that individuals will achieve therapy goals more readily and generalize newly learned behaviors more spontaneously when taught in the context of familiar experiences and activities with supportive communication partners. In CC activities, the client directs the intervention and determines the content, timing, and sequence of therapy. The key steps in naturalistic, or CC, approaches involve *waiting* for the client to initiate a behavior, *interpreting* the behavior as communicative (whether communication was intended), and *responding* to the behavior in a way that places it in a communicative context (Fey, 1986). In contrast to CD approaches, the clinician does not attempt to elicit a predetermined set of responses from the client. Instead, the clinician follows the client's lead and offers consistent and meaningful responses that relate to the client's own actions or utterances. CC approaches are considered highly naturalistic because the client is engaged in enjoyable and meaningful daily activities with a responsive, communicative partner.

The most common CC activity used with children is **facilitative play.** This is an indirect stimulation technique (Owens, 2004; Paul, in press). The clinician arranges the physical environment to encourage the child to generate target responses spontaneously during the natural course of a play sequence. The clinician uses several techniques to promote the child's communicative participation. Examples of some techniques are listed in the following box.

FACILITATIVE PLAY TECHNIQUES

Self-talk: The clinician observes the child's behavior and engages in the same behavior while simultaneously engaging in an animated monologue that describes the clinician's ongoing actions. The monologue stays within the immediate attentional focus of the child.
Example: In the context of the child building a sandcastle at the play table, the clinician builds a sandcastle as well and says "I'm making a castle. A big castle. See how big it is?"

Parallel talk: The clinician produces an ongoing commentary on the child's actions. The commentary stays within the immediate attentional focus of the child.
Example: In the context of the child building a sandcastle at the play table, the clinician watches the child's actions and says, "You're building a castle. It's really big. Look how big your castle is."

Expansions: The clinician reformulates the child's utterances into more grammatically complete versions.
Example:
Child: "Kitty drink water."
Clinician: "Yes, the kitty is drinking the water."

Extensions or expatiations: The clinician enlarges on the child's utterances by adding new semantic information.
Example:
Child: "Kitty drinking water."
Clinician: "Yes, the kitty is very thirsty today."

Recasts: The clinician expands the child's utterances into a different sentence type.
Example:
Child: "Kitty drink water."
Clinician: "Is the kitty drinking water?"

CC intervention also can be used with adult clients. Two primary forms of naturalistic intervention are employed with adults: *functional therapy* and *conversational group therapy.* Functional therapy involves communicative activities of daily living, which the client practices with support and scaffolding from the clinician. Thomas, our fluency client, for example, may work on talking on the telephone with his clinician. The clinician may first conduct some structured activities to encourage easy onset. Thomas would then be asked to use easy onset in a role-playing activity with a telephone. In later phases of therapy, he would be asked to make real telephone calls, with prompts and cues from the clinician that would be systematically faded.

Conversational group therapy is often a form of treatment for adults with neurogenic disorders. Rather than (or in addition to) receiving individual, skill-focused therapy, group members engage in conversations with other clients and a clinician. As in all CC approaches, the clients determine the structure and topics of the conversation. They receive natural feedback on the relevance, intelligibility, and appropriateness of their turns from others in the group. The clinician takes advantage of a set of facilitative techniques, just as the young child's clinician does. These techniques were summarized by Ewing (1999) and are presented in the following box.

Hybrid Approaches

Hybrid approaches represent a midpoint between the two extremes of naturalness. Hybrid approaches use intervention activities that are highly natural, but the clinician maintains control over the therapy environment to maximize learning and generalization. There are three main characteristics of hybrid approaches:

1. Only one or a small set of goals are targeted for intervention.

2. The clinician selects therapy activities and materials, choosing those that promote the client's spontaneous use of the target behaviors.

3. The clinician produces utterance behaviors that are contingent to the client's communication but that also model and accentuate the target forms.

CONVERSATIONAL GROUP THERAPY TECHNIQUES

Attending: Letting participants know their messages are being received (e.g., "I heard Marlene say that she felt happy with that action.")

Facilitating questions: Encouraging participants to query each other (e.g., "Do you need to ask Thomas what he means?")

Negotiating goals: Providing tactful prompts that help participants decide what they want to accomplish, integrate new members, and renew goals (e.g., "Richard, our group has been working to decrease frustration in communication situations. Do you have any personal goals along those lines?")

Rewarding: Giving verbal praise to participants for their group interactions (e.g., "That's a very insightful thought, Marlene.")

Responding to feelings: Providing verbal or nonverbal reactions that show participants that their feelings are understood (e.g., "I can see that it really upsets Thomas to talk about his cancer.")

Focusing: Keeping the group discussion on track by reintroducing the target discussion topic, as needed (e.g., "We were talking about using the telephone, though. Has anyone else had trouble with that?")

Summarizing: Stating a rendition of what the session has covered and providing the next step toward the group's goal (e.g., "It sounds as if everyone has felt frustrated about using the telephone. Should we plan to talk about suggestions to help on this front next time?")

Gatekeeping: Balancing participation between members so that one or a few participants do not dominate the discussion (e.g., "Richard, do you have a thought about what Marlene said?")

Modeling: Using demonstrations to teach conversational skills by example (e.g., "When I feel that way, I sometimes say, 'Hold on! I've got a thought on that!'")

Mediating: Resolving conflicts and encouraging conflict resolution among participants (e.g., "Thomas and Richard have a difference of opinion here; does anyone see some middle ground?")

Acourding to Fey (1986), the five main types of hybrid instruction are

1. Focused stimulation

2. Milieu teaching

3. Script therapy

4. Interrupted behavior chain strategy

5. Conversational coaching

Focused Stimulation The clinician deliberately arranges the verbal and non-verbal environment to increase the likelihood that the client will spontaneously produce the target form. The clinician provides frequent models of the target behavior in meaningful and highly functional contexts to facilitate client success. Although a response is not required from the client, the environmental setup is conducive to the production of the target form. For example, the clinician can increase the salience of a target behavior by presenting it in sentence-final or stressed positions; to elicit the production of the copula *is*, the clinician may respond to the client utterance, "*She tall*" with "*She is*?" or "*Is she tall*?"

There are a variety of language strategies that can be used to accomplish focused stimulation, many of which are given in Crystal, Fletcher, and Garman (1976); Fey, Cleave, Long, and Hughes (1993); Fey, Long, and Finestack, (2003); Owens (2004); and Paul (in press). Some examples include

- *False assertions:* The clinician makes a statement to elicit the copula from the client (e.g, "That's not your hat!" "Yes, it is.").

- *Feigned misunderstandings:* The clinician pretends not to get the message sent by client (e.g., "You want me to 'top'?").

- *Forced choices:* The clinician makes a statement to elicit the negative form from the client (e.g., "You do like it or you don't like it?" "I don't like it").

- *Contingent query:* The clinician asks the client to clarify the message (e.g., "Want gween." "Which crayon do you want?").

- *Violating routines:* The clinician omits an expected action to elicit a response from the client (e.g., when greeting the client, the clinician calls him or her by the wrong name).

- *Withholding objects and turns:* The clinician neglects to provide an expected object to elicit a response from the client (e.g., when playing a card game, the clinician consistently "forgets" to deal the client a card).

Milieu Teaching   Milieu Teaching stresses the use of ongoing activities as the basis for intervention and incorporates the operant principles of imitation, modeling, and reinforcement into naturalistic settings. Incidental Teaching and the Mand-Model method are two specific milieu teaching techniques. The steps involved in the Incidental Teaching approach (Hart & Risley, 1975; Warren & Kaiser, 1986; Yoder & Warren, 2002) are outlined in the following box.

STEPS IN INCIDENTAL TEACHING

1. The clinician arranges the environment so that desired objects or items are visible to the client but out of reach (e.g., a toy, a newspaper).
2. The client initiates the interaction verbally or nonverbally (e.g., pointing to the desired item).
3. The clinician selects the target response to be evoked from the client (e.g., "I want the newspaper so I can read it.").
4. The clinician uses cues to obtain a more elaborated response. The first cue is focused attention, which involves physically approaching the client, making eye contact, or issuing an expectant look. If the client does not respond after a brief waiting period, the clinician then offers a second cue such as a general question (e.g., "What do you want?") If the client's response to the

question contains the target response, the clinician provides a confirmation that includes a model of the target form (e.g., "Yes, you want the newspaper so you can read it?").

5. If the question does not elicit the target response, the clinician issues a prompt in the form of a general request (e.g., "You need to tell me"), a request for partial imitation (e.g., "Say, 'I want the newspaper so . . .' "), or a request for complete imitation (e.g., "Say, 'I want the newspaper so I can read it' "). If the client does not generate the target response even after the prompts, the clinician gives one additional prompt.

6. If the client achieves the target behavior, the clinician provides confirmation that the communicative intent was achieved (e.g., the client is given the newspaper).

7. If the client does not produce the target response, the clinician gives the client the desired item and determines the type of cue that may be more effective for the next session.

The Mand-Model method (Rogers-Warren & Warren, 1980; Warren, 1991) is similar to Incidental Teaching with two exceptions. First, it does not require the client to initiate communication before teaching begins. Rather, the clinician observes the client carefully, and when the client displays interest in an object or some aspect of the environment, the clinician *mands* a response (e.g., "Tell me what you need."). Second, the goals are general (e.g., elicit two-word utterances, elicit well-formed sentences) rather than specific (e.g., elicit agent-object utterances, elicit conjoined sentences). If the client produces an appropriate response, the clinician presents verbal reinforcement and presents the desired item (e.g., "Great! You told me why you wanted the newspaper, and here it is."). If the client's response is inappropriate, the clinician offers prompts such as those used in Incidental Teaching.

Both of these milieu approaches extend the operant procedures of imitation, prompting, and reinforcement to naturalistic activities in which the client accomplishes authentic communication goals with the behaviors being trained. In addition, the reinforcement received is a natural outcome of the communication interaction.

Script Therapy   *Script therapy* is an approach in which target behaviors are taught within the context of a familiar routine or script (Olswang & Bain, 1991; Weismer & Evans, 2002). A script is an ordered sequence of events that depicts a familiar activity such as making dinner, going to a birthday party, or ordering a meal in a restaurant (Nelson, 1985). The clinician and client enact the script, during which the clinician can violate the sequence of activities (e.g., in the birthday party script, the clinician might eat the cake before blowing out the candles), providing a natural opportunity for the client to communicate verbally or gesturally. Other violations may include hiding props necessary for the script and introducing broken or incomplete materials (e.g., using unwrapped gifts in the birthday party script). Once a script is overlearned, the clinician can use it to introduce more complex forms. For example, the client can be told to pretend that the birthday party was yesterday or will be tomorrow to encourage the production of past and future tense markers. The clinician also can have the client pretend that the person who had the birthday received at least two copies of every gift to promote the use of plural tense forms.

Interrupted-Behavior Chain Strategy   *Interrupted-behavior chain strategy* (Caro & Snell, 1989) is a variation of script therapy which utilizes authentic contexts to introduce new intervention targets with structured instructional techniques. In this approach, a new behavior is inserted into an already established behavioral sequence. For instance, Marlene, the adult client with aphasia, may have mastered an instructional strategy for walking her dog, which includes getting the leash, collaring the dog, retrieving house keys, locking the front door, and walking the dog around the block. In the middle of this sequence, the clinician interrupts the behavior chain and asks Marlene to state the dog's name and the address of the dog's owner. If necessary, the clinician models the correct response, prompts Marlene to produce it, and reinforces her attempt.

Conversational Coaching   *Conversational coaching* was developed by Holland (1995) to facilitate functional communication skills of adults with aphasia. This technique simulates conversational interaction in a structured context. The clinician prepares a short written script based on the client's interests, experiences, and level of communication skills. According to Holland (1995), the scripts should be written in a communicative style, consist of short sentences to promote successful communication, and emphasize target communication behaviors. An example script followed by a summary of the recommended procedures is presented in the following box.

SAMPLE SCRIPT AND PROCEDURES
FOR CONVERSATIONAL COACHING

1. I have to change my hairdresser.
2. She always cuts my hair too short.
3. And I always have to wait.
4. This time she made my hair uneven.
5. I need to find someone else.

The client reads the script aloud one sentence at a time. Self-cuing strategies are suggested by the clinician when the client evidences difficulty expressing the scripted information. Common self-cuing strategies include chunking utterances into shorter units and using gestures to communicate meaning. The clinician videotapes the client reading the script to a familiar listener who is unaware of the script's contents. The listener is coached to glean the gist of the script, rather than trying to understand each word. The three participants then evaluate the videotape to determine the success level of the scripted interaction, the aspects that the listener found most and least helpful, and alternative strategies the client and the listener might have used to improve the interaction. The coaching and evaluation format is repeated with increasingly unfamiliar listeners, and new target behaviors are scripted into conversations.

USING THE CONTINUUM OF NATURALNESS

Research evidence supports the use of both naturalistic and structured intervention approaches with a broad range and severity of speech, language, and communication disorders for children (e.g., Conture, 1996; Geirut, 1998; Hemmeter, Ault, Collins & Meyer, 1996; Kim, Yang, & Hwang, 2001; Kouri, 2005; Swanson, Fey, Mills, & Hood, 2005; Yoder & Warren, 2001) and adults (Conture, 1996; Holland, Fromm, DeRuyter & Stein, 1996; Robey, 1998; Ramig & Verdolini, 1998). Some therapy goals are most effectively accomplished through naturalistic strategies although others are more amenable to highly structured clinician-directed approaches.

The degree of naturalness that we use in intervention must be determined by the nature and severity of a client's communication impairment and the client's responsiveness to different intervention strategies. Highly naturalistic activities are preferred only if they bring about improved communication abilities. Less naturalistic activities should be chosen only if they are more effective in eliciting a target behavior. For example, children with language impairments may have difficulty inducing linguistic rules from natural interactions and may require more focused and explicit language input.

The approaches that form the continuum are not mutually exclusive. A combination of strategies may be appropriate for a particular client. For example, one communicative objective may be accomplished most efficiently using a highly structured CD strategy, although another objective may be met more efficiently through naturally occurring activities. Often, programming for the same objective may make use of several activities that can range in naturalness from highly structured to highly natural. Fey (1986) reminded clinicians that only if two activities are equally effective in eliciting a particular linguistic structure or communicative function is the naturalistic one preferred, because it will more likely promote the use of the newly acquired target behavior in everyday speaking situations. Following are examples of intervention activities at various points along the continuum of naturalness for some of the children and adults we have been discussing.

Darrell: a Preschooler
with Unintelligible Speech

Target Behavior: Increase ability to produce three syllable words correctly

Drill: The clinician names a set of picture cards with three syllable words (e.g., tomato, banana). After each label, Darrell is cued to repeat the word. Each time all three syllables are produced, he receives a token. With 40 tokens, he can "buy" a turn throwing darts at a dart board.

Hybrid: The clinician and child play the game I Spy with a picture of fruits and vegetables that Darrell has practiced saying. Darrell chooses which one to name on his turn; the clinician points to the one he names.

Daily: The clinician and Darrell make a Thanksgiving collage together. The cutouts include many of the fruits and vegetables he has been practicing naming. As they work, the clinician names some of these, or asks Darrell to name them. The clinician praises Darrell when he names them correctly, in imitation, in response to the request to name, or spontaneously.

Jonah, a School-Aged Child
with Hearing Impairment

Target Behavior: Improve classroom listening skills using appropriate amplification

Drill: Jonah imitates the clinician's instructions (drawn from those typically used by his classroom teacher) and acts each instruction out as he imitates. The clinician reinforces correct actions.

Hybrid: The clinician and Jonah play "Army," taking turns being "Sarge." Sarge gives instructions (written on slips of paper, following teacher instructions, and drawn from an army hat). The partner must correctly follow the instruction.

Daily: The clinician works with Jonah in class during an instructional activity. Using prompts and cues, the clinician encourages him to write down the instructions, ask questions about what he does not understand, adjust his hearing aid if needed, and so forth.

Anna, a Seventh-Grader
with Learning Disability

Target behavior: Use of *because, if,* and *so* to produce cause/effect complex sentences

Drill: The clinician explains the use of conjunctions, such as *because, if,* and *so* to link ideas in sentences. The clinician presents simple sentences on cards, along with the conjunctions written on paper "hooks." Anna combines each pair with the given conjunction, following the clinician's model.

Hybrid: The clinician reads Anna a cause/effect selection from a classroom textbook. The clinician provides several models of retelling the passage, using sentences with the conjunctions practiced. Anna is then asked a question that she can answer with a similar conjoined sentence.

Daily: The clinician runs a study group with Anna and some other students who are struggling with a classroom textbook selection that discusses cause and effect. The students are encouraged to discuss the selection. The clinician occasionally models sentences using the target conjunctions within the context of the discussion.

Marlene, an Adult with Aphasia

Target behavior: Improve the use of the self-cuing strategy of sentence completion for retrieving verbal labels

Drill: The clinician presents a list of incomplete sentences, such as "We use a broom to sweep the _____," for Marlene to imitate and complete.

Hybrid: Clinician collects several identical pairs of cards depicting objects necessary to perform daily activities and demonstrates the sentence completion strategy for Marlene to imitate. After imitative practice of the strategy, Marlene, the clinician, and some other people play a card game. The clinician shuffles the deck and gives each player five cards. The clinician explains that the goal of this activity is to make pairs for all of the cards in the player's hand by taking turns asking one another, "Do you have a_____?"

Daily: Marlene selects three daily activities (e.g., brushing teeth, making coffee, watering the plants). Marlene and the clinician make a list of items necessary to perform each task. Marlene uses the sentence completion self-cuing strategy, "I need a _____" to request each item.

Richard, an Adult who Wants Esophageal Speech

Target Behavior: Increase the use of appropriate prosody

Drill: The clinician writes pairs of sentences that contain the same subject, verb, and object. Each sentence is written on a separate card with a different word underlined for emphasis (e.g., I want coffee; I want coffee). The clinician points to one card at a time and produces each sentence for Richard to imitate.

Hybrid: Using the same set of cards as above, the clinician places a pair of cards face up on the table and asks a question for Richard to answer using the prosodically appropriate sentence with exaggerated stress (e.g., Q: *Who* wants coffee?; A: *I* want coffee; Q: *What* do you want?; A: I want *coffee*).

Daily: Richard chooses reading passages from magazines or newspapers that interest him, or from which he wants to learn new information. The clinician highlights the words that receive primary stress. The client reads aloud each passage concentrating on emphasizing the appropriate words.

Thomas, an Adult who Has a Fluency Disorder

Target Behavior: Decrease stuttering moments and reduce anxiety associated with dysfluencies

Drill: The clinician reads a presented passage and engages in voluntary stuttering on predetermined words. Thomas imitates each of the voluntary stutters.

Hybrid: The clinician introduces a board game such as Jeopardy! and explains that Thomas is the contestant. After reviewing the technique of pull-outs (Van Riper, 1973), Thomas is instructed to use one or more pseudo or real dysfluencies in response to game questions and to modify stuttering moments using pull-outs.

Daily: Thomas's task is to enter a situation that previously has been identified as mildly fearful and use the pull-out technique. Example situations include: calling a family member on the telephone, making an appointment for a haircut, and asking for directions.

DATA COLLECTION

The collection of data on client performance has three primary purposes.

1. It permits the clinician to track the client's progress from one session to another.

2. It provides documentation of the efficacy of a particular intervention strategy or set of strategies.

3. It maximizes clinician effectiveness.

For naturalistic intervention approaches, videotaping is the data collection procedure of choice because it permits a permanent audio and visual record. Frequently, repeated viewing of an interaction/session is necessary to fully describe and analyze the client's verbal and nonverbal communicative behaviors. Videotaping may not be possible at all times and in all settings, though. Alternative data collection methods include the development of checklists, rating scales, graphs, audiotapes, and use of multiple observers, each focusing on a different behavioral component. Data recording forms can be developed for group as well as individual sessions.

The type of notation system used to chart data yields different kinds of information. A binary system records whether a behavior is correct/appropriate or incorrect/inappropriate. An interval rating scale gives more qualitative information because behaviors are rated on a continuum (e.g., degree of accuracy or appropriateness). It is also desirable to code whether the client's behavior is gestural, vocal, or verbal, or a combination thereof. In addition, data collection procedures should allow the clinician to distinguish between imitative, prompted, self-corrected, and spontaneous responses. Figures 6.2 and 6.3 present two examples of charts that can be used to track client behaviors. You may want to try coming up with your own to track the behaviors elicited in some of the examples we reviewed previously.

Name:	Behavioral objective:
Clinician:	Reinforcement type/schedule:
Date:	Materials:

Trials

Task	1	2	3	4	5	6	7	8	9	10	Percent correct

Figure 6.2. Example of a data log.

Client

Objective _____

										Number of responses					Number of correct responses						Percent correct			
1	2	3	4	5	6	7	8	9	10	11	12	13	14	15	16	17	18	19	20	21	22	23	24	25
26	27	28	29	30	31	32	33	34	35	36	37	38	39	40	41	42	43	44	45	46	47	48	49	50

Client

Objective _____

										Number of responses					Number of correct responses						Percent correct			
1	2	3	4	5	6	7	8	9	10	11	12	13	14	15	16	17	18	19	20	21	22	23	24	25
26	27	28	29	30	31	32	33	34	35	36	37	38	39	40	41	42	43	44	45	46	47	48	49	50

Client

Objective _____

										Number of responses					Number of correct responses						Percent correct			
1	2	3	4	5	6	7	8	9	10	11	12	13	14	15	16	17	18	19	20	21	22	23	24	25
26	27	28	29	30	31	32	33	34	35	36	37	38	39	40	41	42	43	44	45	46	47	48	49	50

Client

Objective _____

										Number of responses					Number of correct responses						Percent correct			
1	2	3	4	5	6	7	8	9	10	11	12	13	14	15	16	17	18	19	20	21	22	23	24	25
26	27	28	29	30	31	32	33	34	35	36	37	38	39	40	41	42	43	44	45	46	47	48	49	50

Figure 6.3. Sample group therapy data sheet.

CONCLUSION

The aim of all intervention is to improve communicative behavior. This means that even though clinicians structure therapy to achieve specific, measurable goals, the true objective is to increase clients' overall ability to use communication in authentic, functional settings. When clinicians assess the effectiveness of intervention, it is this larger goal that needs to be kept in mind. In addition, we need to remember that our job is to help clients communicate better, not to adopt a philosophy of therapy or join a "school" of intervention. We should, in other words, take advantage of ALL of the intervention approaches available to us and match each goal for each client to the most effective technique for that particular objective. Chances are, the appropriate technique will change over time. Although very structured CD intervention may work for some clients early in the course of intervention, the clients are likely to need more naturalistic approaches later. Other clients may require a naturalistic approach early on, while they are still becoming familiar with their clinicians, and may be more willing to tolerate structured formats later. Whatever activities or sequences clinicians decide to employ, the goal is always to maximize communicative effectiveness for the client. Part of the way clinicians do this is by being aware of the range of therapeutic options available and choosing the most appropriate for each situation. Another part is by carefully monitoring the efficacy of the intervention by collecting and analyzing data throughout the course of the therapy. Tracking client behaviors allows us to know when our intervention strategies have achieved their goals so that we can move on to other goals or even, if we are very fortunate, have clients "graduate" from intervention. Performance data also tell us when our strategies are not working and need to be changed to provide a better match to the client's needs. We need to be aware of the standards for EBP and continually update our knowledge of what research tells us about which intervention procedures meet these standards. Communication intervention, then, involves continual and thoughtful monitoring. That is why it takes a clinician, not a technician, to do it.

REFERENCES

Caro, P., & Snell, M. (1989). Characteristics of teaching communication to people with moderate and severe disabilities. *Education and Training in Mental Retardation, 24,* 63–77.

Conture, E.G. (1996). Treatment efficacy: Stuttering. *Journal of Speech and Hearing Research, 39,* 19–26.

Crystal, D., Fletcher, P., & Garman, M. (1976). *The grammatical analysis of language disability: A procedure for assessment and remediation.* London: Edward Arnold.

Dollaghan, C. (2004, April 13). Evidence-based practice: Myths and realities. *The ASHA Leader, 12,* 4–5.

Ewing, S. (1999). Group process, group dynamics, group techniques with neurogenic communication disorders. In R. Elman (Ed.) *Group treatment of neurogenic communication disorders* (pp. 9–17). Boston: Butterworth-Heineman.

Fey, M. (1986). *Language intervention with young children.* San Diego: College-Hill Press.

Fey, M., Cleave, P., Long, S., & Hughes, D. (1993). Two approaches to the facilitation of grammar in children with language impairment: An experimental evaluation. *Journal of Speech and Hearing Research, 36,* 141-157.

Fey, M., Long, S., & Finestack, L. (2003). Ten principles of grammar facilitation for children with specific language impairments. *American Journal of Speech-Language Pathology, 12,* 3–15.

Geirut, J. (1998). Treatment efficacy: Functional phonological disorders in children. *Journal of Speech, Language, and Hearing Research, 41,* 85–100.

Hart, B., & Risley, T. (1975). In vivo language intervention: Unanticipated general effects. *Journal of Applied Behavioral Analysis, 13,* 411–420.

Hemmeter, M., Ault, M., Collins, B., & Meyer, S. (1996). The effects of teacher-implemented language instruction within free time activities. *Education and Training in Mental Retardation and Developmental Disabilities, 31,* 203–212.

Holland, A. (1995, April). *Current realities of aphasia rehabilitation: Time constraints, documentation demands and functional outcomes.* Paper presented at Mid-America Rehabilitation Hospital, Voerland Park, KS.

Holland, A.L., Fromm, D.S., DeRuyter, F., & Stein, M. (1996). Treatment efficacy: Aphasia. *Journal of Speech and Hearing Research, 39,* 27–39.

Kim, Y., Yang, Y., & Hwang, B. (2001). Generalization effects of script-based intervention on language expression of preschool children with language disorders. *Education and Training in Mental Retardation and Developmental Disabilities, 36,* 411–23.

Kouri, T. (2005). Lexical training through modeling and elicitation procedures with late talkers who have specific language impairment and developmental delays. *Journal of Speech, Language, and Hearing Research, 48,* 157–172.

McLean, L. (1998). A language-communication intervention model. In D. Berstein & E. Tiegerman (Eds.). *Language and communication disorders in children* (pp. 208–228). Boston: Allyn & Bacon.

Nelson, K. (1985). *Making sense: The acquisition of shared meaning.* San Diego: Academic Press.

Olswang, L., & Bain, B. (1991). Intervention issues for toddlers with specific language impairments. *Topics in Language Disorders, 11,* 69-86.

Owens, R. (2004). *Language disorders: A functional approach to assessment and intervention* (4th ed.). Boston: Allyn & Bacon.

Paul, R. (in press). *Language disorders from infancy through adolescence: Assessment and intervention* (3rd ed.). St. Louis: Mosby.

Ramig, L.O., & Verdolini, K. (1998). Treatment efficacy: Voice disorders. *Journal of Speech, Language, and Hearing Research, 41,* 101–116.

Robey, R.R. (1998). A meta-analysis of clinical outcomes in the treatment of aphasia. *Journal of Speech, Language and Hearing Research, 41,* 172–187.

Rogers-Warren, A., & Warren, S. (1980). Mands for verbalization: Facilitating the generalization of newly trained language in children. *Behavior Modification, 4,* 230–245.

Roth, F.P., & Worthington, C.K. (2005). *Intervention resource manual for speech-language pathology* (3rd ed.). Clifton Park, NY: Thomson Delmar Learning.

Shriberg, L., & Kwiatkowski, J. (1982). Phonological disorders III: A conceptual framework for management. *Journal of Speech and Hearing Disorders, 47,* 242–256.

Skinner, B.F. (1957). *Verbal behavior.* New York: Appleton-Century-Crofts.

Swanson, L., Fey, M., Mills, C., & Hood, S. (2005). Use of narrative based language intervention with children who have specific language impairment. *American Journal of Speech-Language Pathology, 14,* 131–143.

Van Riper, C. (1973). *The treatment of stuttering.* Upper Saddle River, NJ: Prentice Hall.

Warren, S. (1991). Enhancing communication and language development with milieu teaching procedures. In E. Cipani (Ed.), *A guide to developing language competence in preschool children with severe and moderate handicaps* (pp. 68-93). Springfield, IL: Charles C. Thomas.

Warren, S.E., & Kaiser, A.P. (1986). Incidental language teaching: A critical review. *Journal of Speech and Hearing Disorders, 51,* 291–299.

Weismer, S., & Evans, J. (2002). The role of processing limitations in early identification of specific language impairment. *Topics in Language Disorders, 22,* 15–29.

Yoder, P.J., Kaiser, A.P., & Kaiser, C.L. (1991). An exploratory study of the interaction between language teaching methods and child characteristics. *Journal of Speech and Hearing Research, 34,* 155–167.

Yoder, P.J., & Warren, S. (2001). Relative treatment effects of two prelinguistic communication interventions on language development in toddlers with developmental delays vary by maternal characteristics. *Journal of Speech, Language and Hearing Research, 44,* 224–237.

Yoder, P.J. & Warren, S. (2002). Effects of prelinguistic milieu teaching and parent responsivity education on dyads involving children with intellectual disabilities. *Journal of Speech, language, and Hearing Research, 45,* 1158–1175.

STUDY QUESTIONS

1. What are the three basic purposes of intervention?

2. What are the three components of a behavioral objective?

3. Discuss the sequence of steps used to do a task analysis.

4. Describe three points along the continuum of naturalness of intervention activities.

5. Describe a drill activity to teach correct /s/ production to a 5-year-old client.

6. Describe three types of language used in facilitative play.

7. Name six steps involved in Incidental Teaching.

8. Create an activity for a client with aphasia, using a conversational coaching approach.

9. Compare and contrast two means of clinical data collection.

10. What is meant by hybrid intervention techniques?

CHAPTER 7

Evidence-Based Decision Making in Communication Intervention

MARC E. FEY AND LAURA M. JUSTICE

You are a speech-language pathologist (SLP) working in a public school when Pamela, the parent of one of your clients, comes to you demanding that her child, Adam, receive a new intervention that she has just read about. You have been working with Pamela and Adam for the previous 2 years to address a significant impairment of language. Pamela reports that she read about this intervention in a popular parenting magazine. The article provided data from the intervention developer showing the effectiveness of the new intervention for children such as Adam. The article also included several testimonials from parents regarding the extraordinary benefits of the intervention. Thus, from Pamela's perspective, the intervention is not only appropriate for Adam, but it also represents a cure for Adam's language impairment. You tell Pamela that you are unfamiliar with this new intervention but that you are willing to investigate its merits and the appropriateness of delivering it to Adam. Pamela agrees that you should investigate the intervention, but she indicates that she is not willing to negotiate on its appropriateness. She wants Adam to undergo the desired intervention, even though it is very costly because of the intensity it requires. She informs you that she will not authorize a new individualized education plan (IEP) that does not include the new intervention.

The above example is not intended to portray parents as the "bad guys" in cases in which clinicians must make difficult decisions regarding the provision of new or controversial speech and language interventions. Similar situations that do not involve parents arise all the time:

- What if a supervisor endorses a new technique and believes you and other SLPs should apply it to all clients with certain specific characteristics?

- What if you receive a handout detailing dramatic improvements as a function of a particular intervention at a booth at a professional conference?

- What if you attend a workshop by an international expert at a conference that details an "innovative" and "state-of-the-art" technique designed for clients like many on your caseload?

- What if you read about the results of a clinical trial in a prominent journal that shows a technique to work extremely well for some clients with a particular communicative impairment, albeit not all?

When considering scenarios such as these, it is important to ask: what conditions would prompt you to discontinue an intervention procedure you currently provide for a particular client or group of clients in favor of a new technique? As important, under what conditions would you *not* be willing to change your technique?

Answering questions such as these requires a level of clinical expertise that clinicians develop during graduate training and beyond. This expertise allows clinicians to make knowledgeable and conscientious choices when faced with critical decisions presented by experts, supervisors, clients, and caregivers. Expertise develops not only through clinical experience and theoretical understanding of communication development and disorders, but also through the accumulation of knowledge and understanding of a constantly evolving scientific literature relevant to clinical practice. The conscientious integration of clinical experience, theoretical knowledge, and knowledge of the scientific literature is termed evidence-based practice (EBP).

In this chapter, EBP is considered both for what it is and what it is not. Several methods are described to help SLPs begin taking steps toward the adoption of EBP as a critical aspect of their developing clinical expertise to influence intervention decisions. EBP is also a critical aspect of assessment decision making. For example, when using tests to determine whether a client exhibits a significant problem with language, selections should be based on research demonstrating both **test sensitivity** (i.e., the extent to which a test identifies individuals with real problems in the targeted area of communication) and **test specificity** (i.e., the extent to which a test correctly identifies individuals without real problems). The best test should result in the smallest possible number of **false positives** (i.e., errors in which clients are judged to have problems when they do not) and **false negatives** (i.e., errors in which clients are judged not have problems when they really do). Attention to the scientific literature for decision making in assessment is a crucial part of the assessment process to ensure accuracy in diagnoses and validity of ongoing intervention monitoring. Dollaghan (2004) provided an excellent discussion of the processes of EBP as applied to assessment.

This chapter focuses primarily on EBP as it applies to intervention decisions for clients for whom communication services have been deemed necessary. In it, six steps to follow when using EBP are described and illustrated using a case example.

What Is Evidence-Based Practice?

In many ways, EBP is what its name suggests; that is, it involves solving clinical problems by going to the published literature to find the best available scientific evidence to support the use or disuse of specific speech and language intervention approaches, intensities, procedures, activities, goal attack strategies, and so forth. Nonetheless, integration of evidence from the scientific literature is not as simple as it sounds, as not all evidence is created equal. Just like researchers, clinicians must know what types of studies provide the strongest (and weakest) evidence to support or reject a particular clinical approach. They must also be able to recognize examples of these stronger and weaker types of evidence when they find them in the literature.

It is important, however, to note that published studies are not the only form of evidence to be considered in EBP decisions. An evidence-based decision can only be made confidently when three types of evidence have been carefully considered (American Speech-Language-Hearing Association [ASHA], 2004, 2005; Porzsolt et al., 2003; Sackett, Straus, Richardson, Rosenberg, & Haynes, 2000):

- External evidence from published research

- Internal evidence from careful evaluation of client and family characteristics, their willingness to participate, and their preferences

- Internal evidence from examination of clinician preferences; professional competencies and values; and workplace values, policies, and culture

In short, EBP involves a careful process of decision making that specifies the types of evidence that warrant consideration and types of evidence that do not.

External Evidence in Evidence-Based Practice Decisions

In EBP, the clinical professional consults the available *external evidence* regarding the impact of specific intervention techniques and tools. Some evidence available in published research, however, should have little bearing on decision making, whereas other evidence should be wholly discounted. Dollaghan (2004) identified three propositions concerning how to approach external evidence for use in evidence-based decision making:

1. The opinions of expert authorities (including consensus groups) should be viewed with skepticism and even discounted when they contradict evidence from rigorous scientific research.

2. Not all research is a suitable basis for informing decisions made in clinical practice.

3. Clinicians must be meticulously judgmental about the quality of evidence used to inform clinical practices.

These propositions provide guidelines for considering how to tackle situations such as those posed at the beginning of this chapter.

External Evidence from Experts The first of Dollaghan's propositions notes that the opinions of expert authorities can and should be viewed with skepticism. This proposition makes it clear how to respond to the parent, supervisor, colleague, or designated expert who cites another expert, an authoritative textbook, or even a panel of experts as support for some new or existing approach. These authoritative viewpoints deserve consideration, but history shows that they are often wrong. A good example of this from speech-language pathology is a recommendation by Fey (1986) regarding how clinicians might teach early object words to children for the purpose of commenting, based on the principle of informativeness. According to the principle of informativeness, children are expected to be most likely to imitate and label the names for objects that are novel, or informative, in the context (Greenfield & Zukow, 1978; Leonard, Cole, & Steckol, 1979; Schwartz & Leonard, 1985; Snyder, 1978). In an application of this principle to language intervention, Fey suggested that clinicians might first engage the child in some repetitive activity, such as putting puzzle pieces into their slots. Then, when the child develops accurate expectations of what is coming next (e.g., another puzzle piece), the clinician could present an object or attribute that is new and unexpected (i.e., informative) in the context (e.g., a cup), and say its name. According to Fey, this approach could be used to accelerate object-word learning in young children. (Greenfield & Zukow, 1978; Leonard, Cole, & Steckol, 1979; Schwartz & Leonard, 1985; Snyder, 1978).

Fey's (1986) suggestion, presented in an authoritative textbook, might have seemed useful for evidence-based decision making, but unfortunately, the merits of the suggestion, as described, did not hold up when the procedure was subjected to rigorous empirical testing. When Sorensen and Fey (1992) tested the approach, they found no evidence that it helped children learn words more quickly than another approach that paired the object name with a redundant, and therefore noninformative object. In fact, the informativeness approach failed as a word-teaching procedure possibly because, when the activities were performed repeatedly (as was called for in the approach), the children learned to expect the unexpected. This effectively rendered objects redundant and noninformative when they were presented in contexts designed to make them novel and informative.

The principle of informativeness may still be generally valid and highly useful in language intervention. Clinical implementation of the principle, however, is complex and introduces many factors not present in the experiments and assessment protocols in which it has been used so successfully. And this is the point of the first proposition. Until suggestions proposed by expert authorities are tested clinically under rigorous conditions, clinicians cannot know what effects an expert's recommendation can be expected to have on a client's learning and use of language. Consequently, it is preferable to have direct evidence of the effects of a new intervention instead of an expert's opinion that the new intervention should have desirable effects. Thus, when confronted with expert opinion, clinicians should seek further substantiation of these opinions from more rigorous and preferably experimental evidence, should it be available. If rigorously tested evidence is not available, then such opinions should be greeted with healthy skepticism.

External Evidence from Basic Research   The second of Dollaghan's propositions states that not all research is relevant to decisions about clinical practice. Research is of essentially two varieties: basic and applied (Stokes, 1997). **Basic research** attempts to further knowledge of fundamental processes, and, in the field of clinical communication, it is vital for furthering the understanding of how children develop speech and language. **Applied research** is designed to address specific societal needs, and, in the field of communication disorders, it addresses the needs concerning the impact of various intervention approaches. The latter type of research is particularly relevant to informing EBP, whereas evidence from basic research is less relevant. This is not to say that basic research does not have value; on the contrary, discoveries from basic research often lead to important clinical hypotheses. Clinicians knowledgeable of relevant basic science are likely to have a better understanding of the theoretical principles upon which their interventions are based than do clinicians who have not read the basic literature. With such an understanding, these clinicians are likely to be highly creative and principled when making decisions when evidence from high level, high quality clinical trials is not available. Conversely, EBP practitioners realize that clinical conclusions stemming from basic research are tentative and often incorrect and that clinical practice is best informed by applied research designed to test specific interventions, including their processes and their impacts. Consider an example.

Suppose that a clinician and members of her clinical staff are looking for new ways to teach young children to use object labels in acts of commenting that lead to frequent and consistent spontaneous use in meaningful contexts. A colleague suggests that the clinician try a new approach to teaching object labels that features repetition through picture cards. The clinician points out correctly that the evidence base supplied for the new approach (i.e., the opinions and limited clinical experiences of an expert) is weak and that alternative sources of evidence should be sought. She then counters with evidence from basic research investigations that supports the use of the informativeness technique, as recommended by Fey (1986). In fact, there is considerable support from studies of typical and impaired language development on the principle of informativeness (Greenfield & Zukow, 1978; Leonard, Cole, & Steckol, 1979; Schwartz & Leonard, 1985; Snyder, 1978). Nonetheless, the only experimental examination of informativeness as an intervention principle that is available is the study of Sorensen and Fey (1992), which failed to support the Fey (1986) recommendation. The clinician who advocates for the informativeness approach may still be in a stronger position than her colleague, who supports the new picture technique. This is because the informativeness technique is advocated on the grounds of underlying theory and projections from basic research and the picture card procedure is recommended on the basis of the opinion of an expert. The clinician, however, must realize the tenuous foundation of her argument, unless she can augment the evidence from basic research with other forms of clinical evidence.

Level and Quality of External Evidence   The third of Dollaghan's propositions makes clear that it is the responsibility of the EBP clinician not just to look for external evidence relevant to clinical decisions but also to evaluate and question the level and quality of that evidence. This proposition contends that clinicians must be knowledgeable concerning what constitutes high-level evidence. For example, consider the example of Pamela and Adam from the beginning of the chapter. Suppose that there are two studies reported in the literature indicating that, although the intervention cannot be viewed as a cure for language impairment, it does appear to lead to positive outcomes. One of the studies is a case study of a single child whereas the other is a pretest-posttest research design with no control group. As a knowledgeable clinician, you note to Pamela that, as encouraging as these reports are, the level of evidence they provide must be viewed as weak. Both case studies and pretest-posttest designs that lack a control group show little certainty of the findings, as they do not control for effects of maturation, spontaneous recovery, and other factors unrelated to the intervention. Consequently, even if these types of studies are executed with rigorous attention to measurement and implementation fidelity, they constitute very weak evidence of a cause-effect relationship between the intervention and the observed outcomes. In short, they provide an inadequate rationale for the costly approach demanded by Pamela.

There is an important conundrum in this case, however, in which Pamela asks, "What evidence do *you* have to support continuation of the approach you are now providing to my child?" This is a valid question expressing an important point, and it should always be anticipated by practitioners. EBP requires not only rigorous evaluation of new approaches; it also requires careful self-evaluation of existing approaches that many consider to reflect best practice. In situations such as Pamela's case, you would need to know whether there is equally strong or stronger research evidence supporting your own current methods over the approach advocated by Pamela. In addition, you would need to consider other sources of evidence to determine whether Pamela's desired approach has sufficient merit to warrant a change in programs.

Limitations of the External Evidence SLPs who accept Dollaghan's (2004) three propositions have adopted an EBP attitude or perspective that will serve them well. This is true even if at present these SLPs are unable to search for and find strong evidence to support all of their intervention decisions, which will often be the case. SLPs who have a healthy skepticism toward their own clinical practices recognize that the successes that they observe often are due to factors outside their control rather than due to their clinical procedures. Consequently, they keep careful records about the clients they treat, the intervention options they exercise, and the outcomes they observe. They seek and evaluate external evidence from the research literature that can help them to be more certain about the potential effectiveness of their clinical practices. They question the authors of the articles they read and the experts whose presentations they attend to determine the amount and quality of evidence underlying these individuals' recommendations. They are honest and explicit about the evidentiary bases for their practices when they discuss clinical options with caregivers and other professionals. Finally, they adopt or reject new approaches based on their integration of the best available scientific and clinical evidence following their critical examinations of their own experiences and of the available external evidence.

A concern of many practitioners is that EBP will make them slaves to external research evidence, forcing them to follow certain paths when their experience and expertise and their evaluation of internal evidence, such as particular child and family circumstances, dictate otherwise. Although the risk of this abuse of EBP is real, it is important to note that even the most ardent evidence-based practitioners in medicine recognize the importance of the client and family's values, preferences, and willingness to participate when making evidence-based decisions (e.g., Sackett et al., 2000). Evidence-based practitioners also recognize that the clinician's expertise, experience, and preferences must be taken into consideration.

Internal Evidence Regarding the Child and Family in Evidence-Based Practice Decisions

Any intervention decision that is based on evidence must be based minimally on the client's speech and language status as well as any other characteristics that might influence the response to intervention, such as social, attentional, cognitive, and educational performance. Thus, in any application of EBP to clinical decisions, the clinician must ask, "Does the available research evidence even apply to this particular client?" The clinician answers this question first by examining whether the target client and family resembles the populations sampled in the studies from which support for intervention is based. If the answer to this question is "No," the support for the use of the target approach is weakened on the basis of internal evidence, and the approach may not be applicable. For example, the results from a set of studies demonstrating the efficacy of an intervention approach that improves the language comprehension of adults with aphasia may not be relevant for a clinician working with an adult with dementia and a progressive hearing loss. Similarly, a single good study demonstrating the efficacy of a parent-administered intervention may not be useful to a clinician working with a family in which the caregivers have indicated an unwillingness or inability to deliver the intervention to their child.

In considering the internal evidence regarding a client and the client's family, the clinician also must consider the following questions: What do the client and family see as the client's greatest needs? Are the client's and family's goals consistent with those targeted in the published studies? Are the attitudes of the client and family consistent with the target intervention when considering 1) the level and type of family involvement, 2) the nature of the communication problem, or 3) the intervention intensity and approaches?

EBP clinicians must be cognizant of the potential mismatch between a research-supported approach and the client's and family's values or willingness to participate in the approach (e.g., van Kleeck, 1994). There are four possible implications of a mismatch. First, clinicians can apply the target intervention approach in spite of their awareness of the dissonance between the intervention and family values. Clinicians who neglect client and family desires in this way, however, are likely following a path of greatest resistance. Implementation of and success with the new approach in these cases will likely be limited, even if the evidence in support of the target intervention approach is very strong. Such neglect is not consistent with EBP principles and, therefore, is not recommended.

Second, clinicians can adopt some alternative intervention approach judged to be more consonant with the client's and family's perspectives. This option may often be reasonable and justifiable, even when there is strong research evidence in support of the target intervention approach. This option is strongest, however, when there is similarly strong research evidence supporting the alternative intervention approach. Clinicians can strengthen this decision if they have a documented record of success in administering the alternative intervention approach to other clients.

Third, clinicians can attempt to modify the target intervention approach to reduce the mismatch. Of course, when clinicians modify approaches that have demonstrated efficacy, they could be altering the very components responsible for the effects observed in the published studies. Consequently, clinicians will need to carefully document intervention outcomes, even when the modified intervention approach has a strong foundation in experimental evidence.

Fourth, clinicians can attempt to modify the client's or family's attitude so that a research-supported approach not consonant with that attitude can be implemented. Some clients and families may be willing to cooperate with and even participate in programs that conflict somewhat with their individual values and cultural perspectives. This is especially true if clinicians objectively and unemotionally present evidence that the target intervention approach is the one most likely to bring about the greatest change in the client's performance over the shortest period of time. When clinicians choose to try to modify the family's attitude, however, they must be extremely careful to respect the family's perspectives.

Internal Evidence Regarding the Clinician and School in Evidence-Based Practice Decisions

Internal evidence can also be derived from a clinician's expertise and experience, or clinical craft, as well as from the resources and culture present in the clinician's work environment. This evidence must be weighed carefully in any valid EBP decisions. When considering their own expertise and experience, the most important questions that clinicians must ask are

- What intervention approach would you normally apply in a case *without* the assistance of external research-based evidence?

- Why would you use this approach?

- What level of success have you had with this approach?

- Did you document your results when you applied this approach in other, similar cases?

Consideration of these questions early in the decision-making process can help clinicians better understand their own clinical biases as well as the foundations of those biases. In some cases, for example, a bias may be based on a long history of success that has been well documented in a clinician's records. In these cases, this internal evidence might well outweigh available external evidence for an alternative approach provided in one or more well-implemented clinical trials. Such a decision would be consistent with EBP as long as the clinician has sought out the appropriate external evidence and carefully and fairly weighed it against existing internal evidence. In other cases, a clinician might recognize that his or her standard care is based primarily on the opinions of past instructors and clinical supervisors and from his or her uncontrolled case reports, which are weak forms of evidence for supporting decision making. The clinician should consider changing his or her clinical practice if new evidence from strong clinical trials supporting a new approach is discovered.

A SIX-STEP APPROACH TO INTERVENTION DECISIONS USING EVIDENCE-BASED PRACTICE

Although much has been written recently about EBP in speech-language pathology (ASHA, 2004, 2005; Justice & Fey, 2004), most of the literature on this topic has described the process in broad strokes, focusing primarily on what EBP is and providing rationales for its adoption. Relatively little has been written about what EBP practitioners actually should do. A general six-step model of EBP decision making is provided in this section (see Table 7.1) and illustrated with a case example.

Table 7.1. Six steps crucial to every evidence-based practice decision about intervention

1. Develop a four-part clinical question that explicitly focuses on PICO (i.e., P = the *patient, patient group,* or *problem;* I = *intervention* being considered; C = *comparison* treatment; O = desired *outcome*).

2. Find the internal evidence and answer the question based solely on this evidence, to include 1) attention to client-family values, desires, and circumstances; and 2) the clinician's knowledge of the condition, the clinician's knowledge of the client, the clinician's clinical experience, the clinician's theoretical knowledge, and the institution's attitudes regarding the need for change.

3. Find the external or published research evidence.

4. Critically evaluate the external evidence.

5. Integrate the internal and external evidence.

6. Apply and evaluate the outcome of the decision.

Source: Porszolt et al., 2003.

A Case Example Illustrating Six Steps to Follow when Using EBP

Aaron, who is 5 years and 9 months old, is a kindergartener being evaluated by an EBP clinician, Phyllis. Aaron's kindergarten teacher referred Aaron to Phyllis because his language, social, and prereading skills are not as well developed as those of his peers. Classroom and therapy room evaluations reveal that Aaron rarely communicates with his peers but that he converses with his mother and Phyllis during playtime and shared-storybook reading. In the classroom, Phyllis observes that Aaron uses a lot of pantomime to repair communication breakdowns.

Aaron receives a standard score of 87 on the Peabody Picture Vocabulary Test-3 (Dunn & Dunn, 1997) and a listening quotient of 80 on the Test of Language Development-Primary-3 (Newcomer & Hammill, 1997). His mean length of utterance (MLU) in the richest sample, which was obtained when he was playing with his mother, is 2.5. A developmental sentence analysis reveals a developmental sentence score (Lee, 1975) well below the 10th percentile for his age. Language sample analysis shows that Aaron's sentences are simple (i.e., one verb) and often incomplete (e.g., omission of subject, verb, or object), and they typically omit grammatical functors (e.g., articles, auxiliary verbs, bound morphemes), especially those associated with verbs. Aaron's speech is particularly hard for adults to understand, but some of his peers in the classroom seem to follow his messages, especially when they are accompanied by pantomime. According to his teacher, however, none of his peers interact consistently with Aaron during play or work-times in the classroom.

Based on these results, Phyllis decides to initiate a program of speech and language intervention for Aaron. She selects the basic goals of enhancing Aaron's expressive grammar and his expressive phonology (intelligibility) but does not know which of the two goals to prioritize. Phyllis asks herself, "Do I focus intervention on both areas the whole time, as I usually do in such cases? Or, should I focus solely on grammar, to achieve greater changes in this domain but possibly influencing phonology indirectly? Alternatively, what if I placed my full attention on the intelligibility issue? What would happen to Aaron's grammar? Are there other alternatives I'm not considering?" These are questions often asked by clinicians working with children who simultaneously exhibit significant impairments of both speech sound production and language. This is the type of clinical problem that is tractable using EBP procedures.

Although Phyllis has an extremely limited time to search for the necessary literature, she decides to follow the six-step EBP decision-making process.

Step 1: Develop a Four-Part Clinical Question

Evidence-based practitioners uniformly agree that the first step in making an EBP decision is careful delineation of a clinical question. The system for developing an appropriate question follows the acronym, **PICO** (Centre for Evidence-Based Medicine, 2001a, 2001b; Sackett et al., 2000; see also Table 7.1). In this acronym, **P** represents Patient, Patient group, or Problem, **I** represents the Intervention being considered, **C** represents the comparison intervention (such as the current practice or no treatment), and **O** represents the desired Outcome. In Aaron's case, Phyllis follows the PICO acronym to formulate this question: "Would a 5-year-old kindergartner with primarily expressive specific language impairment affecting grammar and speech (P) show improvement with an intervention that targets both phonology and grammar simultaneously (I) or one that targets phonology and grammar through sequential blocks (C) e.g., a block of phonology followed by a block of grammar), as shown by improvements in grammar and phonology in spontaneous production probes and/or conversational contexts (O)?"

Step 2: Find the Internal Evidence and Answer the Clinical Question Based Solely on this Evidence

In most EBP decision-making schemes, the step following the identification of the question is a search for external research evidence. Porzsolt and colleagues (2003), however, suggested that the insertion of another step prior to examining the external research seemed to help clinicians to better understand the effect of their efforts to identify relevant external research. In this step, the clinician examines the internal evidence to determine what would be his or her typical intervention approach based solely on that evidence without examining the latest research. In effect, the clinician develops his or her own non-EBP solution as the target intervention for the clinical question.

In the example of Aaron, it is useful to consider two possible child-family and clinician-school scenarios and the ways they could affect Aaron's response to intervention. In the first scenario, Aaron is alert and cooperative and transitions easily from one task to another. His parents show a clear understanding of Aaron's speech and language difficulties and their potential effect on his educational performance. They also understand the various options for goal attack strategies (e.g., targeting grammar and phonology simultaneously, alternating targets in blocks), and they have indicated in the Planning and Placement Team (PPT) meeting that they would endorse any approach that shows a clear recognition of Aaron's needs in both grammar and phonology. Phyllis has been uncomfortable with the lack of across-domain progress by children she has treated for problems in both phonology and grammar. In general, she feels that her approach has been inconsistent. She has never felt comfortable targeting phonology or grammar alone, expecting spontaneous generalization to the other area. On the other hand, she is concerned that focusing on both areas simultaneously dilutes the effects of her efforts on each specific domain. In Aaron's case, she decides to target both domains simultaneously because of the parents' interest in addressing both grammar and phonology and because she does have experience with this approach. Her approach targets speech sounds that are difficult for Aaron but that are also important for marking morphosyntactic forms, such as those for plurals; possessives; subject-verb agreement; regular verb tense, such as [s] and [z]; and final word clusters, such as [kt] (e.g., *walked*) and [st] (e.g., *passed*).

In the second scenario, although Aaron is cooperative, he is easily distracted. His teacher reports that he does not change smoothly from one task to the next. His parents do not seem to understand the part of Aaron's problems related to language, and they emphasize that their greatest concern is his speech intelligibility. Furthermore, Phyllis is relatively comfortable with intervention for children with concomitant problems in grammar and phonology. When working with previous clients, Phyllis typically has first targeted the child's intelligibility problem and then has moved on to grammatical problems, if necessary, as the child becomes easier to understand. Phyllis has records from numerous previous clients to document the positive outcomes in grammar and phonology experienced with this sequential blocking of phonology followed by grammar. Consequently, this is the approach she plans for Aaron.

Step 3: Find the External Research Evidence

If Phyllis was practicing from an EBP perspective, she would have to admit that the decision-making processes exemplified in the two scenarios is not evidence-based. To make it evidence-based, she should be prepared to examine the existing evidence to help resolve the clinical question of what intervention approach would be best for Aaron. In medicine, clinicians might search for studies relevant to their PICO-based questions in specialized databases, which are highly accessible. Furthermore, clinicians might find one or more systematic reviews or meta-analyses of studies (primarily randomized controlled trials) related to their clinical questions via Internet-based database projects, such as the Cochrane Collaboration's health care database (http://www.cochrane.org); the Campbell Collaboration's database in social, behavioral, and educational domains (http://www.campbellcollaboration.org); or the What Works Clearinghouse, which focuses on practices in education (http://www.whatworks.ed.gov). These databases also provide critical appraisals (i.e., study reports) of individual clinical trials that enable clinicians to quickly and efficiently ascertain the results and validity of a particular study. In some areas of health care, clinical practice guidelines based on systematic reviews and meta-analyses are available. The Scottish Intercollegiate Guidelines Network (http://www.sign.ac.uk/guidelines) exists primarily to produce such guidelines for clinicians. In these cases, a panel of experts would already have systematically reviewed the experimental literature, made recommendations concerning the clinical problem, and graded those recommendations to specify the level of confidence clinicians might have in putting them into practice.

Unfortunately, the database of studies that evaluate intervention objectively is not nearly as large in speech-language pathology as it is in medicine, nor is it as well organized. The Academy of Neurologic Communication Disorders and Stroke has a project with the goals of producing intervention and diagnostic guidelines and delineating research needs (http://www.ancds.org/practice.html). Several guidelines have been produced and are available for use by EBP clinicians working with adults with neurogenic speech, language, and cognitive disorders. This work illustrates how much progress can be made, but it also shows how far the field of speech-language pathology has to go in developing guidelines for clinicians working with a range of disorders and age groups, if EBP is to become standard clinical practice.

Given this state of affairs, it is reasonable for you to ask, "What can clinicians do now to make use of external evidence as they implement EBP principles to their clients' benefit?" Some of the reasonable answers to this question can be illustrated by returning to the hypothetical case of Phyllis and Aaron and by assuming that Phyllis is interested in making an evidence-based decision.

Phyllis decides to begin her search at Highwire Press (http://highwire.org), which hosts 71 of the 200 most frequently cited journals, including all ASHA journals. Highwire Press not only provides a large repository of articles for Phyllis's search; it also provides free access to articles in all ASHA journals archived back to 1980 for ASHA members and for individuals at subscribing institutions.

Phyllis uses the Highwire Press's search capability to locate articles containing three relevant key words: *phonology, grammar,* and *intervention.* The first 40 results of this search provide a number of encouraging possibilities. After Phyllis reads the titles and brief summaries of these articles, she finds that seven articles seem most pertinent to her question. She reads the abstracts of these articles to determine which are most likely to be useful. Based on the information provided in the abstracts on the participants' ages, problems, the types of intervention provided, and the type of research design used, the following four articles appear highly relevant to Phyllis' clinical question:

1. Tyler and colleagues (2003): "Outcomes of Different Speech and Language Goal Attack Strategies"

2. Tyler and colleagues (2002): "Efficacy and Cross-Domain Effects of a Morphosyntax and a Phonology Intervention"

3. Fey and colleagues (1994): "Effects of Grammar Facilitation on the Phonological Performance of Children with Speech and Language Impairments"

4. Tyler and Sandoval (1994): "Preschoolers with Phonological and Language Disorders: Treating Different Linguistic Domains"

Because she is pressed for time, Phyllis decides to focus on the one article most relevant to her clinical problem, at least at first. She reasons that the most recent of the short-listed articles will yield the most information, partly from the study it reports but also from the literature review that will be included. Thus, she decides to seek information relevant to the clinical question by critically evaluating Tyler and colleagues' article from 2003.

It is important to note that Phyllis's EBP approach is far from ideal. Her review of the external evidence would examine only a single database. A much broader literature needs to be searched. In addition, Phyllis's plan to read and evaluate a single article may be questioned. Ultimately, she should examine all of the experimental literature that is available and relevant to the clinical question. This may only be practical, however, when groups of clinicians focus on common problems and work together. This is not always possible, though, and it can be assumed that this is not possible in Phyllis's present situation. Phyllis realizes that her literature review and critical appraisal will be incomplete. Despite this fact, her review of the external evidence in this example reflects an important first step in integrating external evidence into clinical decisions.

Step 4: Critically Appraise the External Evidence

Any research publication identified as a potential candidate for addressing PICO-inspired questions must be carefully evaluated. This evaluation, or critical appraisal of the topic (CAT; Sackett et al., 2000), grades the article for 1) its relevance to the clinical question; 2) the level of evidence provided by the study in the article based on the study's design and quality; and 3) the direction, strength, and consistency of the study's observed outcomes.

Tyler and colleagues' (2003) article, which Phyllis chose, describes a study in which 47 children participated. The children's ages ranged from 3-0 to 5-11, and they had concomitant speech and language impairment. Forty children were randomly assigned to one of four intervention groups. These children all received a 30-minute individual session and a 45-minute group session every week for 24 weeks. The same approach to speech-language intervention was used in all intervention groups, but the sequencing of intervention targets varied. The first group, which targeted phonology first, received 12 weeks of phonological intervention followed by 12 weeks of morphosyntactic intervention. The second group, which targeted morphosyntax first, received 12 weeks of morphosyntactic intervention followed by 12 weeks of phonological intervention. The third group received alternating cycles of 1 week of phonological intervention and 1 week of morphosyntactic intervention for 24 weeks. The fourth group received intervention that simultaneously addressed both phonology and morphosyntax for 24 weeks. The children's phonological and morphosyntactic gains were measured using percentage consonants correct on the Bankson-Bernthal Test of Phonology (1990) and percentage correct use of a small set of verb morphemes used to mark tense and agreement as measured from a spontaneous language sample.

Relevance to the Clinical Question Critical appraisal of external evidence begins by examining the relevance of the study to the clinical question. Clinicians determine the relevance by examining the study for its description of the individuals who participated, its intervention methods, and its outcome measures. A study found irrelevant for a particular problem or a particular case might not be further considered at all. Clinicians also consider whether the intervention is feasible to implement in a particular setting or with a particular client. For instance, an intervention might not be feasible if it involves a computer program that is not yet commercially available.

Table 7.2 presents specific questions that can be used for determining relevance of a study, and it provides answers to these questions as they relate to Aaron and the Tyler and colleagues (2003) article. The sample of participants in the study appears to include children such as Aaron in age and speech-language profile, although the article provided little information regarding additional features that could potentially influence intervention outcomes. For example, Phyllis would not know if any of the children in the study had attentional or transitional problems as Aaron has in the second scenario. Likewise, the article provides no information on the family characteristics of the children, such as

Table 7.2. Some questions addressing the relevance of clinical questions raised for Aaron (answers apply to the study by Tyler et al., 2003)

	Yes	Unclear	No
Are the participants clearly described and does the sample include patients like the target client?	X	X*	
Is the intervention sufficiently well described that it could be put into practice?	X		
Is the intervention feasible for your practice and client?	X		
Are the outcome measures valid and reliable indicators of clinical significance?	X		

*The clinician in Scenario 1 rated this question as "Yes," but the clinician in Scenario 2 rated this question as "Unclear." In Scenario 2, Aaron was distractible and had difficulty moving to new tasks. The description of the participants in the research report provides no information on participants' attention and ability to transition from one task to another.

parental education and socioeconomic status. In other respects, the study is clearly relevant to Aaron's case, particularly the speech-language characteristics of the sample participants. Also, the intervention approach is well described, especially for a research report; the intensity and structure of the interventions seem feasible for use in Phyllis's school system; and the outcome measures appear valid, reliable, and clinically meaningful. Thus, with some reservations, Phyllis regards the study as relevant to the clinical question in both scenarios.

Level of Evidence Represented by the Study Design and Quality   Critical appraisal of the external evidence involves not only establishing the relevance of professional literature to a particular population or problem, but also judging the level of the evidence, as determined by the study design and the methodological rigor employed. Although there are numerous ranking systems available, the one developed by the Oxford Centre for Evidence-Based Medicine (CEBM) (http://www.cebm.net/levels_of_evidence.asp) is perhaps most frequently used or adapted. Table 7.3 provides an adaptation of this system, which shows how different forms of evidence (e.g., systematic review, randomized controlled trial, expert opinion) are ranked for the level of evidence provided. There are four levels of evidence: 1, 2, 3, and 4, ranging from highest to lowest with several further sublevels.

Categorization of a study involves consideration of three critical features: research design (e.g., case study, clinical trial), methodological quality, and the consistency or strength of observed effects.

Research Design   Each research study is designed in a particular way to answer a specific question or set of questions. For example, a study that determines the validity of a measure of speech intelligibility in children is designed very differently than a study that determines the effects of a parent-implemented speech intervention for preschool children. In evidence-based decision making, the strongest evidence on which an intervention decision can be based is derived from studies featuring **experimental designs.** In true experimental designs, the researcher assigns participants randomly to two or more treatment groups and places rigorous control on all known additional variables that might affect a **dependent variable.** With other variables controlled, the direct influence of the intervention (the **independent variable**) on a particular outcome (the dependent variable) can be assessed.

Experimental designs that involve groups of participants to estimate the relationship between a clinical intervention and an outcome are called **randomized clinical trials (RCTs)**. In an RCT, the researcher assigns participants randomly to two or more groups. Each group then receives a systematic intervention (or, in some cases, no intervention), and the outcomes for each group are compared. In an RCT, all groups are treated identically with the exception of the intervention variable(s) being tested. Because participants are randomly assigned to groups, any differences between groups at the outset of the study are unlikely to be systematic and do not reflect the biases of the researcher. Thus, when one group outperforms another over the course of the intervention, a causal inference connecting the outcome with the intervention is appropriate. High-quality RCTs provide clinicians with the highest level of evidence available from a single study (Level 1b; see Table 7.3). Level 1b evidence is superseded only by the outcomes of systematic reviews that aggregate the findings from two or more RCTs (Level 1a; see Table 7.3).

Other research designs are also pertinent to evidence-based decision making. These designs include quasi-experimental designs, single-subject designs, and case studies. Although **quasi-experimental studies** attempt to estimate the relationship between independent and dependent variables, these designs are not truly experimental because the researcher does not randomly assign participants to different intervention groups. For example, control groups may be formed out of convenience (e.g., participants could not attend all of the intervention sessions), or a new intervention may be compared with one tried in the past, using the performance of some previous group as a historical control. Many of these designs are logically similar to RCTs, but because participants are not assigned to groups at random, there are more opportunities for selection bias to influence the outcomes. Conclusions from quasi-experimental studies about the effects of intervention are generally assumed to be riskier than are conclusions drawn from an RCT. Therefore, the results of even high quality quasi-experimental studies constitute weaker levels of evidence (Level 2b; see Table 7.3) than do those of high quality RCTs.

Single-subject experimental designs are also informative to EBP. Unlike the typical RCT when the researcher focuses on inferences about group performance, single-subject experiments provide a great deal of specific information about the individual participants. These designs are experimental because the researchers systematically manipulate variables so that a relationship between

Table 7.3. Levels of evidence adapted from the system of the Oxford Centre for Evidence-Based Medicine

Level	Type(s) of evidence
1a	A systematic review of randomized controlled trials with consistent study outcomes
1b	A well-conducted single randomized controlled trial (RCT) with a narrow confidence interval
2a	A systematic review of non-randomized quasi-experimental trials or a systematic review of single-subject experiments that document consistent study outcomes
2b	A high-quality quasi-experimental trial or a lower-quality RCT or a single-subject experiment with consistent outcomes across replications
3	A case series or a poor-quality quasi-experimental study
4	An expert opinion that originated without ongoing critical appraisal or based on theoretical knowledge or basic research

Source: Phillips et al., 2001, May.

the intervention and the outcome can be inferred. Single-subject designs have an advantage over group experimental designs in that they allow in-depth monitoring of how individuals respond to interventions over time. Thus, in these designs, causal inferences about the intervention may be applied to specific individuals. In addition, single-subject designs require fewer participants than group experimental designs, which is a significant advantage for clinical research focused on low-incidence disabilities. The greatest liability of these studies is that it is difficult to generalize the results of one or more single-subject studies to a broader population of intervention candidates.

One single-subject research design, called the **multiple baselines across behaviors design,** is commonly used. In this design, intervention begins on a subset of goals, while performance on non-treated goals is monitored. After a criterion is reached on treated targets, intervention begins on another subset of goals, while any remaining untreated goals are still monitored. This pattern may continue over a long period of time. If the gains in a participant's performance for each behavior coincide with the initiation of intervention for that behavior, a causal inference associating the intervention and the improvements becomes appropriate. The Oxford CEBM system does not include single-subject experiments in its strategies for determining levels of evidence. Because these designs are so important in communication disorders, however, strong single-subject experiments can be placed at Level 2b (see Table 7.3). This is consistent with high quality quasi-experimental studies and lower quality RCTs, and it is similar to the level assigned to single-subject experiments by the Section 1 Task Force of the Division of Clinical Psychology of the American Psychological Association (Lonigan, Elber, & Johnson, 1998). Nonetheless, it is important to note that not all intervention researchers would agree that the level of evidence provided by well-controlled single-subject experiments should be so high.

An additional research design used to inform evidence-based decision making is the **case study design.** In a case study, a single individual, event, or context is intensively studied using both qualitative (e.g., interviews, field observations) and quantitative data (e.g., test scores). Case studies can be used to determine how easy or difficult it is to implement an intervention; how well clients tolerate the procedures and intensity of intervention; and whether the intervention has sufficient promise to warrant the planning and execution of additional, more rigorous studies of the intervention's effects. Despite being a type of clinical trial, however, this design provides a very weak form of evidence for intervention effects, because it is impossible to causally link any observed outcomes to the intervention, even if the intervention is expertly implemented and outcomes are rigorously monitored.

A **case series** is simply a collection of case studies in which several participants receive the same intervention and their outcomes are measured following the intervention. Even when a case series involves many participants who all respond similarly, the evidence the series produces can be no higher than Level 3 (see Table 7.3), because the researcher exerts no controls over factors that may be influencing intervention outcomes, and causal inferences of intervention impact are impossible.

To determine the research design used in a relevant study, clinicians must ask a set of questions such as those presented in Table 7.4. As Phyllis critically appraises the Tyler and colleagues (2003) article, she finds that the study is not a systematic review of a particular research design and answers the first two

Table 7.4. Some useful questions for determining the design of a clinical trial (answers apply to the study by Tyler et al., 2003)

	Yes	Unclear	No
Does the study systematically review randomized controlled trials?			X
Does the study systematically review quasi-experimental or single-subject experimental studies?			X
Are two or more groups compared?	X		
Are measures collected before and after therapy?	X		
Are participants randomly assigned to groups?	X		
Are there controls within or across individual participants?			X

Source: Scottish Intercollegiate Guidelines Network, 2004.

questions in the Table 7.4, "No." This means that the evidence from the article cannot be Level 1a or 2a (see Table 7.3). Groups were compared in the article, however, pre- and post-measures were obtained, and participants were randomly assigned to four intervention groups. These are defining characteristics of RCTs. Phyllis recognizes that the study is an RCT but wonders whether to characterize it as Level 1b (single high-quality RCT) or Level 2b (lower-quality RCT). To make this determination, she must evaluate the methodological quality of the study.

Methodological Quality   The level of evidence provided by a study is not based solely on its research design, but also its methodological quality. Examinations of the quality of published studies, even those designs providing the highest level of evidence, show that quality is highly variable (e.g., Troia, 1999), even in highly respected journals. Thus, once clinicians identify a study relevant to an evidence-based question and its research design, they must evaluate its quality. Although it is beyond the scope of this chapter to characterize the quality of different research designs by means of a thorough examination of approaches, several published articles provide excellent descriptions of quality indicators for true experimental and quasi-experimental designs (Gersten et al., 2005) as well as single-subject designs (Horner et al., 2005).

The basic process of appraising methodological quality can be illustrated by posing questions such as those that appear in Table 7.5. These questions provide means for a more in-depth examination of the quality of the evidence provided by RCT studies. The main concern at this stage is to determine whether the researcher has taken sufficient steps to avoid bias and subjectivity. Researchers generally avoid bias and subjectivity by 1) ensuring that before intervention begins, the participant groups are equivalent or arrangements have been made to minimize the effects of group inequalities; 2) individuals who either collect, transcribe, code, or record test data are blind to the participants' group assignments; 3) outcome measures have demonstrated reliability and validity; and 4) either few participants leave the intervention groups before the study has been completed or careful analyses have been conducted to determine that the study results have not been influenced by any changes in group membership. Failures to take these steps make it possible for bias and subjectivity to enter into the results, thus limiting confidence in any conclusions about causal relationships between the intervention and the observed outcomes.

Table 7.5 shows that the Tyler and colleagues (2003) study fares reasonably well on these variables, except that the testers, and perhaps also some transcribers,

Table 7.5. Some useful questions for determining the quality of a clinical trial (answers evaluate the quality of the study reported by Tyler et al., 2003)

	Yes	Unclear	No
Are the participant groups equivalent in regard to dependent variables and other key variables at pretest, or are differences accounted for statistically?	X		
Are assessors blind to group assignments?			X
Are coders blind to group assignments?		X	
Is the implementation of the intervention conditions monitored for fidelity?			X
Are outcome measures reliable and valid?	X		
Are dropouts in all intervention conditions accounted for?	X		

Source: Scottish Intercollegiate Guidelines Network, 2004.

were aware of the participants' group assignments. The concern is not necessarily that the testers and transcribers intentionally favored one participant group over another; rather, the fear is that biases can affect outcomes even when research personnel make strong and conscious efforts *not* to show any kind of favoritism. On the positive side, all participants completed the study, and each group had similarly high proportions of the total number of scheduled sessions. The interventions were well described and the number of sound and morpheme elicitations was reported to have been consistent across groups. Still, there was only limited monitoring of the interventions to ensure that they were delivered as described. Because of those factors, Phyllis rates this study as "Unclear" on this dimension. Although the study was generally well conducted, there is the possibility that bias and subjectivity could have influenced its results to undermine causal inferences. Phyllis ultimately rates the level of evidence for this study as Level 2b (see Table 7.3).

Consistency and Strength of Observed Effects   An available study may implement the most rigorous research design, and it may also exhibit strong methodological quality; nonetheless, it is possible that the effects of the intervention are weak or inconsistent. For example, a well-conducted RCT may find that group intervention for people with aphasia has little advantage over an individual intervention program, or it may find that the group intervention influences one area of language, such as word finding, but not sentence length, suggesting that effects of the intervention are small or inconsistent. It is important to consider the strength and consistency of observed outcomes across dependent measures. The strength of the intervention effect is typically examined by studying **statistical significance** and **effect-size estimates.** In experimental and quasi-experimental designs, statistical significance is the probability that differences between groups observed over a course of intervention resulted from the manipulation of the independent variable. Researchers typically use a probability threshold of .05 to differentiate results attributable to chance ($>.05$) from those attributable to experimental manipulation ($<.05$).

An intervention effect that is statistically reliable, however, is not necessarily clinically meaningful. For example, a memory intervention for clients with dementia may have a statistical advantage over a control condition because the members of the intervention group show more consistent change on the dependent variable over time than the members of the control group. At the same time, the actual improvement in memory performance of participants in the intervention group could be very small, suggesting that in reality the interventions are similar in their effect or that the small advantage attributed to the intervention is not worth the costs of implementing it. To estimate the magnitude of intervention effects, researchers calculate *size of the effect*. The most common measures of the size of the effect estimate the magnitude of an intervention's effect in standard deviation units.

To thoroughly appraise the Tyler and colleagues (2003) study for their EBP purposes, Phyllis must answer the questions as shown in Table 7.6, which review the size and consistency of the observed effects in the study. Phyllis' answers indicate that the study yielded some significant differences between groups. After 24 weeks, the participants in the alternating group made greater gains in morphosyntax than the participants in the other three groups. These differences were not only statistically reliable; the effects were large. In fact, after 24 weeks of intervention, the mean correct use of finite verb morphemes for participants in the alternating group was approximately one full standard deviation higher than the gains made by the participants in the other groups (i.e., size of effect = 1). In contrast, although the study provided some evidence that the participants in each group made gains in the percentage of target and generalization sounds produced correctly, there were no differences between group gains in phonology at 24 weeks when comparing the phonology-first and the morphosyntax-first groups. Thus, Tyler and colleagues appropriately concluded that their study supported the use of a strategy that alternates morphosyntactic and grammatical goals on a weekly basis compared to the tested alternatives. Tyler and colleagues also noted that their study needs to be replicated by other researchers.

To summarize Phyllis's critical appraisal of the Tyler and colleagues (2003) study, the study is a Level 2b RCT that, although generally well implemented, had some characteristics that might have allowed bias and subjectivity to influence the results. The observed effects in favor of the alternating sequence approach, however, were large and clinically meaningful. This Level 2b evidence surpasses a number of other types of evidence (e.g., expert opinion, theory, basic research, case study, poor quality quasi-experimental research). After determining this, Phyllis must ask herself, "How should the evidence influence what I do in my management of Aaron's speech and language problems?" Answering this question requires her to merge the external evidence with the internal evidence.

Table 7.6. Some useful questions for determining the strength and consistency of observed effects (answers apply to the study by Tyler et al., 2003)

	Yes	Unclear	No
Were experimental effects statistically significant?	X		
If more than one measure was used, were the effects across measures consistent?			X
Is the magnitude of the observed effects (i.e., effect size) reported and interpreted?	X		
Were the effects clinically meaningful?	X		

Source: Scottish Intercollegiate Guidelines Network, 2004.

Step 5: Integrate the Internal and External Evidence

The extent to which the results of Tyler and colleagues' (2003) study should influence Phyllis's intervention decision cannot be determined solely by ascertaining the level and quality of the external evidence. An evidence-based decision depends on the way in which a clinician consolidates the available internal and external evidence. For example, in the first scenario, Phyllis is actively searching for a reason to adopt a more consistent approach to goal attack for children exhibiting both speech and language deficits, Aaron is alert and cooperative, and his parents have advocated the use of an approach that targets their son's phonological and grammatical difficulties. In addition to the Level 2b evidence provided by Tyler and colleagues' study, a number of internal factors are also present that further encourage Phyllis to adopt the alternating goal attack strategy.

Now consider Phyllis's approach in the second scenario. She is much more comfortable with her current intervention approach in that she frequently targets intelligibility directly until the child is significantly easier to understand, at which time she focuses on grammatical and other deficits. Although she recognizes it as a relatively weak form of evidence, Phyllis has pre-/post- information in her own treatment records that document the success of this approach with children similar to Aaron. Perhaps more importantly, Aaron in this scenario is arguably not as good a fit to the alternating strategy as he is in the first scenario, as it is not clear that the evidence from Tyler and colleagues (2003) is applicable to children with Aaron's attentional challenges. Phyllis must ask herself, "Would Aaron's attentional difficulties and problems moving from one task to another complicate the application of the alternating intervention? Would his parents' desire for the intervention to focus on intelligibility negatively influence attempts to employ the alternating strategy?" Based on her clinical experience, Phyllis argues that the answer to both of these questions is "Yes." Taking all of these factors into consideration, she decides to maintain her typical approach with an emphasis on intelligibility, despite her awareness of the Level 2b evidence available to support an alternating approach. In Aaron's PPT meeting, she tells the parents about the evidence from Tyler and colleagues' study that supported the alternating strategy and explains her rationale for adopting a strategy other than the alternating approach. Her awareness of the evidence supporting an alternative strategy would make her especially vigilant with respect to Aaron's developing grammar as his speech begins to improve.

These two scenarios illustrate how an evaluation of the same external evidence may not always result in the same clinical decision. Actions that might be recommended based on the results of a review of external evidence may be deemed less suitable or even inappropriate after a careful integration of the external and internal evidence.

Step 6: Evaluate the Decision by Documenting Outcomes

There are very few studies in which all members of a treatment group completing an intervention study responded precisely to the same extent and in the same positive manner. In the same way, some clients enrolled in clinical interventions can be expected to show little or no progress despite receiving the same intervention as those who make dramatic gains. Consequently, inferences based on evidence from research must be questioned, even when the external and internal evidence is uncharacteristically supportive of a particular intervention option. Clinicians must carefully measure participant outcomes during interventions selected through evidence-based decision making. When intervention outcomes support evidence-based decisions, clinicians should continue to implement them, and they may even attempt to apply the decision to a broader set of intervention candidates. When outcomes do not measure up to the evidence-based predictions, EBP clinicians must ask why? and they must seek the answers to this question from their own internally generated evidence as well as from new and extant findings provided in the research literature.

CONCLUSION

This chapter has introduced many important concepts related to EBP in speech-language intervention. In addition, guidelines for what clinicians might do to begin their EBP initiatives in the short term have been recommended. This presentation should lead readers to three broad conclusions.

1. EBP principles do *not* limit SLPs to the use of clinical practices shown by the external evidence to be efficacious and effective. At this stage of the profession's development, the evidence that clinicians need to support their clinical decisions often is simply unavailable. In these cases, principled decisions based on a comprehensive understanding of relevant theory and basic research and careful attention to available internal evidence are likely to be of greatest benefit to the clients and families served. In fact, new ideas concerning intervention possibilities are most likely to emanate from such understanding.

2. EBP principles *do* require SLPs to critically examine their own practices to determine what types and what amounts of evidence support current practices. Recognizing situations in which extant practices are *not* supported by strong clinical studies is equally as important as identifying those practices that are well grounded in research.

3. EBP principles *do* require SLPs to be skeptical about the use of all intervention practices. This conclusion is especially true when practices in speech-language pathology generally do not have a strong body of evidentiary support. In such cases, clinicians must be particularly vigilant with respect to monitoring the outcomes of their interventions, they should actively seek evidence in the literature that is relevant to their clinical questions, and they should encourage members of the research community to design studies that address their most important and pressing clinical questions. This conclusion is *most especially* true when there is less external evidence for a selected approach relative to some alternative. In all cases, knowledge and understanding of the literature relevant to clinical decisions puts clinicians in the best position to make and defend their decisions, to evaluate the outcomes of those decisions, and to deal effectively with parents, professionals, and policy-makers who have a vested interest in ensuring that SLPs are accountable for what they do.

REFERENCES

American Speech-Language-Hearing Association. (2004). *Evidence-based practice in communication disorders: An introduction.* [Technical report]. Retrieved July 15, 2006 from http://www.asha.org/NR/rdonlyres/B36BF8F8-C4C3-4E86-8FAD-26D76F130CBF/0/ebpTR.pdf

American Speech-Language-Hearing Association. (2005). *Evidence-based practice in communication disorders.* [Position statement]. Retrieved July 15, 2006 from http://www.asha.org/NR/rdonlyres/4837FDFC-576B-4D84-BDD6-8BFF2A803AD3/0/v4PS_EBP.pdf

Bankson, N., & Bernthal, J. E. (1990). *Bankson-Bernthal Test of Phonology.* Austin, TX: PRO-ED.

Centre for Evidence-Based Medicine (2001a). *Focusing clinical questions.* Retrieved July 15, 2006, from http://www.cebm.net/focus_quest.asp

Centre for Evidence-Based Medicine. (2001b). *Levels of evidence and grades of recommendation.* Retrieved July 15, 2006, from http://www.cebm.net/levels_of_evidence.asp

Dollaghan, C.A. (2004). Evidence-based practice in communication disorders: What do we know, and when do we know it? *Journal of Communication Disorders, 37,* 391–400.

Dunn, L.M., & Dunn, L.M. (1997). *Peabody Picture Vocabulary Test.* (3rd ed.). Circle Pines, MN: AGS Publishing.

Fey, M. (1986). *Language intervention with young children.* Boston: Allyn & Bacon.

Fey, M., Cleave, P.L., Ravida, A.I., Long, S.H., Dejmal, A.E., & Easton, D.L. (1994). Effects of grammar facilitation on the phonological performance of children with speech and language impairments. *Journal of Speech and Hearing Research, 37,* 594–607.

Gersten, R., Fuchs, L.S., Compton, D., Coyne, M., Greenwood, C., & Innocenti, M.S. (2005). Quality indicators for group experimental and quasi-experimental research in special education. *Exceptional Children, 71,* 149–164.

Greenfield, P., & Zukow, P. (1978). Why do children say what they say when they say it?: An experimental approach to the psychogenesis of presupposition. In K.E. Nelson (Ed.), *Children's language* (Vol. 1, pp. 287–336). New York: Gardner Press.

Horner, R.H., Carr, E.G., Halle, J., McGee, G., Odom, S., & Wolery, M. (2005). The use of single-subject research to identify evidence-based practice in special education. *Exceptional Children, 71,* 165–179.

Justice, L.M., & Fey, M.E. (2004). Evidence-based practice in schools: Integrating craft and theory with science and data. *The ASHA Leader, 4-5,* 30–32.

Lee, L. (1975). *Developmental sentence analysis.* Evanston, IL: Northwestern University Press.

Leonard, L., Cole, B., & Steckol, K. (1979). Lexical usage of retarded children: An examination of informativeness. *American Journal of Mental Deficiency, 84,* 49–54.

Lonigan, C., Elber, J., & Johnson, S. (1998). Empirically supported interventions for children: An overview. *Journal of Clinical Child Psychology, 27,* 138–145.

Newcomer, P.L., & Hammill, D.D. (1997). *Test of Language Development-Primary (TLDP).* (3rd ed.). Austin, TX: PRO-ED.

Phillips, B., Ball, C., Sackett, D., Badenoch, D., Straus, S., Haynes, B., et al. (2001, May). *Oxford Centre for evidence-based medicine levels of evidence.* Retrieved July 1, 2006, from http://www.cebm.net/levels_of_evidence.asp

Porzsolt, F., Ohletz, A., Thim, A., Gardner, D., Ruatti, H., Meier, H., et al. (2003). Evidence-based decision making-the six step approach. *EBM Notebook, 8,*(November-December), 165–166.

Sackett, D.L., Straus, S.E., Richardson, W.S., Rosenberg, W., & Haynes, R.B. (2000). *Evidence-based medicine: How to practice and teach EBM.* New York: Churchill Livingstone.

Schwartz, R., & Leonard, L. (1985). Lexical imitation and acquisition in language-impaired children. *Journal of Speech and Hearing Disorders, 50,* 141–149.

Scottish Intercollegiate Guidelines Network (2004). *Sign 50: A guideline developers' handbook. Annex C.* Retrieved July 16, 2006, from http://www.sign.ac.uk/guidelines/fulltext/50/annexc.html

Snyder, L. (1978). Communicative and cognitive abilities and disabilities in the sensorimotor period. *Merrill-Palmer Quarterly, 24,* 161–180.

Sorensen, P., & Fey, M.E. (1992). Informativeness as a clinical principle: What's really new? *Language, Speech, and Hearing Services in Schools, 23,* 320–328.

Stokes, D.E. (1997). *Pasteur's quadrant.* Washington, DC: The Brookings Institution Press.

Troia, G. (1999). Phonological awareness intervention research: A critical review of the experimental methodology. *Reading Research Quarterly, 34,* 28–53.

Tyler, A.A., Lewis, K.E., Haskill, A., & Tolbert, L.C. (2002). Efficacy and cross-domain effects of a morphosyntax and a phonology intervention. *Language, Speech, and Hearing Services in Schools, 33,* 52–66.

Tyler, A.A., Lewis, K.E., Haskill, A., & Tolbert, L.C. (2003). Outcomes of different speech and language goal attack strategies. *Journal of Speech, Language, and Hearing Research, 46,* 1077–1094.

Tyler, A.A., & Sandoval, K.T. (1994). Preschoolers with phonological and language disorders: Treating different linguistic domains. *Language, Speech, and Hearing Services in Schools, 25,* 215–234.

van Kleeck, A. (1994). Potential cultural bias in training parents as conversational partners with their children who have delays in language development. *American Journal of Speech-Language Pathology, 3*(1), 67–78.

STUDY QUESTIONS

1. Define *evidence-based practice* in your own words.

2. What is meant by external evidence? Internal evidence?

3. Describe how the acronym PICO is used in evidence-based decision making.

4. What are the six steps used to make evidence-based clinical decisions?

5. Name and discuss three critical features used to categorize studies according to the levels of evidence.

6. Describe a hypothetical study with each of the following designs: randomized clinical trial, quasi-experimental, single subject experimental, case study, and case series.

7. Define *dependent* and *independent variables* in your own words.

8. Give two ways in which the strength of intervention impact can be examined.

9. Does evidence-based practice limit clinicians to using only practices shown by external evidence to be effective? Why or why not?

10. Define *sensitivity, specificity, false positive* and *false negative* in your own words.

CHAPTER 8

Interviewing, Counseling, and Clinical Communication

KEVIN M. MCNAMARA

As audiologists and speech-language pathologists (SLPs), we need to be effective in sharing information with clients across the entire continuum of clinical services: interviewing and counseling clients; documenting evaluation findings; developing intervention plans; recording outcomes; and educating family members, teachers, medical personnel, and caregivers regarding clients' communication needs. In each of these tasks, information must be conveyed clearly and understandably to clients, families, educators, other care providers, and administrators. To success-fully accomplish this, we need to learn sensitive and efficient strategies for sharing information with the people that we serve. Our effectiveness in commu-nicating information will contribute a good deal to the quality of the therapeutic relationships that we establish with our clients. It will influence our ability to advocate for appropriate services and equipment for those that we serve, as well as obtain adequate funding for those services. Poorly written clinical documen-tation can severely compromise a clinician's professional credibility (Roth & Worthington, 2005), and a poor oral communication style can negatively influ-ence the ability of a clinician to establish trusting relationships with clients and to relate vital clinical information to them. Part of our job as clinicians for people with communication disorders is to be skilled communicators ourselves.

BASIC PRINCIPLES OF ORAL AND WRITTEN CLINICAL COMMUNICATION

As clinicians, we rely on a set of principles governing effective communication in order to exchange information with those who we serve in a manner that is sensitive and appropriate to their needs. Information shared either orally or in writing should be presented in a manner that is concise, well organized, and related to a clearly stated topic. Sensitivity must be shown to issues such as a client's language style, emotional needs, and level of familiarity with the topic being discussed. In the case of written reports, audiologists and SLPs write for a mixed and sometimes unknown audience of readers, many of whom will differ from the author in terms of educational backgrounds, language styles, and cultural perspectives. Unlike direct verbal exchanges, in which a listener has an opportunity to provide verbal and nonverbal feedback in order to clarify or expand the information being presented, there is not always an immediate opportunity for readers to ask for clarification or to confirm their understanding of written information. To increase our effectiveness in both oral and written communication, some general principles of effective clinical communication follow.

PRINCIPLES OF EFFECTIVE CLINICAL COMMUNICATION

In both oral and written presentations

Clearly introduce the topic about which you are writing or speaking.

Organize all information in a logical, cohesive manner by subtopic.

Avoid using technical language whenever possible. Use vocabulary and a language style easily understood by a wider audience.

When you cannot avoid using technical terms, explain them parenthetically or by stating examples.

Whenever possible, use objective terms such as *observed, completed,* or *demonstrated*; avoid vague or judgmental terms such as *appears* or *seemed*.

Avoid redundancy unless you are summarizing key concepts.

Use "person first-language" ("a man with aphasia" or "a person who stutters") rather than referring to people as disabilities ("an aphasic" or "a stutterer").

During direct verbal exchanges

Attend to the comfort of your listener.

Explain the purpose of your discussion.

Organize questions and informational statements in an orderly, sequential manner.

Establish trust by being an active, empathetic, and nonjudgmental listener.

Allow the people with whom you are communicating to be active participants in the conversation, ensuring opportunities for them to respond to questions, make comments, and ask questions of their own.

Remember that individuals comprehend information differently. Provide sufficient time for your listener to process and react to your statements.

Be sensitive to and respectful of cultural differences and their impact on interpersonal communication. Avoid imposing your own cultural values, especially if they appear to conflict with those of your listener.

Watch for both verbal and nonverbal cues from your listener to see if you are presenting your message in a way that is understandable and culturally acceptable. Rephrase, expand, or eliminate statements and questions based on these cues.

Enlist the assistance of interpreters to assist in situations in which you must verbally communicate with people who speak a language different from yours. Exercise extra caution in these situations to ensure that your message is being translated appropriately and that you accurately comprehend the information being conveyed to you via an interpreter.

The information that you convey to people during the course of their engagement with you can at times be difficult or even painful for them to hear. A family in the initial phase of identifying their child's hearing loss or communication impairment or an adult faced with a newly acquired communication disorder due to neurological damage or a disease process must come to terms with a new and unfamiliar disability. This change in anticipated abilities may have a significant influence on a family's hope and expectations for their child or an individual's own perception of self-worth (Shames, 2000). As a new clinician, you may be tempted to avoid confronting your clients with "bad news" regarding their prognoses for improvement or limited achievements in therapy. In addition, clients or administrators may at times ask you to provide information that you do not have or pressure you into saying or writing statements that you do not believe or cannot substantiate through research or clinical data. Above all else, clinicians are bound by ethical practice to be honest in all interactions with their clients, as well as with those people and agencies that support their clients. The Code of Ethics of the American Speech-Language-Hearing Association (ASHA) and the American Academy of Audiology clearly emphasizes your responsibility for truthfulness in all aspects of your clinical practice. The ASHA Code of Ethics states

> Individuals shall honor their responsibility to the public by promoting public understanding of the professions, by supporting development of services designed to fulfill the unmet needs of the public, and by providing accurate information in all communications involving any aspect of the professions. (ASHA, 2003, p. 2; see Chapter 2)

It is possible, however, to share difficult information with your clients in a manner that is supportive, sensitive, and truthful if you employ the basic principles of effective clinical communication.

Maintaining Confidentiality of Information

Clients, or their legal guardians, ultimately control to whom information is released, and the principle of confidentiality applies to both oral and written communication between clients and clinicians (Silverman, 2003). The Health Insurance Portability and Accountability Act (HIPAA) of 1996 (PL 104-191) requires that virtually all health care organizations, including speech-language pathology and audiology providers, adopt and maintain rigorous standards and procedures to ensure the protection and restriction client information. HIPAA levies severe financial and legal consequences on organizations that fail to keep confidentiality. This public law legally mandates what had been standard ethical practice in our profession for many years; that the information we obtain and record about our clients be kept confidential and restricted to those directly working with those clients unless our clients provide us with written permission to release such information to others. ASHA's Code of Ethics states

> Individuals shall not reveal, without authorization, any professional or personal information about identified persons served professionally or identified participants involved in research and scholarly activities unless required by law to do so, or unless doing so is necessary to protect the welfare of the person of the community or otherwise required by law. (ASHA, 2003, p. 14)

As SLPs and audiologists, it is essential that you become knowledgeable of and adhere to the information protection policies of the facilities in which you practice.

STRATEGIES USED TO GATHER AND CONVEY CLINICAL INFORMATION

It is essential to gather as much pertinent background information regarding your clients as you can when you start the process of evaluating their communication needs. You may acquire information through a combination of methods, such as reviewing existing records, conducting interviews, and using written questionnaires. You should be as thorough as possible in exploring all relevant sources of information to which you have been granted access.

Reviewing Existing Records

You have an obligation as a clinician to consider the needs of the clients you serve in the context of their home, school, work, family, and social interactions (Tomblin, 2000). A review of existing records can provide vital clues revealing clients' communication needs in those settings. Other audiologists or SLPs, as well as other medical, therapeutic, or educational service providers, may have already seen the clients who now seek your assistance. These previous contacts may yield medical reports, educational records, previous speech-language and audiological evaluations, and documents summarizing past interventions. You can gain knowledge of previous medical, cognitive, psychological, or psychiatric diagnoses, as well as information regarding clients' social, adaptive, and educational functioning. This information can allow you to make more appropriate decisions relating to evaluation and intervention strategies and avoid recommending interventions that may have been contraindicated by medical status or previously unsuccessful therapies. Remember that clients or their guardians ultimately control to whom information is released, and that "the confidentiality precept applies to both oral and written communication between clients and clinician and includes reports and other clinical records" (Silverman, 1999, p. 15).

CASE EXAMPLE 1

Mr. Rodrigues, a 78-year-old man, has just been transferred from an acute care unit in a local hospital to a short-term rehabilitation unit of a skilled nursing facility. He experienced a stroke approximately 2 weeks ago and received speech therapy in the hospital setting prior to his transfer. He has been admitted to the rehabilitation unit with doctor's orders for speech therapy evaluation and intervention of residual communication and swallowing problems secondary to his stroke.

If you were the SLP evaluating Mr. Rodrigues in the skilled nursing facility you could, theoretically, assess both his communication and swallowing status without looking first at the information available from his previous stay in the hospital acute care unit. By doing so, though, you would miss vital information essential to the safe and effective management of this client. For example, it would be important for you to review information regarding his ability to swallow safely, as determined by a modified barium swallow (MBS) study performed in the hospital setting, prior to initiating dysphagia (swallowing) therapy. Implementing therapy procedures or diet modifications and feeding protocols based on insufficient information about the client's functioning in this area may put him at risk for aspiration or other related and potentially life-threatening medical complications such as pneumonia. Specific information regarding the nature of the client's brain damage, as revealed through a computed topography scan, and more general medical information regarding the client's overall health status will help you to determine a realistic prognosis. Access to this information would allow you to understand the etiology of the client's impairment better and to make more appropriate intervention decisions that are consistent with his medical status and potential for improvement.

CASE EXAMPLE 2

Susan, a 7-year-old girl with a severe bilateral sensorineural hearing loss, has recently moved with her family to a new home in a different state. She currently wears two be-hind-the-ear hearing aids. She has been referred to a local audiologist's office for an audiological reassessment and to explore the possibility of being fitted with an FM System to enhance her classroom listening skills.

In Susan's example, it is essential that the new audiologist has an opportunity to review previous findings regarding this client's hearing status in order to monitor for potential deterioration of hearing across time. A review of previous audiological evaluations, recommendations for hearing aids and other assistive listening devices, and follow-up documentation of audiological intervention will allow the audiologist to make better decisions regarding the assessment and management of the client's audiological needs. In addition, reviewing related educational and speech-language pathology records will allow the audiologist to understand the functional, social, and academic communication needs of the client and to offer recommendations for equipment and audiological management strategies that are appropriate for those needs and settings.

As you review existing records, you must remember that "information from other professionals can potentially lead to a biased view of your client's condition" (Shipley & McAfee, 2004, p. 65). It is essential to balance your own clinical observations and findings with the information reported from other sources when making diagnostic and intervention decisions.

Conducting Interviews

One of the most useful ways we can gain insight into the needs and backgrounds of our clients is by directly interviewing them and the people who care for them. An **interview** is an organic, fluid, and multifaceted process that is guided by the clinician and constructed by all participants (see Figure 8.1). It is a vehicle for gathering relevant information and educating people on issues related to communication disorders. It is also the first opportunity to begin to establish a trusting and cooperative relationship with clients and their families. It is a task that requires you to employ active listening skills (Luteman, 2001; Shames, 2000); to be sensitive to individual personal, cultural, and linguistic styles (Battle, 2002; Coleman, 2000); and to exercise flexibility in questioning and responding to the

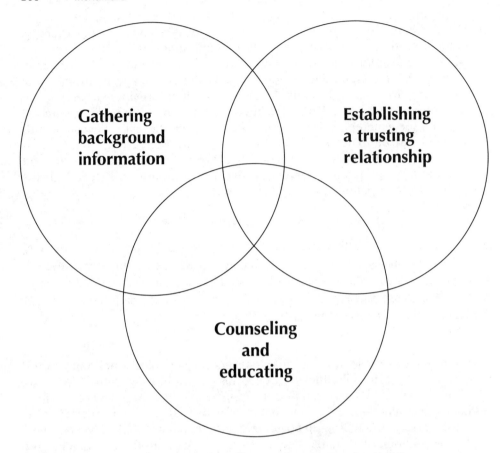

Figure 8.1. The interrelationship of counseling, questioning, and trust building in a clinical interview.

information being shared. In addition to your clients and their families, you may interview doctors (e.g., general practitioners, otolaryngologists, neurologists, pediatricians), nurses, caregivers, classroom teachers, special educators, social workers, vocational counselors, and clinicians from other disciplines including physical and occupational therapists and psychologists.

Establishing Trust

Shapiro (1999), in his discussion of interviewing parents of children who stutter, noted the importance of beginning a clinical interview in a positive and support-ive manner. He stated that

> Too often the communication problem becomes the immediate focus rather than the people with whom we are interacting. A social greeting enables clini-cians and clients to begin the journey as co-equal participants in a shared process, and helps to establish a social and personal foundation. Before we can respect and respond to each other's roles and responsibility as clients or clinicians within the clinical process, we must first value each other as people. The importance of establishing positive rapport cannot be overstated. (p. 225)

Rollin (2000), in his discussion of facilitating a counseling relationship, further encouraged us to value our clients as individuals first, and to "separate the disorder from the person" (p. 24). Being sensitive to differences in cultural styles can help clinicians better establish respect and trust during an interview (Lynch and Hanson, 2004). For example, Latino clients and their families may view an initial period of informal talking as an appropriate prelude to more serious discussions, whereas an attempt to discuss such issues immediately may be considered rude (Anderson & Fenichel, 1989; Zungia, 2004). Members of many other cultural groups, however, may find it disrespectful if too casual an approach is taken during an interview. Professionals are cautioned to address family members in a formal manner, using titles and surnames, unless specifically invited to do otherwise, or risk impeding the establishment of respect and trust (Willis, 2004).

Maintaining Appropriate Professional Boundaries

As we establish trusting and empathetic relationships with our clients through effective interview and counseling strategies, we may set the stage for those individuals to engage in the process of *transference*. From a psychodynamic standpoint, this concept refers to the process by which "the counselor becomes the object for, target of, and the symbol of the client's emotional expressions" (Shames, 2000, p. 79). Shames noted that this transference was a natural result of establishing a trusting relationship between client and clinician. These emotional expressions from a client can take many forms, from personal questions to romantic inclinations, and Shames cautioned clinicians to try to understand the function of these expressions and to not view them as necessarily a personal threat. Clinicians, however, may share their own personal feelings only if the expression of those feelings will facilitate the therapeutic process. Stone and Olswang (1989) noted the importance of establishing limitations on the content, focus, and style of the counseling efforts of SLPs and audiologists. They suggested that the expression of attitudes and questions relating to the presenting communication disorder is within an appropriate content boundary for audiologists and SLPs, but other topics not related to communication disorders are out of bounds and may necessitate referring the client to other sources of support.

Using Appropriate Question Formats to Elicit Information

Clinicians rely on a variety of question types to elicit information during an interview. Open-ended questions, or comments, are typically used to initiate an interview, allowing the person being questioned to establish the direction of the interview and express issues that he or she holds as priorities. These questions encourage the client to be an active participant rather than a passive respondent in the interview process. Hall and Morris (2000) noted that by using open-ended questions, clinicians, although controlling the general background areas being explored, do not control the range of responses elicited from the person or how extensively the person responds. Questions or statements such as "How can I help you today?" or "Tell me about the trouble you're having hearing" allow you to relinquish some of the control held in an interview to the respondent, leading to increased trust and willingness to share information about sensitive and important issues.

After the client has had an opportunity to express priority concerns by responding to open-ended questions, you may find it necessary to use closed questions that narrow the range of responses and elicit more specific information. There are a finite number of possible answers to questions such as "How much did your son weigh when he was born?" or "When was your last hearing evaluation?" The use of such question forms allows the interviewer to regain more control of the interview and focus on specific clinical issues. A particularly narrow form of closed questions is one that requires only a "yes" or "no" response. This type of questions requires the respondent to confirm or deny statements made by the clinician and allows the client no control over the intent or direction of the question.

As with all interpersonal interactions, cultural values and styles may affect how a person responds to certain question forms. For African American clients, direct questions may, at times, be seen as rude or overly personal (Shipley & McAfee, 2004), and disagreement by an African American listener may be conveyed through silence. Latino clients, out of respect for people in professional roles, may refrain from openly expressing disagreement with a clinician's statements, even though they may not agree with the clinician (Langdon & Cheng, 1992). Members of some Asian cultures, to avoid offending a person, may say what they think the listener wants to hear, rather than what they themselves believe (Shipley & McAfee, 2004; Roseberry-McKibbin, 2002). Gender differences also play a part in how a respondent may answer questions, and this especially may be the case with some Middle Eastern cultures that place restrictions on the content and format of interactions between people of different genders. Even within the broader collective American culture, differences in communication styles often demonstrated by both genders may lead to miscommunication. This can be seen in a woman's affirmative head nod to indicate active listening and empathy and a man's use of the same gesture to convey agreement (Maltz & Borker, 1982). A more comprehensive discussion of multicultural issues related to communication disorders can be found in Chapter 11.

Case History Questionnaires

A written **case history questionnaire** is a tool that is used to gather and organize information regarding the nature of speech, language, and hearing concerns; general developmental and health history; educational background; and history of related support services. By presenting both general and specific questions, it attempts to elicit a client's opinion of the communication disorder and its affect on daily communication needs. Case history questionnaires may be broad in their scope of questions related to communication or may be customized to include questions related to specific issues such as hearing loss, auditory processing disorder, fluency or voice disorders, and augmentative communication needs. Separate formats are typically used for adults and children (see Figure 8.2 for an adult format).

In some practice settings, clients or caregivers are asked to complete a case history questionnaire prior to arriving or a few minutes before the start of their initial diagnostic evaluation. You must be cautious, however, that you do not make your clients' first task the completion of a long, jargon-filled, and often confusing and intimidating questionnaire form, thereby creating a barrier for people who are attempting to gain access to clinical services. Alternatively, case history questionnaires may serve as a flexible guide for topics during person-to-person

Name: _____ Date: _____

1. How old were you when your hearing loss was first identified?

2. What have you done about your hearing loss?

3. What do you feel is the cause of your hearing problem?

4. Has a physician examined your ears?
   Who?   Date of last examination?

5. Have you experienced pain in either of your ears?   When?
   Describe.

6. Have you ever had ear infections (running ears)?
   Which ear?   When?

7. Have there been any changes in your hearing in the last 6 months?

   Last year?

   Last 2 years?

8. Do you have any allergies?
   Describe.

9. Do you ever feel dizzy?   How often?

10. Does your hearing seem better on some days than on others?

11. Have you ever worn a hearing aid?

Figure 8.2. Sample questions found on an audiological case history form for adults.

diagnostic or intake interviews. You may find the structure offered by such forms useful as you develop skills in the areas of interview and evaluation, but you should not rely too much on the rigid format of written case history question-naires during client interviews. Inflexible use of these forms may interfere with efforts to modify individual interpersonal styles and language to better meet the needs of the people being interviewed (Haynes & Pindzola, 2004; Shapiro, 1999).

FORMATS FOR CONVEYING CLINICAL INFORMATION

The formats you use to share information with your clients and those individuals and agencies that support your clients are influenced by a number of factors. The type of information being conveyed, as well as the audience with whom the in-formation is being shared, may in part determine whether you use a structured versus informal format or a written versus oral format. Specific speech-language pathology or audiology programs or facilities may follow policies that dictate the use of particular formats for documenting evaluation results, intervention pro-grams, and outcome data. For example, early intervention programs for children birth to 3 years old, school-based services for children 3 to 21 years old, and geri-atric speech-language pathology and audiology services funded by Medicare all have documentation requirements, formats, and timelines influenced by federal, state, and local policies.

Evaluation Reports

Written **diagnostic evaluation reports** are used to summarize information obtained in both audiological and speech-language evaluations. These reports serve as an official record of assessment findings, diagnoses, and recommendations (Meitus, 1983) and as a written description of the hearing and communication profiles of the individuals who are being evaluated. They are legal documents that, as is the case with all written documentation, may be called into legal pro-ceedings to determine service provision and liability issues. The actual format for an evaluation report will vary across settings and sometimes by individual clini-cian. The format may include specific outlines for individually written reports or, in some cases, prewritten forms or checklists into which the details and interpre-tations from a client's evaluation are inserted. There are even software programs that, after the clinician inserts individual details, will generate a written sum-mary report. Regardless of the format, most evaluation reports contain specific sections presenting identifying and background information, a summary of test results and diagnostic observations, interpretations of findings, prognosis for improvement, and recommendations. A well-written diagnostic report is one that presents all information in an organized and sequential manner and effi-ciently integrates all diagnostic data, interpretations, and recommendations. The structure of a diagnostic report will be examined in greater detail later in this chapter.

Oral Reports and Conferences

Interactions with clients may involve sharing information orally as well as in writing. You will continue to answer questions from your clients and their family members and caregivers regarding intervention procedures and outcomes. With their written permission, you may share information concerning your clients' communication needs with teachers, program administrators, and insurers in order to advocate for the materials, resources, or funding necessary for adequate intervention of their communication disorders. The expanding role that SLPs and audiologists play in providing collaborative intervention has increased the frequency and importance of orally reporting information regarding clients' communication needs (ASHA, 1991, 2002).

Case conferences are focused opportunities to present information to or about your clients. During these exchanges, you may follow a more systematic approach to sharing information than you do in more casual oral reports. The specific content may be dictated by the purpose of the conference as well as by the needs of the participants. Examples of formal case conferences include individual meetings with clients and their families and conferences with teachers to discuss their students' communication needs in the classroom setting. Clinicians working in hospitals or rehabilitation centers may meet with other therapists, medical personnel, caregivers, and family members to discuss their clients' progress in therapy and service needs. Regardless of the setting, audiologists and SLPs are responsible for presenting information in a succinct and organized manner that is easily understood by clients as well as those individuals who support them.

Intervention Plans

After an initial assessment of speech, language, and/or hearing, the need for intervention is determined. This decision is based on evaluation findings, client and family priorities, program eligibility requirements, and other related factors. Once the decision is made to begin an intervention, a formal **intervention plan** is developed. The formats and required terminology for intervention plans may be determined by both federal and state regulations governing a particular type of service delivery program. Examples of comprehensive intervention plans that outline a broad range of supports and outcomes include school-based **individualized education programs (IEPs)** and **individualized family service plans (IFSPs)** for children from birth to 3 years old who are enrolled in early intervention programs. In medically based rehabilitation settings funded by Medicare, specific intervention plans outline the skilled services that only a certified SLP may perform, although **functional maintenance plans** are developed to identify nonskilled communication supports that are provided by noncertified support staff, family members, and other caregivers.

In your initial clinical training, you may be asked to develop intervention plans that outline individual sessions of speech, language, and audiology intervention in detail. These plans usually include long-term goals and short-term objectives related to speech, language, hearing, and other communication needs. Targeted communication behaviors are identified, as well as the conditions under which they are expected to occur, and measurable criteria for success are stated for each behavior. Intervention techniques, activities, and materials are listed as well. Such plans serve as a guide from which we organize and implement individual therapy sessions and are similar in purpose to the lesson plans developed by classroom teachers. During your clinical training, you may be asked to develop intervention plans that offer a large amount of detail in order to facilitate your understanding of intervention and documentation processes.

INDIVIDUAL INTERVENTION PLAN
FOR SPEECH-LANGUAGE THERAPY

Long-term goal(s)

José will increase his recognition and use of picture communication symbols in order to express needs and participate in classroom activities.

Short-term objective(s)

1. José will match 10 newly introduced picture symbols depicting classroom materials with the actual objects they represent.
2. José will point to the above-mentioned picture symbols presented on a picture symbol communication board when named by the clinician.
3. José will request a minimum of two items needed during a classroom activity by pointing to an appropriate picture symbol on a picture symbol board with no more than verbal prompting from the clinician.

Procedures

Verbal instruction, visual modeling of the targeted behavior, physical cuing, verbal reinforcement

Activities

1. Object/picture matching using the "Treasure Hunt" game
   A. Short-term objective(s) targeted during activity: 1
   B. Materials needed: Picture symbol cards, corresponding objects
2. Arts and crafts project based on curriculum-based reading theme
   A. Short-term objective(s) targeted during activity: 2, 3
   B. Materials needed: Picture communication board, corresponding objects, craft material, storybook

SOAP Notes

Therapeutic intervention is a dynamic process in which continual changes to therapy objectives and activities are made in response to a client's performance and to new information revealed through ongoing assessment. The **SOAP note**—with the acronym standing for Subjective, Objective, Assessment, and Plan—is a format often used in medical settings and other settings to record and analyze data specific to a client's ongoing performance in therapy (Golper, 1998). SOAP notes are documents summarizing the clinician's observations regarding a client's level of attention and participation in therapy (i.e., subjective), specific data regarding performance on therapy tasks (i.e., objective), interpretation of those subjective observations and objective data (i.e., assessment), and recommendations for future action based on that interpretation (i.e., plan). SOAP notes may be quick handwritten entries in a client's chart in a hospital or rehabilitation setting or may take the form of more extensive reports summarizing a client's progress in therapy. The SOAP note format may also be used for reporting more detailed diagnostic findings.

A BRIEF PROGRESS REPORT IN A SOAP FORMAT

Subjective: Mr. Smith was alert and oriented during today's session. Nursing staff reported an increase in the number of hours he was awake and in his general orientation to surroundings since yesterday evening. Mrs. Smith (his wife) was present during the last half of therapy, and she reported that he was frustrated the night before at his inability to "find the right words."

Objective: Mr. Smith pointed to pictures of familiar household items with 75% accuracy (15/20) when named by the clinician and with 80% accuracy (8/10) by function. He named 20% (2/10) of the same pictures with maximum cuing from the clinician. Severe dysarthria persisted, negatively affecting speech intelligibility. Imitation of lingual movements (tongue tip elevation, lateralization, and tongue retraction) was slow and labored.

Assessment: Mr. Smith continues to demonstrate severe word finding problems negatively influencing functional communication, as well as limited speech intelligibility secondary to oral motor weakness. An increase in word recognition and overall alertness and orientation to communication partners was noted since last intervention session.

Plan: Continue speech therapy for 30 minutes per day, targeting increased word finding and speech intelligibility. Provide a picture board of common objects to facilitate Mr. Smith's word finding when he is conversing with his wife and the staff. Counsel Mrs. Smith regarding strategies to facilitate word finding and to repair communication breakdowns.

Progress Reports

At periodic intervals throughout the course of your clients' intervention, you will be required to summarize and document their cumulative progress toward achieving targeted intervention goals and to make recommendations regarding their need for continued therapy. These intervals are typically determined by the regulations governing the specific program in which the service is provided and the funding source requirements, and these intervals may vary from 1 month or less to 1 year or more. In these days of increasing demands on clinicians' time and increasingly limited funding for clinical services, it has become critical for clinicians to make carefully documented decisions regarding the continued need for intervention based on client outcome data. Progress reports are used as vehicles to summarize and review a client's cumulative achievement of intervention goals and objectives across a specific period and to outline the future direction of intervention. Typically, such reports contain brief background information, a summary of specific goals and objectives, a data-based analysis of the client's progress, an interpretation of the data, a prognosis for change, and a recommendation regarding the need for and direction of future intervention.

Discharge Summaries

Discharge from audiology and speech-language pathology services is based on a number of interrelated factors. These may include a client's progress (or lack of progress) toward targeted objectives, achievement of functional communication status, successful fitting and use of hearing aids or other assistive listening devices, and changing priorities regarding communication intervention (ASHA, 2004). A **discharge summary** is a written report of a client's cumulative progress from the initiation of therapy to his or her discharge. As in the case of a progress report, a summary and interpretation of a client's accomplishments and continued needs are made based on a review of cumulative client performance data, our judgment regarding the client's prognosis for further change, and other related variables. Recommendations for necessary post intervention supports or services are typically offered.

Professional Correspondence

SLPs and audiologists often exchange information regarding clients with other professionals serving those same individuals. A variety of written correspondence formats are used to share client information, including **referral letters** to other service providers, **follow-up letters** to those professionals referring clients, and requests for the release of information from other service providers. At times, we write **letters of justification** to advocate for diagnostic or therapy services, hearing aids, FM Systems, communication devices, and other supports for our clients. In accordance with HIPAA and the ASHA Code of Ethics (ASHA, 2003) written permission must be obtained from a client before any information can be released between practitioners or agencies, and clients have the final decision about what information, if any, may be released and to whom.

REPORTING DIAGNOSTIC FINDINGS

It is essential for SLPs and audiologists to share diagnostic assessment findings in a manner that is efficient, well organized, and clearly understood by all who need access to this information. This process begins with a verbal review shared with your client and his or her family or caregivers immediately after the completion of the evaluation and continues with a written summary of findings that becomes a permanent record of this information.

Evaluation Feedback

Anyone seeking the help of professionals generally expects to have at least some feedback regarding findings immediately following an evaluation. Think about your last trip to your general physician for a comprehensive physical examination. Although you know that your doctor will not have the results of blood tests, throat cultures, biopsies, or other lab tests immediately following your examination, you would expect him or her to take a few minutes to summarize the general findings and their implications regarding your overall health status. Failure to do so would certainly leave you in a state of uncertainty and anxiety, potentially reducing your confidence in the physician's ability to effectively evaluate and manage your health needs. Individuals who seek a clinician's help in diagnosing hearing loss, swallowing, speech, language, and other communication disorders have a similar need for immediate feedback, and they experience many of the same concerns if a summary of the findings at the conclusion of the evaluation is not provided.

How can you immediately summarize your evaluation findings before you have had time to score tests, transcribe language samples, or carefully analyze the relationship between all of the diagnostic data collected during the course of an evaluation? First, clearly state that all comments made during follow-up counseling sessions are only your first impressions of diagnostic findings and will be subject to possible revision after you have had time to carefully analyze the information that you have collected. Second, review the purpose of the assessment activities and your initial impression of the outcomes of each in order to help the client begin to understand both the reasons for those activities and their implications concerning his or her communication status. Such a review provides you with a systematic and sequential structure through which to begin to relay your findings and helps you to convey information in smaller segments more easily processed by your client.

In addition to providing a mechanism to summarize evaluation results, engaging in post evaluation feedback presents an opportunity for audiologists and SLPs to continue the process of educating clients about communication disorders that began during the preassessment interview, a very important step in developing a partnership between the client and clinician. As is the case during an initial interview, the style in which you present information when counseling a client after an evaluation is as important as the content. Haynes and Pindzola (2004) cautioned to "refrain from being didactic; do not lecture your clients. Focus on sharing options rather than giving advice" (p. 43). You should begin your discussion with a summary of strengths demonstrated by the client and transition to areas of weakness in measured increments based on your perceptions of his or her ability to accept and process that information. Incorporate information about normal processes of hearing and communication, and relate this information to the profile of communication strengths and needs that you have identified for your client. Again, as in all clinical interactions, use language that is readily understood by clients, their family, and their caregivers. You must be alert to both verbal and nonverbal signals from your listeners regarding their level of understanding and you should paraphrase or modify the style and content of your statements accordingly. Remember that the counseling following a diagnostic assessment often takes place immediately after a long and sometimes arduous evaluation session that may leave the participants fatigued and emotionally drained. Too much technical information, information presented in a rapid and confusing manner, or information that is presented in a style inconsistent with the clients' cultures may be difficult to understand. Because some individual and cultural interaction styles may preclude listeners from letting you know that they do not understand what you are saying, you must not assume that your clients have comprehended your message simply because they nodded their heads or verbally agreed. You should allow opportunities for follow-up questions, and you should listen carefully to these questions to judge the listeners' comprehension of the information that you have presented.

By maintaining a flexible style in which you encourage ongoing comments and questions from your clients as you present diagnostic findings, you will create a two-way flow of communication rich with opportunities for further clarification of information and the establishment of a trusting therapeutic relationship. Remember that counseling remains an ongoing dynamic process woven into the continuum of clinical activities and does not end with the reporting of diagnostic findings. You must be prepared to develop and maintain an appropriate counseling role throughout the entire course of intervention.

Diagnostic Evaluation Reports

A diagnostic evaluation report serves as a tool for organizing, integrating, and interpreting information regarding a client's hearing and communication skills. A thorough report summarizes background information pertaining to a client's presenting concern, gives results of evaluation measures and observations, and allows for a discussion of the implication of those findings as related to the person's communication needs and potential. Such as all clinical records, diagnostic reports serve as legal documentation of assessment activities and findings long after the diagnostic event has passed. Both audiology and speech-language pathology reports are divided into subsections to more clearly organize information. The exact format and section headings of reports may vary from setting to setting but typically include background information, test results and other diagnostic data and observations, a summary, and recommendations based on the findings of the evaluation. In some settings, these sections follow the SOAP format. Figure 8.3 shows an example of a format for a speech-language diagnostic report from a university speech and hearing clinic.

Identifying Information   All reports begin with a section identifying the client who was evaluated, as well as other pertinent information regarding the type, setting, and date(s) of evaluation. The name(s) of the clinicians who conducted the evaluation, as well as their credentials, must be clearly listed. Other identifying information includes the client's address and telephone number, primary languages, parents or guardians if appropriate, and referral source. It is extremely important to list complete and accurate identifying information to facilitate record keeping and assure confidentiality.

Background History   Most diagnostic evaluations are at best a snapshot in time, reflecting the test data and observations collected during a limited period and often under conditions that do not represent the functional communication environments of the person being tested. One way that you can attempt to compensate for this partial view of your client's communicative competency is to summarize background information collected through written case histories, record reviews, and personal interviews with the client and his or her family members, educators, or other caregivers. This summary should be a succinct overview of medical and developmental diagnoses related to the presenting communication concerns; findings of previous speech, language, and audiological evaluations; and evaluations from other disciplines and reviews of any past or current speech, language, or audiological intervention. In the case of children, background summaries typically include a birth and developmental history and information regarding educational placement and related support services. In the case of adults, educational and vocational history is usually summarized. The individual's primary and any secondary languages should be identified, as well as any other considerations unique to the person that may influence the interpretation of evaluation findings.

Evaluation Conditions and Results   In the results section of a diagnostic report, all standardized tests and nonstandardized assessment procedures are listed, along with a brief explanation of what each test or procedure attempted to

Initial Communication Evaluation

Name: _____

Date of birth: _____ Chronological age: _____

Address: _____

Telephone (home): _____ (work):_____

Parent/guardian/spouse:_____ Relationship to client:_____

Referral source:_____ Date of evaluation: _____

Supervisor: _____ Clinician:_____

Background

• State referral information/reason for evaluation.

• Summarize birth/developmental history as appropriate.

• Identify primary language(s).

• Comment on findings of previous communication evaluations and other related evaluations.

• List medical/developmental diagnoses that relate to presenting communication disorder.

• Identify educational placement/modifications (children).

• Summarize history of past and current speech-language intervention; contacts made with other service providers.

Evaluation conditions

• Describe testing conditions (location, length of time, use of interpreter, augmentative communication, etc.).

• Describe client behavior during evaluation (attentiveness, cooperation, etc.).

• State your level of confidence in your findings, based on the above factors.

Figure 8.3. Initial communication evaluation.

(continued)

Results

• List standardized tests used, describe their purpose, and list scores obtained.

• List observed and derived data from nonstandardized evaluation tasks (MLU, frequency of stuttering, summary of language strengths and weaknesses, etc.).

Interpretation

• Describe findings related to presenting communication concerns (receptive language, expressive language, oral motor skills, speech production, voice, fluency, hearing, etc.).

• Synthesize data listed in the *Results* section.

• Answer diagnostic questions you posed when planning the evaluation.

• Conclude with a short statement summarizing findings, diagnosis, and contributing factors.

• State prognosis for improvement.

Recommendations

• State all recommendations as options to consider, not mandates to follow.

• Present a menu of options to achieve same result, if possible.

• Include suggestions for additional evaluations and related services, when appropriate.

• Provide suggestions for therapy goals and objectives, as well as frequency and duration of therapy, when appropriate.

John Doe, B.A.
Graduate Student Clinician

Jane Smith, M.A.
Supervising Speech-Language Pathologist

Figure 8.3. *(continued)*

accomplish. Normative test scores, data from nonstandardized evaluation tasks, and behavioral observations are listed in a brief narrative or table format. In speech-language evaluation reports, this section may contain a summary of communication strengths and weaknesses, whereas an audiological evaluation might report the results of a client's response to trial fittings of hearing aids, FM Systems, and other assistive listening devices. A description of the testing conditions, duration of testing, adaptations to standardized test administration protocols, and the level of cooperation and attention demonstrated by the individual being assessed is typically included to assist in appropriately interpreting evaluation results. Detailed analysis of evaluation findings, however, is usually reserved for the *interpretation* section of the report.

Interpretation   Once you have successfully summarized all of the data, you must then interpret those data to draw conclusions regarding the communication status of the individual. Similar to research projects, all communication evaluations begin with the evaluator framing a series of questions regarding the client's communication and hearing status (Tomblin, 2000). These questions guide the evaluator and provide the foundation for interpreting all evaluation results. In the interpretation section of an evaluation report, the clinician compares and interprets the data collected in relation to these questions or hypotheses. Because the data collected during an evaluation do not always point to the same conclusions, you must consider these data in relation to client behavior, evaluation conditions, pertinent background information, and other related factors in order to make a thoughtful interpretation of their meaning and draw conclusions relevant to your initial questions. You will not always be able to definitively answer the questions that you initially set out to explore during the evaluation. Based on careful interpretation of diagnostic data, however, you should be able to integrate and summarize the knowledge you have gained through the evaluation process and identify if any diagnostic questions remain fully or partially unanswered. Based on this summary, you must also include a statement of prognosis, estimating the likelihood that the individual can improve (or maintain) communication or hearing skills.

EXAMPLE OF A PROGNOSTIC STATEMENT

Prognosis for improvement of Jon's speech intelligibility through the elimination of speech sound errors appears fair to good, given his ability to imitate developmentally appropriate speech sounds and his strong family and educational support systems.

Recommendations   The recommendations section of a diagnostic report is often the first, and sometimes the only, section to be read by the numerous individuals who will review this document. In this section, recommendations regarding the need for follow-up intervention are stated based on the data collected during the evaluation and the conclusions outlined in the preceding interpretation section. The recommendations section reflects the culmination of the diagnostic process and serves as an important tool for determining an individual's need and eligibility for service. You may make recommendations for additional testing, either within the domain of the current evaluation or by professionals in other disciplines. Recommendations for equipment needs such as hearing aids and other assistive listening devices, augmentative and alternative communication devices, or educational materials can be stated. Recommendations are also sometimes included for modifications to home, educational, and vocational routines to better enhance communication skills in those settings. Potential intervention goals and objectives and the suggested frequency, duration, and model of intervention may be outlined. Realistic recommendations should be offered based on the individual client's needs and the priorities and values held by the client, his or her family members, and their community. Other factors necessary to implement the recommendations include the client's health status and the availability of time, money, and other resources. Recommendation statements usually take the form of numbered or bulleted statements but may at times include more narrative descriptions of recommended intervention strategies, adaptive equipment, or environmental or educational modifications.

EXAMPLES OF RECOMMENDATION STATEMENTS

1. Anita will benefit from speech-language intervention targeting the development of age-appropriate language and speech skills necessary for her successful participation in academic tasks and social routines. Specific focus should be placed on
   A. Increased speech intelligibility through the elimination of the sound error patterns of fronting and final consonant deletion
   B. Increased use of age appropriate syntax, including auxiliary verb forms, prepositions, and the possessive marker /s/
   C. Increased comprehension of vocabulary related to curricular and social demands
2. Anita should continue to be monitored regularly for signs of middle-ear infection and receive medical intervention as needed to minimize the risk of transient hearing loss due to middle-ear infection.
3. The SLP should collaborate with the classroom teacher to develop intervention activities that can be supported in the context of classroom-based activities.

CONTRIBUTING TO COMPREHENSIVE SERVICE PLANS

SLPs and audiologists often serve as contributing members of interdisciplinary and/or transdisciplinary service teams comprised of service providers from multiple disciplines, as well as of clients, of families, and of other stake holders. In this capacity, you will be called on to assist in the development of comprehensive service plans outlining the educational or rehabilitative supports offered to your clients. The formats of these plans will vary based on the age of the client and the service delivery setting. Regardless of their format, all comprehensive service plans serve as a legal mechanism for detailing the supports to be offered to a client, the time lines for delivery of these services, the people responsible for providing these supports, and the mechanisms for evaluating outcomes.

Individualized Family Service Plans

When the Education for All Handicapped Children Act of 1975 (PL 94-142) was reauthorized as the Education of the Handicapped Act Amendments of 1986 (PL 99-457), it introduced Part H in order to create a federally supported mechanism for the provision of early intervention services for children from birth to 3 years of age who demonstrated substantial and measurable delays in key developmental areas. More recently, the Individuals with Disabilities Education Improvement Act (IDEA) of 2004 (PL 108-446) has reauthorized that legislation, continuing a mechanism for early intervention as Part C. Early intervention services include adaptive/self-help skills (e.g., bathing, feeding, dressing), cognitive skills, physical development (e.g., gross and fine motor skills, hearing, vision), social and emotional development, and receptive and expressive communication skills. Services provided through this program are based on the concept of family-centered practice (see Chapter 13), with the child's family members serving as key team members and determiners of the type and focus of the intervention services. Assessment and intervention are implemented in the child's natural environment, and a major focus is placed not only on the specific developmental needs of the child but also on the needs of the child's family members.

Upon referral, a child undergoes a transdisciplinary developmental evaluation by two or more members of the birth-to-3 team. If the child meets eligibility requirements, team members will meet with the family members to develop an Individualized Family Service Plan (IFSP). Throughout this process, the child's family is encouraged to identify their child's likes, dislikes, strengths, and areas of need. A written IFSP document is developed to capture this information and will ultimately serve as the comprehensive guide to the family's individualized support (see Figure 8.4).

More global family needs, such as access to health care or adequate shelter or the needs of other siblings, are also discussed in recognition of the influence that such considerations have on the child's development. Early intervention specialists assist the family in identifying their priorities for support and then aid in developing a plan to meet those needs, helping the family to access needed services both within and outside of the birth-to-3 program. At times, the priorities stated by the family may differ with the priorities set by other team members, including the SLP and audiologist, but family-generated priorities always take precedence. This information is documented in the written IFSP document (see Figure 8.5). Once the child's strengths and needs and the family's priorities are identified, a plan of services and supports is developed. The team outlines in the plan the type of supports the team will need, the service providers responsibilities, and the location and schedule of the intervention services (see Figure 8.6). The completed IFSP document becomes the working guide to the child and family's participation in the birth-to-3 program. The document will be reviewed by the early intervention team periodically throughout the period the child is enrolled in the program and revised as needed. As is the case with all of the clinical intervention and documentation formats, you must rely on a style of presenting

---

Name: <u>Tonya Williams</u>   Date: <u>2/19/01</u>

1. Indicate the dates and types of evaluations or assessment reports that were used to develop this plan.

Eligibility evaluation of 2/14/01 and 2/16/01, parent interview, and family assessment of 2/16/01

2. Summarize additional observations by family and other team members of the child's abilities, strengths, and needs in day-to-day routines. Areas to include:

• Your child's likes and dislikes

• Your child's frustrations

• Daily routine/activities

• Bathing, feeding, dressing, and toileting (adaptive self-help skills)

• Thinking, reasoning, and learning (cognitive skills)

• Moving, hearing, vision, and health (physical development)

• Feelings, coping, and getting along with others (socioemotional development)

• Understanding, communicating with others, and expressing self with others (communication skills)

Tonya spends most of the day at home with her mother and grandmother, where she often plays in her room alone. In addition, she spends 3 hours each morning in a home-based child care center where she reportedly separates herself from the other children. She enjoys playing with stuffed animals. She likes to line them up in neat rows, move them, and line them up again. Tonya also spends time repeatedly stacking plastic rings on a post. She becomes quickly frustrated when someone tries to move her stuffed animals or other toys out of the order in which she placed them. At these times she will vocalize loudly and quickly restore her toys to their original order. Tonya becomes agitated when her mother and grandmother cannot figure out what she wants. She does not, however, appear to change strategies in order to make her needs known. Tonya is beginning to feed herself soft foods with a spoon and prefers cold foods to hot foods. She has not yet shown a readiness for toilet training.

See background information contained in eligibility report for more detailed developmental information.

Figure 8.4. Summary of a child's present abilities, strengths, and needs. (Courtesy of the Connecticut Birth to Three System, December 1999.)

information that is clear, supportive, and respectful to the needs of the families with whom you are working.

Individualized Education Programs

The Education for All Handicapped Children Act was passed in 1975, ensuring a free and appropriate public education and related services for all children regardless of their disability. This act has been amended and reauthorized several times

---

Family information for the individualized family service plan

Tonya lives with her mom and grandmother. The family enjoys watching television and visiting Tonya's aunt at her home across town. They are very involved in church activities and turn to their church for emotional support. Both mother and grandmother state that they "have not slept well since Tonya was born" and constantly worry over her well being.

What would be helpful for you or your family in the months and year ahead? (family outcome)

- Help in learning how to teach Tonya to "play like other kids"

- Assistance in finding safe, affordable housing

- Medical resources when family members are sick

What assistance or information will you need to achieve this outcome?

- Help in applying for financial assistance for housing and health care

- Someone to show the family how to play with Tonya

- Toys and books

Figure 8.5. Summary of a family's concerns, priorities, and resources as they relate to enhancing their child's development. (Courtesy of the Connecticut Birth to Three System, December 1999.)

Name: Tonya Williams   Date of birth: 2/3/98   Date: 2/19/01

What is going to happen	Delivered by (discipline responsible)	Location	How often	How long	Start date
Instructional home visit	Early intervention specialist (teacher)	Family's home	Once per week	1 hour	3/5/01
Speech therapy consultation	Speech-language pathologist	Family's home	Once per month	1 hour	4/2/01
Nursing consultation	Nurse	Family's home	Twice per month	1 hour	3/12/01

Figure 8.6. Early intervention services and supports. (Courtesy of the Connecticut Birth to Three System, December 1999.)

over the ensuing years and is currently encompassed in IDEA'04, which specifies that educators develop an annual IEP for children ages 3–21 who are determined eligible for special education services. An IEP is a comprehensive written document identifying the specialized resources needed to maximize the academic success of students who have met eligibility requirements due to academic-based learning impairments, such as speech, language, and hearing disorders. The process leading to the development of an IEP begins with the informal identification of children with special needs by classroom teachers; parents; family members; or specialists such as SLPs, psychologists, or social workers. A prereferral screening process is used to estimate the nature and extent of the child's problems and their potential influence on academic success. If, after an initial period in which trial strategies and modifications to academic tasks and classroom routines are implemented, the child continues to exhibit problems that are likely to have a negative influence on academic success, a more formalized evaluation process is initiated. In this phase, the SLP serving the school may be asked to complete and document a more comprehensive speech-language evaluation if communication problems appear to contribute to the child's academic difficulties. This evaluation may include both standardized testing and nonstandardized assessment and observation of the student communicating in classroom or other social settings. An interdisciplinary **planning and placement team (PPT)** reviews the results of this evaluation, along with the results from evaluations by educators and professionals in other disciplines who may have been called into the process. The PPT determines the appropriateness of special education services based on state and federal eligibility criteria. If eligible, an IEP is developed at a PPT meeting to outline specific educational services and modifications designed to meet the student's individualized learning needs. The IEP document is typically handwritten on a prepared fill-in-the-blank form and is completed by the conclusion of the PPT meeting.

The components of an IEP are clearly specified in IDEA'04. The IEP document begins with a cover sheet with identifying information regarding the child, his or her family members, the participating team members, and the reason for the PPT meeting. Subsequent sections summarize the child's present level of educational performance in the areas of health and development (e.g., vision, hearing); academic, cognitive, and social/emotional/behavioral skills; motor and communication abilities; activities of daily living; and vocational domains. These summaries are generated from observations of classroom performance, parent reports, and direct assessment results. Not all domains may be reviewed, given the age and presenting concerns of the child. The SLP participating on the planning and placement team may be called upon to contribute both formalized evaluation findings and more incidental observations of the child's communication skills. As part of this discussion, the SLP should employ the principles of effective oral and written communication discussed earlier in this chapter. Based on this cumulative information, the team ultimately decides if the child's disability affects his or her involvement and progress in the general academic or preschool curriculum and if the child's intervention may be eligible for federally funded special education services.

Once eligibility has been determined, the team proceeds to formulate and record annual goals and short-term objectives based on the child's needs. Broad-based goals, including those in the communication domain, are written in functional terms that directly relate to the child's success in an academic environment and are followed by measurable short-term objectives that support those goals. Methods of evaluating progress and a schedule and place for reviewing and recording the child's outcomes are also included in this section (see Figure 8.7).

☐ Academic/cognitive	☐ Social/behavioral	☒ Communication	☐ Gross/fine motor	☐ Employment/postsecondary education
☐ Self help	☐ Community participation	☐ Independent living	☐ Health	☐ Other: (specify) _____

☐ **Check here if the student is 15 years of age.**

Measurable Annual Goal Number (linked to present levels of performance) ____1____

Eric will demonstrate improved _receptive language skills allowing him to participate in grade level_

curricular activities

	Enter Dates For Evaluating and Reporting Progress in Boxes Below			
	9/30	10/31	11/28	1/5
	2/2	3/3	4/30	6/1

Eval. Procedure: _10_

Perf. Criteria: _A_

(%, Trials, etc.): _75%_

Report Progress Below (Use Reporting Key)

9/30	10/31	11/28	1/5
S	S		
2/2 S	3/3 S		

Short Term Objectives/Benchmarks (linked to achieving progress towards annual goal)

Obj. 1 ___Eric will___ _demonstrate understanding of 2-step directions related to academic routines_

by listening to each complete direction, restating the direction, and correctly following the instruction

Eval. Procedure: _10_

Perf. Criteria: _A_

(%, Trials, etc.): _75%_

Report Progress Below (Use Reporting Key)

9/30	10/31	11/28	1/5
S	S	M	
2/2 S	3/3 S		

Obj. 2 ___Eric will___ _demonstrate comprehension of later developing "wh" questions "when", "why", and "how"_

by producing correct verbal responses to targeted question forms in the context of curriculum based

activities

Eval. Procedure: _10_

Perf. Criteria: _A_

(%, Trials, etc.): _75%_

Report Progress Below (Use Reporting Key)

9/30	10/31	11/28	1/5
S	S		
2/2 S	3/3 S		

Figure 8.7. Example of goal and objective documentation on an individual education plan (IEP). (*Key:* Eval. = evaluation, Perf. = performance, Obj. = objective, % = percentage, CMT = Connecticut Master Test, CAPT = Connecticut Academic Performance Test.) (Courtesy of the Connecticut State Department of Education. [2005]. *IEP Manual and Forms.* Retrieved March 3, 2006, from http://www.state.ct.us/sde/deps/Special/IEPManual.pdf)

(continued)

Obj. 3   Eric will demonstrate comprehension of prepositions "under", "behind", "in front of",
and "next to" by pointing to appropriate picture stimuli or manipulating objects during classroom-based
activities _____

Eval. Pocedure: 1,3

Perf. Criteria: A

(%, Trials, etc.:) 75%

Report Progress Below (Use Reporting Key)

NS	S	S

Evaluation Procedures		Performance Criteria	
1. Criterion-referenced/curriculum-based assessment	7. Behavior/performance rating scale	A. Percent of change	F. Duration
2. Pre and post standardized assessment	8. CMT/CAPT	B. Months growth	G. Successful completion of task/activity
3. Pre and post base line data	9. Work samples, job performance or products	C. Standard score increase	H. Mastery
4. Quizzes/tests	10. Achievement of objectives (Note: use with goal only)	D. Passing grades/score	I. Other: (specify) _____
5. Student self-assessment/rubric	11. Other: (specify) _____	E. Frequency/trials	J. Other: (specify) _____
6. Project/experiment/portfolio	12. Other: (specify) _____		

Progress Reporting Key: *(indicating extent to which progress is sufficient to achieve goal by the end of the year)*   **M** = Mastered   **S** = Satisfactory progress— likely to achieve goal   **U** = Unsatisfactory progress—unlikely to achieve goal   **N** = No progress—will not achieve goal   **NI** = Not introduced   **O** = Other: (specify)

Figure 8.7.   *(continued)*

228

SUMMARY: SPECIAL EDUCATION, RELATED SERVICES, AND REGULAR EDUCATION

Special education	Goal	Hours/ week	Staff responsible	Start date	End date	Site
Reading instruction	5,6	5	Special education teacher	9/1/00	6/5/00	2
Related services						
Speech-language pathology	1,2,3	2	Speech-language pathologist Speech assistant	9/1/00	6/5/00	1,4
Occupational therapy	4		Occupational therapist	9/1/00	6/5/00	1

Instructional site (indicate all that apply)
1. Regular classroom   2. Resource room   3. Self-contained classroom   4. Related service office/classroom
5. Community-based   6. Other: (specify) _____

Figure 8.8. Identifying educational support services on an individual education plan (IEP). (Courtesy of the Connecticut State Department of Education. [2005]. *IEP Manual and Forms.* Retrieved March 3, 2006, from http://www.state.ct.us/sde/deps/Special/IEPManual.pdf)

The team then documents the specific education resources allocated to the child. These include services such as speech-language therapy, physical therapy or other supports, the hours each week that those services will be delivered, beginning and ending dates, and the parties responsible for implementing the service (see Figure 8.8). The instructional site (e.g., regular classroom, resource room, related services office) for each service is identified, and the need for assistive technology (e.g., communication devices, FM Systems) is identified as well. Any modifications to the child's academic schedule are listed, as are accommodations for hearing and vision impairments, behavior challenges, or limited English proficiency.

A placement summary outlines the rationale for the type and location of educational placement chosen, as well as exit criteria from special education. IDEA'04 mandates that school systems provide education for all students in the least restrictive environment. Modifications and adaptations in general education settings are indicated, including specialized instructional strategies; organizational supports; behavior management support; testing procedures; and adaptations to materials, books, and equipment (see Figure 8.9).

Individualized Transition Plans

Under IDEA'04, the focus of educational goals and objectives for students 16–21 years old shifts to include training in independent living and employment-related skills. An effort is made to involve members from the client's educational team and representatives from adult support agencies in this transitional planning process. An **individual transition plan (ITP)** may be developed as an integrated component of the client's IEP and is designed to identify the specific skills and supports that the client will need to make a successful transition. The focus of goals and objectives may shift somewhat at this point from academic development to independent living, community participation, and prevocational

Program Accommodations and Modifications—INCLUDING NONACADEMIC AND EXTRACURRICULAR ACTIVITIES/COLLABORATION/SUPPORT FOR SCHOOL PERSONNEL	
Accommodations and Modifications to be Provided to Enable the Child	**Sites/Activities Where Required and Duration**
To advance appropriately toward attaining his/her annual goals To be involved in and make progress in the general education curriculum To participate in extracurricular and other non-academic activities To be educated and participate with other children with and without disabilities	
Accommodations May Include Assistive Technology Devices and Services	
Materials/books/equipment:	
Supplementary visuals, frequency modulation (FM) systems auditory trainer, access to computer in classroom	Regular classroom, resource room
Tests/quizzes/assessments:	
Alternative tests, extra time, preview test procedures, simplify test wording, allow extra response time	Regular classroom, resource room
Grading:	
Base grade on ability	
Organization:	Regular classroom, resource room
Provide study outlines, give one paper at a time, assist student to make daily assignment and homework lists, post routines and assignments near students work areas	

Environment:

Preferential seating away from sources of noise and visual distractions

Regular classroom, resource room

Behavioral interventions and support:

Daily feedback to student regarding performance, visual progress charts, alert student prior to transitions

Regular classroom
All settings

Instructional strategies:

Check work in progress, use manipulatives, employ a multi-sensory learning approach with emphasis on visual information, verbal and

visual reinforcement, preteach content with emphasis on key vocabulary

Regular classroom, resource room

Other:

Note: When specifying required supports for personnel to implement this IEP, include the specific supports required, how often they are to be provided (frequency) and or how long (duration)

Frequency and Duration of Supports Required for School Personnel to Implement This IEP Include:
Speech-language pathologist to train classroom teachers and instructional aid in use of Frequency Modulatory System during the first 2 weeks of term;
Special education teacher and speech-language pathologist to consult with regular classroom teacher regarding multimodality teaching strategies

Figure 8.9. Educational modifications as outlined on an individual education plan (IEP). (Courtesy of the Connecticut State Department of Education. [2005]. *IEP Manual and Forms.* Retrieved March 3, 2006, from http:-/www.state.ct.us/sde/deps/Special/IEPManual.pdf)

231

Transition Planning

1. ☐ NA: Student has not reached the age of 15 and transition planning is not required or appropriate at this time.

2. ☒ This is the first IEP to be in effect following the child's 15th birthday (or younger if appropriate and transition planning is required).

3. Student Preferences/Interests: (document the following)
   a) Was the student invited to attend his or her PPT meeting? ☒ Yes ☐ No
   b) Did the student attend? ☒ Yes ☐ No
   c) How were the student's preferences/interests, as they relate to planning for Transition Services, determined?
      ☒ Age appropriate informal/formal assessment ☒ Functional vocational evaluations
      ☒ Personal interviews ☐ Other: (specify)
      ☒ Comments at meeting

   d) Summarize student preferences/interests as they relate to planning for Transition Services:

      Jamal's preferences include physical activities, social interaction, and being outdoors

4. Anticipated Post Secondary Outcomes: (check all that apply)
   ☐ Post-secondary education ☐ Adult services
   ☐ Vocational education ☒ Independent living or community participation
   ☐ Integrated employment

5. Agency Participation: ☐ NA
   a) Were any outside agencies invited to attend the PPT meeting? ☐ Yes ☐ No (if no, specify reason) _____
   b) If yes, did the agency's representative attend? ☒ Yes ☐ No
   c) Has any participating agency agreed to provide or pay for services/linkages? ☐ Yes ☒ No, (if yes, specify)

6. Summary of the Transition Services recommended in this IEP and settings(s) where these services will be provided: (complete the items below that apply)
   a) ☐ An Employment/Post Secondary Education goal and related objectives will be developed and implemented in the following setting(s): (check each that applies)
      ☐ School based instruction/activities ☐ Community based experiences/activities
   b) ☐ An Independent Living Goal and related objectives will be developed and implemented in the following setting(s): (check each that applies)
      ☐ School based instruction/activities ☐ Community based experiences/activities
   c) ☒ A Community Participation Goal and related objectives will be developed and implemented in the following setting(s): (check each that applies)
      ☒ School based instruction/activities ☒ Community based experiences/activities

7. If the student has transition goals and related objectives, respond to the following: ☐ NA
   a) The course of study needed to assist the child in reaching the transition goals and related objectives will include: (e.g. Student will be enrolled in college prep courses/student will participate in career awareness exploration classes):

   Jamal will participate in vocational preference assessment and individual and small group community-based instruction

   b) The related services needed to assist the child in reaching the transition goals and related objectives will include:

   Speech-language pathology consultation, social skills training

   c) The assistive technology devices and/or services needed to assist the child in reaching the transition goals and related objectives will include:

   Voice-output augmentative communication device, assistive technology assessment/consultation

8. At least one year prior to reaching age of 18, the student must be informed of their rights under IDEA which will transfer at age 18.
   ☒ NA (student will not be 17 within one year)
   ☐ The student has been informed of her/his rights under IDEA which will transfer at age 18
   ☐ No IDEA rights will transfer

9. For a child whose eligibility under special education will terminate the following year due to graduation with a regular education diploma or due to exceeding the age of eligibility, the Summary of Performance will be completed on or before: (specify date) _____ ☐ NA

   Parents please note: Rights afforded to parents under the Individuals with Disabilities Education Act (IDEA) transfer to students at the age of 18, unless legal guardianship has been obtained.

Figure 8.10. Individual Transition Plan. (*Key:* NA = Not applicable, PPT = planning and placement team, IEP = individual education plan, IDEA = Individuals with Disabilities Education Improvement Act of 2004 [PL 108-4660].) (Courtesy of the Connecticut State Department of Education. [2005]. *IEP Manual and Forms.* Retrieved March 3, 2006 from http://www.state.ct.us/sde/deps/Special/IEPManual.pdf)

skills. The transition plan is recorded as part of the overall IEP document (see Figure 8.10).

An SLP's role in the IEP process continues after the development of the initial plan and involves subsequent implementation and review of the components of the IEP. Audiologists, although not always physically present during planning and placement team meetings, also contribute to the development and implementation of IEPs through consulting with the team, writing diagnostic reports, and communicating to the team via the school-based SLP.

CONCLUSION

The act of obtaining, relaying, and documenting clinical information is a multifaceted task that requires you to integrate writing abilities, interpersonal skills, cultural sensitivity, and clinical knowledge in order to serve clients, their families, and their caregivers effectively. It is a process in which form does not follow function but rather blends with it to create an effective format for information sharing. It is a process that we refine throughout the entire course of our clinical education and subsequent professional practice as audiologists and SLPs. We will serve our clients most effectively if we remember that, in addition to increasing their communication skills, we have an obligation to refine our own.

REFERENCES

American Speech-Language-Hearing Association (1991). A model for collaborative service delivery for students with language-learning disorders in the public schools. *ASHA, Supplement, 5,* 44–50.

American Speech-Language-Hearing Association (2002). *A workload analysis approach for establishing speech-language caseload standards in the schools: Guidelines.* Rockville, MD: Author.

American Speech-Language-Hearing Association (2003). Code of ethics (revised). *ASHA Supplement, 23,* 13–15.

American Speech-Language-Hearing Association (2004). Admission/discharge criteria in speech language pathology. *ASHA Supplement, 24,* 65–70.

Anderson, P.P., & Fenichel, E.S. (1989). *Serving culturally diverse families of infants and toddlers with disabilities.* Washington, DC: National Center for Clinical Infant Programs.

Battle, D.E. (2002). *Communication disorders in multicultural populations* (3rd ed.). Boston: Butterworth-Heinemann.

Coleman, T.J. (2000). *Clinical management of communication disorders in culturally diverse children.* Boston: Allyn & Bacon.

Connecticut State Department of Education. (2005). *IEP Manual and Forms.* Retrieved March 3, 2006, from http://www.state.ct.us/sde/deps/Special/IEPManual.pdf

Education for All Handicapped Children Act of 1975, PL 94-142, 20 U.S.C. §§ 1400 *et seq.*

Education of the Handicapped Act Amendments of 1986, PL 99-457, 20 U.S.C. §§ 1400 *et seq.*

Golper, L.G. (1998). *Sourcebook for medical speech pathology* (2nd ed.). San Diego: Singular Publishing Group.

Hall, P.H., & Morris, H.L. (2000). The clinical history. In J.B. Toblin, H.L Morris, & D.C Spriestersbach (Eds.), *Diagnosis in speech-language pathology* (2nd ed., pp. 65–82). San Diego: Singular Publishing Group.

Haynes W.O., & Pindzola, R.H. (2004). *Diagnosis and evaluation in speech pathology* (6th ed.). Boston: Allyn & Bacon.

Health Insurance Portability and Accountability Act of 1996, PL 104-191, 42 U.S.C. §§ 201 *et seq.*

Individuals with Disabilities Educational Improvement Act of 2004, PL 108-466, 20 U.S.C. §§ 1400 *et seq.*

Langdon, H.W., & Cheng, L.L. (1992). *Hispanic children and adults with communication disorders: Assessment and intervention.* New York: Aspen Publishers.

Luteman, D.M. (2001). *Counseling the communicatively disordered and their families* (4th ed.). Austin, TX: PRO-ED.

Lynch, E.W. & Hanson, M.J. (2004). *Developing cross-cultural competence: A guide for working with children and their families* (3rd ed.). Baltimore: Paul H. Brookes Publishing Co.

Maltz, D., & Borker, R. (1982). A cultural approach to male-female miscommunication. In J.J. Gumperz (Ed.), *Language and social identity: Studies in international sociolinguistics* (pp. 146–216). New York: Cambridge University Press.

Meitus, I.J. (1983). Clinical report and letter writing. In I.J. Meitus & B. Weinberg (Eds.), *Diagnosis in speech-language pathology* (pp. 287–301). Boston: Allyn & Bacon.

Roseberry-McKibbin, C. (2002). *Multicultural students with special language needs: Practical strategies for assessment and intervention* (2nd ed.). Oceanside, CA: Academic Communication Associates.

Rollin, W.J. (2000). *Counseling individuals with communication disorders psychodynamic and family aspects* (2nd ed.). Boston: Butterworth-Heinemann.

Roth, F.P., & Worthington, C.K. (2005). *Treatment resource manual for speech-language pathology* (3rd ed.). Clifton Park, NY: Thomson Delmar Learning.

Shames, G.H. (2000). *Counseling the communicatively disabled and their families: A manual for clinicians.* Boston: Allyn & Bacon.

Shapiro, D.A. (1999). *Stuttering intervention: A collaborative journey to fluency freedom.* Austin, TX: PRO-ED.

Shipley, K.G., & McAfee, J.G. (2004). *Assessment in speech-language pathology: A resource Manual* (3rd ed.). Clifton Park, NY: Thomson Delmar Learning.

Silverman, F.H. (2003). *Essentials of professional issues in speech-language pathology and audiology.* Long Grove, IL: Waveland Press.

Stone, J.R., & Olswang, L.B. (1989). The hidden challenge in counseling. *ASHA, 31,* 27–31.

Tomblin, J.B. (2000). Perspectives on diagnosis. In J.B. Tomblin, H.L. Morris, & D.C. Spriestersbach, (Eds.), *Diagnosis in speech-language pathology* (2nd ed., pp. 3–33). San Diego: Singular Publishing Group.

Willis, W.O. (2004). Families with African American roots. In E.W. Lynch & M.J. Hanson (Eds.), *Developing cross-cultural competence: A guide for working with children and their families* (3rd ed., pp. 141–177). Baltimore: Paul H. Brookes Publishing Co.

Zungia, M.E. (2004). Families with Latino roots. In E.W. Lynch & M.J. Hanson (Eds.), *Developing cross-cultural competence: A guide to working with children and their families* (3rd ed., pp. 179–217). Baltimore: Paul H. Brookes Publishing Co.

STUDY QUESTIONS

1. Describe at least four principles of effective oral and written communi-cation.

2. Discuss the advantages of using an in-person interview rather than a written case history questionnaire to gain background information from your clients.

3. Name three cultural factors that may influence a person's responses to interview questions.

4. Explain the importance of follow-up counseling as a component of diag-nostic assessment.

5. What criteria are used to determine if a particular topic is appropriate for an audiologist or SLP to address during a clinical counseling session?

6. Describe the components of an individual intervention plan for speech-language therapy.

7. Compare and contrast the purpose of the following documents: individ-ual intervention plan, SOAP note, progress report, and discharge summary.

8. Describe the purpose and format of at least one comprehensive service plan.

CHAPTER 9

Public Policies Affecting Clinical Practice

NICKOLA W. NELSON, YVETTE D. HYTER, AND MICHELE A. ANDERSON

Public policies influence clinical service provision at all age levels, from early infancy through late adulthood. They play a significant role in determining how clinical decisions are made, where and when clinical services are provided, and how (and if) clinical expenses are reimbursed. Public policies vary with and are related to the broader systems in which clients are assessed and treated—home, educational, employment, or health care settings. Moreover, public policies can change at any time, which is both good and bad news. The good news is that ineffective policies can be modified, which can be reassuring when a policy clearly has negative effects. The bad news is that effective policies can be modified, which has the possibility of changing a policy with clearly positive effects in negative ways. Therefore, vigilance must be maintained, and professionals clearly should be ready to advocate on behalf of individuals with communication disorders and the services that they need.

What makes a good, effective policy? As clinical practitioners, we coauthors take the position that a good policy is one that leads to increased access to services and other communication opportunities for individuals whose communication disorders put them at risk for educational, vocational, or social disadvantage. Such definitions, however, are sometimes ambiguous. Policies can limit the access that individuals have to interventions, with possible negative effects on individuals' potential for recovery from acute or chronic conditions. For example, Medicare periodically has placed a $1,500 reimbursement limit on fees for speech-language pathology and physical therapy services. This policy has the potential to negatively affect individuals who cannot afford to pay for services. Although from a societal perspective, a reimbursement limit may be an essential step toward keeping Medicare solvent, from the perspective of an individual's access to care, the policy is a bad one because it may force a choice as to whether the ability to walk or talk should be the priority for treatment. Another example is the No Child Left Behind Act (NCLB; PL 107-110). Although it raises the expectation for all children to develop literacy abilities, which is clearly an admirable goal, it could have unintended negative consequences on schools that are penalized if students with disabilities do not meet the law's expectation.

This chapter provides an overview of key public policies that have implications for clinical service provision. Clinicians who are knowledgeable about policies can implement them accurately, recognize when variations are allowable within policy boundaries, and decide when and how to advocate actively for changes if necessary. This overview emphasizes each policy's major features rather than its specific details. As public policies change frequently, it is recommended that professionals also review updated policy versions, which are readily accessible on web sites maintained by policy-making agencies, professional associations, and other advocacy groups.

DEFINING PUBLIC POLICY

Public policy has been defined as any action (or lack thereof) taken by local, state, or federal officials to address a given problem or set of problems (Dye, 1998). Public policies may be established at federal, state, and local levels and can occur in many forms, such as laws, regulations, guidelines, and court decisions. Policies may apply to the development of programs, the distribution of money or benefits, or the levying of taxes (Dye, 1975, 1998; Lieurance, 1993).

Laws begin as bills that move through legislative committees. After they are passed by legislative bodies, they are reconciled as necessary and signed into law by executive officials, who then become responsible for implementing them. **Regulations** are generated by executive agencies charged with interpreting and implementing particular laws. Before passage, proposed regulations are generally opened for a period of public comment. Both laws and regulations require action by the regulatory and legislative bodies that originated them before they can be changed. **Guidelines** are developed by entities such as communities, school districts, health care agencies, hospitals, or professional associations to provide interpretations of how legislative and regulatory mandates are to be implemented in specific settings. Guidelines carry less legal weight than laws and regulations, but they also are easier to change. Finally, court decisions, known as **case law**, influence how policies are implemented when disputes are taken to court and result in decisions that have implications broader than the single case.

EDUCATIONAL LAWS: HISTORICAL ROOTS

Policies evolve along with shifts in social priorities. Educational policy is one case in point. The 1960s were a period in the history of the United States of America that saw changes associated with civil, human, and educational rights for groups of people who were economically marginalized. During this time, several education laws were passed, many of which derived from the Elementary and Secondary Education Act of 1965 (ESEA'65; PL 89-10). ESEA'65 was aimed at improving the educational opportunities for children living in poverty by providing resources for instruction (Title I) and for educational research and training (Education Trust, 2003). The subsequent amendments to ESEA'65 supported programs for children with disabilities and for bilingual education. Three critical amendments to the ESEA were made during the 1960s: 1) ESEA Amendments of 1966 (PL 89-750) assigned funds for states to provide educational services to children with disabilities in state-operated schools and institutions; 2) ESEA

Amendments of 1968 (PL 90-247; also known as Title VI, the Rural Education Initiative) authorized educational services for children with disabilities at the local, rather than state, level and established the Bureau of Education for the Handicapped (BEH) and National Council on Disability; 3) the Bilingual Education Act (BEA) of 1968 (PL 90-247; also known as Title VII) supported programs for children with disabilities through funding for research and training of educational personnel, and also supported programs for bilingual education. The BEA offered support to school districts for meeting the needs of English language learners (ELLs) including those with limited English proficiency (National Dissemination Center for Children and Youth with Disabilities [NICHCY], 1996). The BEA expired in January 2002, the same month in which the NCLB act was put into place. The co-occurrence of these events is particularly noteworthy because the BEA emphasized support for the development of the students' proficiency in the English language by teaching in tandem with the students' native language (Crawford, 2002); whereas the NCLB act, which is discussed in the following section, emphasizes the development of English proficiency and requires that students be tested in English.

NO CHILD LEFT BEHIND ACT

On January 8, 2002, President George W. Bush signed into law the NCLB act. NCLB emphasizes that schools are accountable for providing "high-quality" education that results in adequate educational achievement for all children. The law consists of four primary components: 1) how schools are held accountable for their students' academic results, 2) the flexibility that schools have in meeting the law's requirements, 3) the methods that are emphasized as effective, and 4) the options parents can take if their children do not show adequate educational improvement within their schools (U.S. Department of Education, 2002).

Accountability is defined as the legal requirement of educational agencies to ensure that students in all racial and ethnic groups, including students with disabilities and students affected by socioeconomic disadvantage, achieve academic proficiency. Accountability is measured through the annual statewide testing of all students in third through eighth grade. Scoring goals set by the state define adequate yearly progress (AYP) for each school. Schools and school districts that meet AYP are eligible for State Academic Achievement Awards; those that do not meet AYP are targeted for corrective action and improvement. The student population that provides the scores on which the AYP is based includes many subpopulations. Of the subpopulations that are classified as high risk, the scores of at least 95% of students within those subpopulations must contribute to the AYP. The subpopulations classified as high risk are: 1) economically disadvantaged students, 2) students from major racial or ethnic groups, 3) students with disabilities, and 4) students with limited English proficiency. The U.S. Secretary of Education, issued an interpretation in April 2005 in which she indicated that 3% (a revision of the originally specified 1%) of students with disabilities (largely students with developmental disabilities) would be allowed to take alternate annual assessment tests without penalizing the AYP result of the school or school district (U.S. Department of Education, 2005). Accommodations, modifications, or alternative assessment tests for students with disabilities must also be consistent with the requirements of the current version of IDEA (Annett, 2003).

School districts are permitted by law to apply federal education monies to improve student outcomes and a portion of the funds for special education may be used to support general education activities. *Flexibility* is defined as the school districts' ability to use these federal monies with discretion in ways that are tailor-made for their particular contexts. Flexibility, for example, allows schools to use special education monies to hire speech-language pathologists (SLPs) to take part in preventive and identification activities in general education that will affect students with disabilities (Annett, 2003). For schools that fail to make AYP, the SLPs potentially could then be approved as supplemental education service contractors, which are not considered part of special education.

Effective methods are methods that have been satisfactorily demonstrated to have a positive effect on student education. NCLB identifies *five essential components* that should be targeted within reading instruction: 1) *phonemic awareness,* which involves noticing, thinking about, and working with individual sounds in spoken words; 2) *phonics instruction,* which involves associating written language letters (graphemes) with spoken language speech sounds (phonemes); 3) *fluency,* which involves reading a text quickly as well as accurately; 4) *vocabulary,* which affects fluency, comprehension, and formulation for listening, speaking, reading, and writing; and 5) *text comprehension,* which involves purposeful and active construction of text meaning. Federal funding also is available through NCLB for a variety of special programs—Reading First, Early Reading First, Even Start Family Literacy, and Even Start Migrant Education Program. Grants for these initiatives can be obtained through competitive federal and state application processes (Moore-Brown & Montgomery, 2005).

Parental choice permits the parents of students who are attending schools that fail to meet AYP for two consecutive years to elect to send their children to different schools of their choice. In such instances, school districts are required to spend up to 20% of their Title I monies to provide alternative school options for qualified families.

Several critics have raised concerns about the ability of the NCLB legislation to address educational needs for all children adequately and fairly (see e.g., Metcalf, 2002; Meyer, 2004). Concerns include that: 1) the law is under-funded; 2) testing in a "one size fits all" model focuses on limited skills; 3) the English language tests "leave behind" students who have limited English proficiency; 4) the government's interpretations of the research contain discrepancies, which also may be biased by the close relationships among policy makers, research funders, and test and curriculum developers (see Metcalf, 2002). An even more basic concern is that schools in impoverished communities are unlikely to achieve AYP goals without extensive changes in unequal socioeconomic structures.

INDIVIDUALS WITH DISABILITIES EDUCATION ACT

In the 1970s, the previous laws and amendments of the ESEA for students with special needs were united into one act, which became known as Part B of the Education of the Handicapped Act of 1970 (EHA; PL 91-230)—the antecedent to the Education for All Handicapped Children Act of 1975 (EAHA; PL 94-142; Education Trust, 2003; NICHCY, 1996). The EHA was the first iteration and predecessor to the Individuals with Disabilities Education Act when it was reauthorized in 1990 and became known by the acronym IDEA (PL 101-476). In 2004, the act was reauthorized once more as the Individuals with Disabilities

Education Improvement Act (PL 108-446), although it still carries the official designation IDEA. This law took effect July 1, 2005, but the *code of federal regulations (CFR)*, with implementation specifications for the revised act, were not approved until the summer of 2006. The term *improvement* in the title of the law signaled the lawmakers' goal to align IDEA with provisions of NCLB (Moore-Brown & Montgomery, 2005).

The purpose of IDEA, from the time it was originally passed in 1991 until IDEA'04, has been to ensure that all children with disabilities have access to a *free appropriate public education (FAPE)* in the *least restrictive environment (LRE)*. IDEA has four major parts:

- *Part A* includes definitions and general provisions

- *Part B* specifies how services are to be provided to preschool and school-age students

- *Part C* specifies requirements for service provision to infants and toddlers and their families

- *Part D* includes provisions for supporting research, personnel preparation, technical assistance, support, and dissemination of information for improving the education of children with disabilities

As noted, Part B regulates the provision of services for children with disabilities aged 6–21 years and includes *Section 619,* which provides grant funding to states for services for preschool children aged 3–5 years. With IDEA '04, families who have been receiving services under Part C may elect to continue receiving services from their Part C provider using an Individualized Family Service Plan (IFSP). Alternately, families could begin to receive services through Part B, in which case they would have an Individualized Education Program (IEP) with services provided by a public education agency.

IFSPs define the service unit as the family rather than the child. Development of IFSPs requires decisions to be made about a family's service needs and mandates family representation in the decision-making process. IFSPs include statements of: 1) the present development level of the infant or toddler; 2) the family's resources, priorities, and concerns; 3) the major outcomes expected; 4) the specific early intervention services; 5) the natural environments in which services shall occur; 6) the projected dates of initiation of services and length thereof; 7) the identification of the service coordinator, and 8) the steps to be taken to support the transition to preschool or other educational levels. IFSPs must be revised at least every six months. Figure 9.1 contains a sample IFSP that shows how one school district interpreted these components.

Alternately, depending on state-level decisions for implementing IDEA, families could begin to receive services through Part B when their children reach 3 years of age, in which case they would have an IEP with services provided by a public education agency. Identification of students with disabilities under Part B of IDEA'04 must involve consideration of whether the child has had appropriate instruction in reading, including the essential components of reading instruction as defined in NCLB. In determining eligibility, IEP teams must review existing evaluation data, including local and state assessments. A major change in IDEA'04 is that IEP teams are no longer required to consider a severe discrepancy between achievement and intellectual ability in determining whether a child has a specific learning disability. As an alternative, they may use a process that determines

Referral date: 2/11/06

Person referring: D. Smith

Today's date: 2/12/06

Agency initiating IFSP: Public School

Child Information   Social security number: 111-11-1111

Child's legal name: Janna Johnson   Nickname: Janna   Date of Birth: 11/1/03   Sex: Female

Address: 123 Main Street   Telephone (home): 500-555-5555   Telephone (child care): 500-555-5554

Great Falls, USA   Medical insurance number: 123456789

School district of residence: Sussex   County: Columbia   Ethnic heritage: African American   Native language: English

Child's Family Members

Name	Relationship to child	Birth date (optional)	Address	Telephone (home)	Telephone (work)
Mike Johnson	Father		Same as above	Same	500-555-1212
Sharika Johnson	Mother		Same	Same	500-555-1234
Isaac Johnson	Brother	7/13/01	Same	Same	N/A

If parent/guardian needs an interpreter, list language:

Agencies and Person Working with the Family (fill in anytime)

Start date	Agency	Contact Person	Telephone	Type of service or title	End date	Send copy of IFSP?
11/5/05	Health Services Hospital	Isabel Jones	500-222-2222	Audiologist		Yes
1/5/06	Sussex Public School	Diane Smith	500-333-3333	Speech-language pathologist		

Child's Strengths and Needs

Child's name: Janna Johnson   Birth weight: 7.2 pounds   Birth date: 11/1/03   Number of weeks premature: N/A

Area	Present level of development		Date	Name or type of evaluation	Person doing evaluation	Agency
	Parent input	Professional input				
General	Very expressive, and "laid back;" a good baby	Speech therapy, continues hearing impairment services after a Cochlear implant	1/15/04	Cognitive screening	Developmental psychologist	Sussex Public School
Hearing	Does not respond to sound but does to gestures	Profound bilateral hearing impairment	11/5/04 12/15/05	Neonatal screening ABR	Audiologist	Health Services Hospital
Communication	Follows eyes, coos, and makes sounds	Age appropriate so far		Rossetti Infant-Toddler Scale	Speech-language pathologist	Sussex Public School

Child Eligibility

Part C of IDEA: X Yes   No   Unknown   Based on: X Established condition (deafness)   Developmental delay

Service Plan

Service coordinator: D. Smith   Services coordinator telephone: 500-333-3333

Interim   Initial X   Review   Annual   Transition (90 days before entry into new program or third birthday—whichever comes first)

Outcomes	Who & What	Where, When, & How	Date Service		Payor	Review
What would we like to have happen, by when, and how will we know when it happens	What service or activity is needed and who will do it?	When will the services occur, how often, how long each time, individual or group?	Begins	Ends	Who will pay for it?	Date/ rating/ comments
1. Cochlear implant (3/5/06) 2. Understand and say words by age 2 (at least 50) 3. Take part in family discussions by age 3 (make comments and ask questions) 4. Play normally with other children by age 4	1. Universal Hospital 2. Speech-language pathologist, speech language therapy 3. Hearing impaired teacher consultant 4. Early intervention coordinator	1. Implant programming 2. Parent-toddler group (60 minutes, twice a week), individual therapy with family (20-30 minutes) 3. Home visit (once a month), individual therapy (45 minutes) 4. Weekly home or clinic consultation by hearing impairment consultant	1. 3/5/06 2. 2/17/06 3. 1/18/03 4. 11/1/03	1. When complete 2. When complete 3. When complete 4. Ongoing	1. Private insurance and Medicaid 2. Sussex Public School 3. Sussex Public School 4. Sussex Public School	

Figure 9.1.   Sample individualized family service plan. (*Key:* IFSP = Individualized Family Service Plan, ABR = auditory brainstem response, IDEA = Individuals with Disabilities Education Improvement Act [PL 108-446].)

if the child responds to scientific, research-based interventions. This change has resulted in the development of a variety of responsiveness to intervention (RTI) initiatives (Graner, Faggella-Luby, & Fritschmann, 2005; Moore-Brown, Montgomery, Bielinski, & Shubin, 2005), which may involve SLPs in preventive instructional activities. Such approaches also could change the manner in which students with language impairment are identified and whether language impairments are linked to specific learning disabilities (Ehren & Nelson, 2005; Staskowski & Rivera, 2005). The following case example provides an illustration of how an IEP team might lead to advocacy efforts on the part of a school-based SLP.

Case Example 1

As an SLP who works in a school district, you are concerned about the district's long-standing policy that students with language delays are not eligible for services unless formal tests show a discrepancy between IQ scores and language quotient scores. Brian is a 6-year-old child in the first grade with a history of preschool language problems involving phonology and syntax. He is struggling with phonemic awareness, reading decoding, and spoken and written language comprehension, but he has cognitive skills in the low-normal range which are not significantly above his language test scores. Although you have done some research, you can find no support for the cognitive referencing policy in the professional literature. You also notice that changes in the IDEA '04 method of identifying students with disabilities prohibit schools from requiring discrepancy measures to determine eligibility for specific learning disability services. You advocate for a program that allows you to work with Brian and determine his responsiveness to intervention as part of the NCLB activities. Eventually, Brian is found eligible for services on the basis of language impairment and becomes a client on your caseload.

The LRE requirements of Part B specify that, whenever appropriate, children with disabilities must be educated with children without disabilities. The IEPs for students with disabilities must include statements of:

1. The child's present levels of academic achievement and functional performance

2. The measurable annual academic and functional goals designed to meet needs that result from the child's disability, support the child's progress in the general education curriculum, and meet each of the child's other educational needs resulting from the disability

3. The special education, related services, modifications, and supports that are designed to help the child advance toward attaining the annual goals, be involved in and make progress in the general education curriculum, participate in extra-curricular and other nonacademic activities, and participate with other children with and without disabilities

4. To the extent practicable, an explanation of how special education, related services, and supplementary services are based on peer-reviewed research

5. The accommodations necessary for state and districtwide assessments and, as needed, an explanation for how benchmarks and short-term objectives are aligned to the alternate achievement standards on the IEP

6. The transition goals and services that must be implemented by the time the child is 16 years old

7. The plans for periodic reports of the child's progress toward annual goals provided concurrent with report cards. Changes in IDEA '04 also specify procedures for excusing selected professionals from IEP meetings (e.g., if their area or service is not being reviewed, if their written input is deemed sufficient) and for modifying IEPs in writing rather than in periodic face-to-face meetings if team members agree that such procedures are acceptable at the annual meeting.

In developing each student's IEP, the team members must consider, in addition to the evaluation or reevaluation of the student, the strengths of the student; the concerns of the parents for enhancing the education of their child; and the academic, developmental and functional needs of the student indicated by state and district testing. The IEP team should consist of one or both parents, at least one general education teacher, and at least one special education teacher or service provider, one of whom may serve as representative of the local education agency (LEA), who also must be knowledgeable about the general education curriculum. A sample portion of an IEP appears in Figure 9.2.

THE REHABILITATION ACT

Section 504 of the Rehabilitation Act of 1973 is civil rights legislation that preceded IDEA legislation and other nondiscrimination policies. It specified that an otherwise qualified individual with a disability cannot be excluded from participation in, denied the benefits of, or subjected to discrimination under any program or activity receiving financial assistance from the federal government-including public elementary, secondary, and postsecondary schools. To qualify for accommodations under Section 504, individuals must be identified as having a physical or mental impairment that substantially limits one or more of their major life activities. Section 504 covered conditions that currently do not qualify as disabilities under IDEA, including attention deficit/hyperactivity disorder (although ADHD can be considered an "other health impairment" under IDEA'04). Section 504, however, carried no funds to pay for its provisions, whereas IDEA does.

Protection from discrimination in education agencies means that schools must make reasonable accommodations, such as structural alterations and modifications of classroom materials and procedures. Educational agencies must ensure that students with disabilities have access to nonacademic services as well. At the postsecondary level, this might include providing students with disabilities access to housing comparable to housing for students without disabilities. Other modifications in academic programs might include extra time to complete assignments, adjustments in the length of assignments, the use of peer tutors, provision of visual aids, the ability to audio record lectures, or the use of specialized curricular materials. Modification of tests might include permission to receive testing orally or from an audio recording, extra time to complete tests, permission to dictate test answers, an altered test format, or a test printed in an enlarged type. Provision of auxiliary aids and devices might include interpreters, frequency modulated amplification systems, and other forms of assistive technology. In requiring schools to be accessible, Section 504 does not require every part of a school to be modified in compliance with Section 504 as long as the school's

Sample Individualized Education Program: Measurable Annual Goal with Benchmarks

Student: __Sam Miller__   Date of birth: __7/25/98__   Today's date: __10/2/2006__

☒ Academic/cognitive   ☐ Social/behavioral   ☒ Communication   ☐ Gross/fine motor   ☐ Health   ☐ Self help   ☐ Other: (specify)

☐ **Check here if the student is 13 or older.** (If checked, **IEP/28-R99**, the transition-planning summary must be completed.)

Measurable Annual Goal Number: 1	Method of evaluation	Performance criteria	Report of progresses*			
			Nov.	Jan.	April	June
Sam will show story reading, writing, and retelling abilities that are comparable to those of his second grade general education classmates.						
Benchmarks for Annual Goal						
1a: Sam will use a planning template to organize a story with characters, a problem, and cause and effect when writing and for stories written by others to use in retelling.	Probe stories and stories produced in language arts	Demonstration of new behaviors independently				
1b: Sam will show ability to combine sentences using a variety of structures to yield average lengths that exceed his baseline levels (MLTU at baseline was 3.5, two sentences were simple incorrect, three were simple correct, zero were complex).	Same	An MLTU of >4.0 At least 1 complex sentence				
1c: Sam will increase the number of different words in his written and retold stories from baseline levels (10 different words, 20 total words) and, with scaffolding help, will add at least 2 novel in teresting words" when editing.	Same	New stories will average 25 words and include 15 different words				

Evaluation procedures

1=Criterion-referenced/curriculum based assessment
2=Pre & post standardized assessment
3=Pre & post base line data
4=Quizzes/tests
5=Student self-assessment/rubic
6=Observation
7=Work samples/project/experiment/portfolio
8=Job performance or products
9=Behavior/performance rating scale
10=CMT/CAPT
11=Achievement of objectives **(note: use with goal only)**
12=Other: (specify) _____

Performance criteria

A =100%
B =90%
C =80%
D =70%
E =Standard score increase: _____
F =Months growth increase: _____
G =Passing grades/score: _____
H =Frequency/trials: (e.g., 9/10) _____
I =Duration: (e.g., 15 min, 1 per) _____
J =Successful completion of task/activity
K =Other: (specify) _____
L =Other: (specify) _____

Report of progress key*

M=Mastered
S=Satisfactory progress (likely to achieve)
U=Unsatisfactory progress (unlikely to achieve)
NP 1 =No progress (will **not** achieve) lack of prerequisite skills
NP 2 =No progress (will **not** achieve) need more time
NP 3 =No progress (will **not** achieve) inadequate assessment
NP 4 =No progress (will **not** achieve) excessive absences/tardiness
NI =Not introduced
O=Other: (specify) _____

Indicating extent to which progress is sufficient to achieve goal by the end of the year

Figure 9.2. Sample individualized education program form. (*Key:* IEP/28-R99 = individualized education program form section for beginning transitional living, MLTU = mean length of T-unit, SLP = speech-language pathologist, IEP = individualized education program, CMT = Connecticut Master Test, CAPT = Connecticut Academic Performance Test, Nov. = November, Jan. = January, min = minutes.)

(continued)

Sample Individualized Education Program (continued)

Modifications and Adaptations in Regular Education Including Nonacademic and Extracurricular Activities and Collaboration and Supports for School Personnel

Student: _Sam Miller_   Date of birth: _7/25/1998_   Today's date: _10/2/2006_

Modifications and Adaptations in Regular Education Including Nonacademic and Extracurricular Activities	Sites and Activities Where Required and Duration	Required Supports for Personnel and Frequency and Duration of Supports
Materials/books/equipment: ☐ Alternative text ☐ Consumable workbook ☐ Modified worksheets ☐ Manipulatives ☒ Access to a computer ☐ Tape recorder ☐ Supplementary visuals ☐ Large print text ☒ Spell check ☐ Calculator ☒ Assistive technology (specify): _Software with synthesized speech_ ☐ Other: (specify)	During Writing Laboratory times: Tuesday/Thursday for 1 hour each	SLP will work in classroom with teacher on Tuesday, teacher will provide support on Thursday
Tests/quizzes/time: ☐ Prior notice of tests ☐ Preview test procedures ☐ Test study guide ☐ Simplify test wording ☐ Oral testing ☐ Limited multiple choice ☐ Student writes on test ☐ Shortened tasks ☐ Hands-on projects ☐ Reduced reading ☐ Alternative tests ☐ Objective tests ☐ Extra credit options ☐ Extra time on written work ☒ Extra time on tests ☐ Extra time on projects ☐ Extra response time ☐ Modifies tests ☐ Pace long-term projects ☐ Rephrase test questions and directions ☐ Other: (specify)		
Grading: ☒ No spelling penalty ☐ No handwriting penalty ☐ Grade effort and work ☐ Grade improvement ☐ Course credit ☐ Base grade on IEP ☐ Base grade on ability ☐ Modified grades ☐ Pass/fail ☐ Audit course ☐ Other: (specify)	Any formal graded activities	
Organization: ☒ Provide study outlines ☐ Desktop list of tasks ☐ List sequential steps ☐ Post routines ☐ Post assignments ☐ Give one paper at a time ☐ Folders to hold work ☐ Pencil box for tools ☐ Pocket folder for work ☐ Assignment pad ☐ Daily assignment ☐ List daily homework ☐ List worksheet formats ☐ Extra space for work ☐ Assign partner ☐ Other: (specify)		SLP will work with student in therapy sessions
Environment: ☒ Preferential seating ☐ Clear work area ☐ Study carrel ☐ Other: (specify)	Any formal instruction	
Behavioral management: ☐ Daily feedback to student ☐ Chart progress ☐ Behavior contracts ☐ Parent/guardian sign homework ☐ Positive reinforcement ☐ Collect baseline data ☐ Set/post class rules ☐ Parent/guardian sign behavioral chart ☐ Cue expected behavior ☐ Structure transitions ☐ Break between tasks ☐ Time out from positive reinforcement ☐ Proximity/touch control ☐ Contingency plan ☐ Other: (specify)		
Teaching strategies: ☒ Check work in progress ☐ Immediate feedback ☐ Pre-teach content ☒ Have student restate information ☐ Extra drill/practice ☐ Review sessions ☐ Review directions ☐ Provide lecture notes and outline to student ☐ Use manipulatives ☐ Modified content ☐ Assign study partner ☐ Computer assisted instruction ☐ Monitor assignments ☒ Provide models ☐ Repeat instructions ☐ Support auditory presentation with visuals ☐ Multi-sensory approach ☐ Highlight key words ☐ Oral reminders ☐ Display key vocabulary ☐ Visual reinforcement ☐ Pictures/charts ☐ Visual reminders ☒ Provide student with vocabulary word bank ☐ Mimed clues/gestures ☐ Concrete examples ☐ Use mnemonics ☒ Personalized examples ☐ Number line ☐ Other: (specify)	During Writing Laboratory times and any other times when teacher deems appropriate	SLP will work in classroom with teacher on Tuesday during Writing Laboratory sessions

Figure 9.2. (continued)

educational programs as a whole are accessible. Evaluations under Section 504 must be conducted with procedures that are 1) validated for the specific purpose for which they are used, 2) administered by trained personnel, 3) tailored to assess specific areas of educational need, and 4) selected to ensure that, when a test is administered to a student with impaired sensory, manual, or speaking skills, the test results reflect the student's aptitude or achievement accurately rather than reflecting the student's impairment.

The Rehabilitation Act of 1973 also is a major legislative influence behind programs under the Rehabilitation Services Administration (RSA), a branch of the Office of Special Education and Rehabilitive Services (OSERS) within the U.S. Department of Education. Under this policy, both adults and children with disabilities may qualify for SLP services. Qualification occurs when an individual with a disability applies to his or her state office of vocational rehabilitation for the purpose of identifying a plan to procure or enhance a work opportunity. In the case of an adult with new onset of traumatic brain injury or stroke, SLP services may be provided for the restoration of or compensation for the language or cognitive skills that would enhance the individual's chances of successfully attaining or returning to gainful employment (OSERS' Rehabilitation Services Administration Legislation Page, 2005).

AMERICANS WITH DISABILITIES ACT

The *Americans with Disabilities Act (ADA) of 1990* (PL 101-336) has three basic purposes. These are to ensure that individuals with disabilities enjoy equal opportunity to 1) participate fully in society, 2) live independently, and 3) have access to economic self-sufficiency through removal of barriers. The legislation is divided into five areas, or *titles,* addressing employment, public services, public accommodations operated by a private entity, telecommunications, and miscellaneous other issues.

Title I applies to *employment.* It requires employers with 15 or more employees, employment agencies, labor agencies, and labor-management committees to make accommodations for qualified employees. Qualified employees include individuals who have a disability in one or more area but who can still perform the essential functions of an employment position with or without reasonable accommodation. Title I prohibits discrimination in the following areas: job application procedures; hiring, advancement, or discharge of employees; employee compensation; job training; and other terms, conditions, or privileges of employment. Reasonable accommodations include restructuring of the job; modification of work schedules; acquisition or modification of equipment or assistive devices; adjustment or modification of examination materials, training materials, or policies; and provision of qualified readers or interpreters. Procedures for determining reasonable accommodations include analyzing the requirements of the job, identifying potential accommodations in consultation with the individual with the disability, and considering the preferences of the individual when deciding which options to pursue.

Title II applies to *public services* in such entities as schools, colleges, and universities. It ensures that policies are in place to protect the educational opportunities of individuals with disabilities and to guard against discrimination.

Title III applies to *public accommodations operated by a private entity.* It protects the rights of individuals with disabilities to gain access to places of lodging, exhibition or entertainment, recreation, education; places where social services are offered; and stores, shopping centers, bars, and restaurants. For example, architectural accessibility modifications must be made to remove architectural and structural barriers in existing facilities when the modifications are readily achievable. If they are not readily achievable, the private entities must provide alternative methods for gaining access to the public accommodations. New buildings are required to comply fully with ADA accessibility requirements. Some strategies for removing architectural barriers include installing ramps, repositioning shelves, adding raised markings on elevator control buttons and lowering elevator control panels, designating parking spaces, installing accessible door hardware, widening doors and doorways, and installing grab bars in toilet stalls.

Title IV applies to *telecommunication services*. It requires the provision of technical support for persons with hearing and speech impairments. This title is responsible for making telephone systems with teletypewriter (TTY) devices available to the public in places such as airports and restaurants.

Title V applies to **due process** provisions. It includes notice that states are not immune from the law's provisions. States, as well as other public or private entities, may be sued for noncompliance. Other provisions allow courts to award attorney's fees to prevailing parties and indicate that the law prohibits retaliation and coercion against people with disabilities who are seeking enforcement of the policy. Although the ADA is enforced through court actions, parties are encouraged to resolve disputes through methods other than litigation if possible.

MEDICARE, MEDICAID, AND THE BALANCED BUDGET AMENDMENTS

Prior to 1961, public policies aimed at assisting older adults consisted primarily of retirement supplements and benefits for individuals of low socioeconomic status. In 1961, President John F. Kennedy sponsored a "Conference on Aging" to build national awareness of issues important to older adults. This conference identified the problems ("want-get gaps") that were distressing to older adults, such as health and income maintenance; opportunity to retire with dignity; and issues pertaining to housing, transportation, and social isolation (Brown, 1996). This conference set the stage for the development of several key pieces of legislation, including the Older Americans Act of 1965 (PL 89-73) which was reauthorized in 2000 as the Older American Act Amendments (PL 106-5011), as well as Medicare and Medicaid (Brown, 1996). The purpose of the Older American's Act of 1965 was to help older individuals by providing funds to states for programs and services such as education about nutrition, hot meals, transportation, legal assistance, and materials to train service providers in the area of gerontology (Gelfand, 1999). Medicare and Medicaid policies later extended this legislation (Brown, 1996; Rigby & Kipping, 2000).

Medicare

The Social Security Act (SSA) of 1935 (PL 74-271), which was originally passed under the leadership of President Franklin D. Roosevelt, was designed to alleviate conditions of poverty. **Medicare** was established in 1965 as Title 18 to the SSA. It was an initial attempt by the government to assist individuals to meet costs of adequate health care. Medicare assistance is administered by the Centers for Medicare and Medicaid Services (CMS), a federal agency. Medicare is available to individuals older than 65 years of age who are eligible for benefits or disability based on their employment before retirement. It also is available to individuals younger than age 65 who have renal disease or a disability (Gelfand, 1999). Medicare has two parts: *Part A* provides prepaid hospital insurance and *Part B* offers additional optional medical insurance.

Part A finances hospital insurance through payroll tax. Consequently, those who are eligible for Medicare do not pay additional premiums for hospital insurance, which covers inpatient care in hospitals, **skilled nursing facilities (SNFs)**, and a limited number of days for hospice care in any benefit period. A **benefit period** includes the time from when an individual enters into a hospital up to and including the day of discharge. The longer the stay in the hospital, more out-of-pocket costs are charged to the individual and less costs are covered by Medicare. For example, Medicare covers the first 60 days after the individual has paid a deductible, which is typically equivalent to 1 day's stay in the hospital. For days 61-90, the individual is responsible for a copayment for each day of hospital stay (Dye, 1998).

Part A benefits also cover limited days in SNFs. SNFs (previously known as *nursing homes*) are identified as such because they include a percentage of residents who require services from skilled professionals such as nurses and rehabilitation specialists. For the first 20 days in a SNF, Medicare pays 100% of the costs. For days 21–100 there is a copay (e.g., Medicare pays 80% of costs and the individual pays 20%). After 100 days, the individual must have a pay source other than Medicare. Such pay sources include private pay, Medicaid, or other supplemental insurance plans.

Part B of Medicare consists of medical insurance that is financed through a monthly premium paid by the individual. As of 2006, the Medicare Part B monthly premium was $88.50 (http://www.cms.hhs.gov/apps/media/press/release.asp?Counter=1557). After an annual deductible of $100 is met, Part B pays 80% of "reasonable and necessary charges" for covered services. Part B covers such services as home health services, physician medical and surgical services, supplies (including drugs that cannot be self administered), diagnostic services, physical therapy, home dialysis, X-rays, surgical dressings, casts, orthopedic devices, oxygen tanks, wheelchairs, ambulance services, prosthetic devices (but not dentures), and immunizations. Part B does not cover hearing aids, but augmentative and alternative communication (AAC) coverage was added in January 2001 for individuals with a documented severe expressive impairment that is not expected to improve. In order to qualify for funding as a form of medical durable equipment, the AAC device must be appropriate for the individual's cognitive and physical abilities. In addition, the sole purpose of the device must be for speech (i.e., laptops or personal digital assistants do not qualify) (Augmentative and Alternative Communication-Rehabilitation Engineering Research Center, 2001).

Some programs are designed to fill gaps in Medicare services for older adults of low socioeconomic status and for individuals with disabilities. For example, **Medigap** offers an array of 10 supplemental insurance policies designed to fill gaps in Medicare (Gelfand, 1999). Each supplemental policy offers a different benefit package, but some services are common to all of them. These core services include coinsurance for Part A, 365 days of hospital coverage after Medicare benefits end, 20% of doctors' fees not covered by Medicare, and the first 3 pints of blood needed each year (Gelfand, 1999).

Managed care organizations (MCOs) provide additional forms of supplemental insurance to Medicare recipients. MCOs manage or control health care expenditures by closely monitoring how service providers (e.g., hospitals, physicians) treat their patients and by evaluating the necessity, appropriateness, and payment efficiency of the health services. **Health maintenance organizations (HMOs)** are examples of MCOs that provide a range of care on a prepayment basis. Individuals continue to pay Part B premiums, and the HMO receives payment from the federal government for each HMO member equivalent to 95% of the average Medicare costs. HMOs may cover costs that are not covered by Medicare. For example, HMOs may contract with or employ service providers and pay for a *minimum* of two months or 60 visits (whichever is more) per condition for a combination of speech-language pathology, occupational therapy (OT), and physical therapy (PT) services. Some HMOs interpret these visits as the *maximum* rather than the minimum, however, resulting in inadequately provided services. Some SLPs also have experienced problems with HMOs when attempting to get approval for necessary services, as illustrated in the following case example.

Case Example 2

Mrs. Robinson, an outpatient at Cedar Rehabilitation Services, was referred to you for voice therapy by an ear, nose, and throat specialist following a medical treatment for vocal nodules. For each of the next 6 months after receipt of the referral, however, the HMO refused to approve the voice therapy treatment. When the treatment was approved, it was approved for three visits only. Based on past records, you know that three visits are insufficient to serve Mrs. Robinson adequately. You provide the HMO with evidence that additional sessions are likely to be more effective in retraining Mrs. Robinson's vocal behaviors so that the vocal nodules are less likely to recur. You also work with Mrs. Robinson to write to her legislators about problems in the health care financing system that are affecting their constituent's access to adequate health care.

The Balanced Budget Act and Medicare Modernization Act

On August 1, 1997, President William J. Clinton signed into law the *Balanced Budget Act (BBA) of 1997* (PL 105-33). The BBA, as its name implied, was designed to balance the national budget. Thus, it included provisions to reduce overall spending on Medicaid and to slow the growth of Medicare spending over 5 years. These reductions included limiting the funds designated for preventive benefits not previously covered, such as mammograms, self-management of diabetes, and prostate and colorectal cancer screening. Funding limits also were placed on spending under the BBA, which resulted in some programs receiving more funds and other programs receiving less, causing agencies and providers to compete for limited resources. This new competitiveness had the effect of denying Medicare funds to individuals who most needed them (ASHA, 2005).

One result of the spending limits was the $1,500 cap on Medicare outpatient rehabilitation services, which has affected the provision of speech-language pathology, PT, and OT services. Specifically, this cap required SLPs and physical therapists to share a maximum of $1,500 for Medicare Part B services for each individual. Several problems arose from this cap, but two primary concerns were that: 1) the shared cap forced people to choose between two vital services, and 2) that individuals in SNFs or rehabilitation agencies who had reached their $1,500 limit would have to leave their current placements in order to seek help in potentially less accessible hospital outpatient facilities.

The *Balanced Budget Refinement Act of 1999* (BBRA; PL 106-113) was signed into law on November 29, 1999, also by President Clinton, with a two-year moratorium on the $1,500 cap on Medicare Part B services for combined outpatient speech-language pathology and PT services from January 2000 through December 2001. Through this refined act, speech-language pathology service was reinstated as an independent service no longer linked with PT; this made it possible for SLPs and physical therapists to be reimbursed separately. The BBRA was initiated through the actions of legislators and the advocacy of professional groups such as the American Speech-Language-Hearing Association (ASHA), the American Occupational Therapy Association (AOTA), and the American Physical Therapy Association (APTA). The $1500 cap limits were not in effect from 2000–2002, but they remain a subject of controversy that requires constant vigilance.

Significant modifications in Medicare occurred in 2003 when President George W. Bush signed the *Medicare Prescription Drug Modernization Act of 2003* (*MMA;* PL 108-173). The MMA added provisions for prescription drug coverage and for improved healthcare access for rural Americans and increased existing coverage for preventive care services, including flu shots and mammograms. Businesses also were offered incentives to keep prescription drug coverage in their benefit packages for retirees. Section 624 of the MMA extended the hold on funding limits for outpatient therapy from December 8, 2003 through December 31, 2005.

Medicaid

Congress established Medicaid in 1965 under Title 19 of the SSA. Funding for Medicaid comes from state, federal and city taxes. Hence, it is a *federal/state matching program* because both the state and federal governments must contribute to it. Medicaid is run by state governments under guidelines from the federal government, resulting in variability in eligibility benefits from one state to the next.

Medicaid was created by Congress to pay medical bills for persons of low socioeconomic status who have no other financial means to pay for medical care. It is an **entitlement program** in that Congress has set eligibility criteria based on age, income, retirement, disability, or unemployment, which entitle those individuals who qualify to its benefits (Dye, 1998). Most Medicaid spending goes to older individuals and to individuals with disabilities. Additionally, anyone receiving public assistance through **Supplemental Security Income (SSI)** or **Temporary Assistance for Needy Families (TANF)** is automatically eligible for Medicaid.

Medicaid covers such services as payment to hospitals, prenatal and delivery services for those with no other insurance, and services to families of low socioeconomic status who do not receive cash assistance. It is possible to obtain Medicaid coverage for rehabilitation for individuals of low socioeconomic status without insurance, but this requires an evaluation and the completion of the appropriate Medicaid Prior Approval form. The Medicaid Prior Approval form includes information on expected duration, short-term objectives, and the projected outcome of treatment, but the form has a waiting period for approval. In a similar manner, coverage for AAC devices may be obtained if the appropriate codes are used (Higdon, 2003). Medicaid also covers long-term SNF care, but only after beneficiaries have exhausted all other income and forms of payment. Most benefits are limited to long-term rehabilitative care.

The federal government does not mandate states to provide speech-language pathology and audiology services under Medicaid, but there is an exception for providing services to Medicaid-eligible children under the age of 21. These children are mandated to receive comprehensive benefits including periodic screenings and wellness checks through the Early and Periodic Screening, Diagnostic, and Treatment Services (EPSDT). As part of the required medical screening, speech-language pathology and audiology services are included to identify and diagnose children with speech or language impairments, provide speech and language services, make referrals to other medical professionals as needed for rehabilitation, and offer counseling and guidance to parents and teachers. In addition, Medicaid can reimburse school districts for the provision of school-based speech-language pathology and audiology services required by Part B of IDEA in an IEP (ASHA, 2003). The services must be compliant with the Medicaid requirements for coverage of services including frequency, duration, scope, comparability, medical necessity, prior authorization, and provider requirements.

ADVOCACY

It is difficult to imagine how practitioners could be effective and ethical without being actively involved in understanding, implementing, and influencing public policy. Thinking of professional roles in **advocacy** may conjure up intimidating images of visits to Capitol Hill in Washington, D.C. This is one important avenue and not nearly as scary as it may seem at first, but active advocacy roles also may be assumed at the level of the individual client.

As discussed in this chapter, policies are in place to govern who is eligible for service and who will pay for it, as well as how services are to be delivered. SLPs and audiologists are responsible for seeing that individuals receive services according to the policies written to address their needs. This means that professionals must know how to conduct assessments and write reports that maximize their ability to deliver high quality services. For example, this includes the responsibility to advocate for individuals who at first might appear not to qualify for services because of overly strict interpretation of eligibility guidelines. It also refers to advocacy efforts in calling and writing to third party payers on behalf of individual clients who have been denied funding for needed services.

Advocacy at the individual client level also may include working with others to make policy implementation effective. For example, one of the provisions of IDEA is that children with disabilities should be involved in learning the general curriculum and participating in extracurricular and other nonacademic activities. Implementation of this policy may require personal advocacy efforts by SLPs and audiologists with school district and building teams to increase opportunities for individual clients to participate with peers and be active in the general education curriculum.

Case Example 3

You have been working as an SLP for a year in an elementary school in which the students with disabilities traditionally have been served in separate classrooms or pulled out of general education classrooms for speech-language therapy. You are concerned that this approach is not meeting the students' needs and begin to work with the early and later elementary special education teachers to bring more aspects of the general education curriculum into the special education room and to explore more ways for the students with disabilities to participate actively with their peers in the general education classrooms.

Advocacy at the individual client level also includes the responsibility to instruct clients and their families about how to advocate for themselves. This includes informing them about relevant public policies, helping them acquire strategies for communicating their needs to others consistent with those policies, and providing consultation about due process for remedying problems if they arise. Consultation also may be provided to individuals and families who want to know how to play an active role in advocating for policy change.

In addition to being an advocate for individuals, it is important to consider extending advocacy efforts to broader issues of practice. Local, state, and federal policies govern such areas of professional certification and licensure as well as access to care for people with disabilities and other aspects of clinical decision making. When policies (or the lack thereof) have negative effects on how professional services are provided, it is the responsibility of professionals to advocate for changes in those policies. Case example 4 illustrates such a situation.

Case Example 4

Mr. Rivers resided in a SNF 2 years prior to having a stroke. Following the stroke, you conducted an assessment of his abilities and found that Mr. Rivers required dysphagia treatment. You recommended treatment for 5 days per week for 3 weeks. Mr. Rivers' HMO, however, approved treatment for only 5 days for 1 week. You provided this treatment and trained the nursing staff to feed and support Mr. Rivers during meal times. His records, however, show that the limited time approved for therapy was insufficient to establish and monitor a routine with the nursing staff charged with managing Mr. Rivers' care. Consequently, the staff often forgot to use the food and liquid thickener and frequently did not assist Mr. Rivers during meal times. He experienced several episodes of aspiration and eventually reverted to his original swallowing problem. You continued to advocate with the HMO to justify more treatment sessions and communicated with Mr. Rivers' legislators about the dangers inherent in the current system, some of which were life threatening.

Advocacy Strategies

Grassroots advocacy involves efforts of groups of individuals. Such efforts are particularly effective because it is individuals who are eligible to vote for policy makers. Professional associations often guide the process, however, making it less daunting.

Associations serve as a resource for clarifying issues, keeping individuals informed, and establishing opportunities to communicate with key policy makers.

Understanding Current Policy and How to Change It   The first step for individuals who wish to influence existing policy is to obtain a copy of the actual wording of the current policy. This involves a series of steps to find out: 1) where the policy is printed (this usually can be done through Internet research), 2) which government body or agency made the policy or rule, 3) whether the policy might have flexibility that was previously not noticed, and 4) whether the employer or reimbursement agency might have room to negotiate a variation that will overcome the particular problem or concern. If current policy still presents a problem, professionals have three choices (Nelson, 1998):

- *Study the rationale for the policy and decide to accept it.* In some cases, investigating the rationale for a policy may lead to greater understanding about why the policy was established, and professionals may decide there is no need to influence change.

- *Seek approval for a policy exception.* If a policy includes any room for negotiation or for exceptions, professionals may pursue such options. Obtaining permission for an exception to the rule may make it possible to gather additional data, which then can be used to make a case for more widespread change if it still seems desirable.

- *Work to change the official policy.* If a policy clearly needs changing, professionals have an obligation to work within official systems to advocate for change.

Communicating Directly with Policy Makers   The framing of a new bill requires direct involvement with legislators, particularly those on the committee where the bill first will be considered. Professional associations often employ legislative specialists who are familiar with this complicated process and know how to influence it. If the change needed is at the level of regulation rather than legislation, it may be more appropriate to start by communicating with the agency of the executive branch of government that is responsible for implementing the policy. One important question in such cases is whether the agency expects the regulations to be opened for change any time soon.

When communicating directly with policy makers, it is important to note that most employers do not want their employees to write letters with political implications on agency stationery. Political advocacy messages should be conveyed as personal communication by individuals. This makes it clear that a constituent's views do not necessarily represent the official position of the individual's employer. In fact, personal communication coming from constituent's home addresses to legislative representatives and senators (state or national) generally have the most meaning for policy makers. Table 9.1 summarizes considerations for writing advocacy letters or composing email messages.

Working within Professional Associations   Some of the most effective efforts occur when members of professional associations work together. ASHA, for example, keeps its members informed of policies and their implications, through both its web site (hpp://www.asha.org) and its publications, particularly *The ASHA Leader.* ASHA's Government Relations and Public Policy Board is responsible

Table 9.1. Checklist for advocacy letters

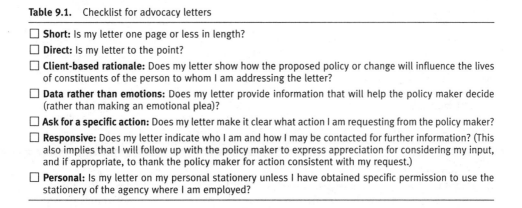

☐ **Short:** Is my letter one page or less in length?

☐ **Direct:** Is my letter to the point?

☐ **Client-based rationale:** Does my letter show how the proposed policy or change will influence the lives of constituents of the person to whom I am addressing the letter?

☐ **Data rather than emotions:** Does my letter provide information that will help the policy maker decide (rather than making an emotional plea)?

☐ **Ask for a specific action:** Does my letter make it clear what action I am requesting from the policy maker?

☐ **Responsive:** Does my letter indicate who I am and how I may be contacted for further information? (This also implies that I will follow up with the policy maker to express appreciation for considering my input, and if appropriate, to thank the policy maker for action consistent with my request.)

☐ **Personal:** Is my letter on my personal stationery unless I have obtained specific permission to use the stationery of the agency where I am employed?

for developing an annual public policy agenda to prioritize the advocacy activities of the association. The goal is to address issues that are of major concern to speech-language-hearing scientists, SLPs, audiologists, and the individuals whom they serve. Two examples of the effectiveness of this agenda setting strategy (Moore, 2000) were observed in 1999 when 1) a campaign of letters, phone calls, emails, and visits to Capitol Hill by consumers and ASHA members in 1999 led to the suspension of the $1,500 funding limit for rehabilitation outpatient services that could be covered by Medicare Part B; and 2) a similar campaign, fortified by an ASHA-led coalition of 20 organizations, resulted in the passage in 1999 of the federal *Newborn and Infant Hearing Screening and Intervention Act* (PL 93-406; Boswell, 2000).

At a minimum, professionals who pay their dues to professional associations help to maintain professional organizations so that they can monitor public policy and communicate with their members, the public, and the policy makers. At a level of slightly greater involvement, professionals can make voluntary contributions to political action committees, which are in a position to lobby directly for change. At the most active level, professionals can become personally involved by writing letters, sending email messages, and making telephone calls or personal visits to policy makers. Individual SLPs and audiologists have played important roles in the development and modifications that have been made over the years in many of the key pieces of legislation discussed in this chapter.

CONCLUSION

Public policies guide many aspects of clinical decision making. It is the responsibility of professional practitioners to understand how public policies are generated, legislated, and regulated. Although professionals are expected to implement public policies, they also can question the wisdom of some policies, and when problems are evident, it is professionals' responsibility to advocate for change. Effective advocacy involves gathering and presenting data in a way that communicates a need clearly to policy makers at the level of the policy and individuals affected by the policy. Among the policies that are important for the practice of speech-language pathology and audiology are ESEA '65, including its latest iteration as the NCLB act, IDEA, Section 504 of the Rehabilitation Act, the ADA, Medicare, Medicaid, the BBA, and the MMA.

REFERENCES

American Speech-Language-Hearing Association. (2003). *Medicaid and third party payments in the schools.* Retrieved November 2, 2005, from http://www.asha.org/members/issues/reimbursement/medicaid/thirdparty-payment.htm

American Speech-Language-Hearing Association. (2005). *Therapy cap advocacy center: Background on therapy cap.* Retrieved May 1, 2006, from http://www.asha.org/about/legislation-advocacy/federal/cap

Americans with Disabilities Act (ADA) of 1990, PL 101-336, 42 U.S.C. §§ 12101 *et seq.*

Annett, M.M. (2003 December 16). No Child Left Behind: A key focus of 2003 schools forum-ED officials address law, students with disabilities. *The ASHA Leader, 3,* 33.

Armbruster, B.A., & Osborn, J. (2001). *Put reading first.* Washington, DC: National Institute for Literacy.

Augmentative and Alternative Communication-Rehabilitation Engineering Research Center. (2001). Medicare. In *Medicare AAC device coverage guidance* (National Coverage Decision #50.1). Retrieved May 1, 2006, from http://aac-rerc.com/pages/Medicare/RMRP.htm#ncd

Balanced Budget Act of 1997, PL 105-33, 111 Stat. 251.

Balanced Budget Refinement Act of 1999, PL 106-113.

Boswell, S. (2000). Congress funds newborn hearing screening. *The ASHA Leader, 5*(1), 1.

Bilingual Education Act of 1968, PL 90-247.

Brown, D.K. (1996). *Introduction to public policy: An aging perspective.* Lanham, MD: University Press of America.

Crawford, J. (2002). *Obituary: The Bilingual Education Act—1968–2002.* Retrieved May 1, 2006, from http://ourworld.compuserve.com/homepages/JWCRAWFORD/T7obit.htm

Dye, T.R. (1975). *Understanding public policy* (2nd ed.). Upper Saddle River, NJ: Prentice Hall.

Dye, T.R. (1998). *Understanding public policy* (9th ed.). Upper Saddle River, NJ: Prentice Hall.

Education Trust (2003). *Elementary and Secondary Education Act (ESEA).* Retrieved May 1, 2006, from http://www2.edtrust.org/edtrust/esea

Education for All Handicapped Children Act of 1975, PL 94-142, 20 U.S.C. §§ 1400 *et seq.*

Education of the Handicapped Act of 1970 (EHA), PL 91-230, 84 Stat. 121-154, 20 U.S.C. §§ 1400 *et seq.*

Ehren, B., & Nelson, N. (2005). The responsiveness to intervention approach and language impairment. *Topics in Language Disorders, 25*(2), 120–132.

Elementary and Secondary Education Act Amendments of 1966, PL 89-750, 80 Stat. 1191, 20 U.S.C. §§ 873 *et seq.*

Elementary and Secondary Education Act Amendments of 1968, PL 90-247, 20 U.S.C. §§ 877b *et seq.*

Elementary and Secondary Education Act of 1965, PL 89-10, 20 U.S.C. §§ 241 *et seq.*

Finn, C.E. (2002). Leaving education reform behind. *The Weekly Standard, 7*(17), 14–16.

Gelfand, D.E. (1999). *The aging network: Programs and services* (5th ed.). New York: Springer-Verlag.

Graner, P.S., Faggella-Luby, M.N., & Fritschmann, N.A. (2005). An overview of responsiveness to intervention: What practitioners ought to know. *Topics in Language Disorders, 25*(2), 93–104.

Higdon, C. (2003) CPT Coding for AAC/SGDs. *The ASHA Leader Online.* Retrieved May 1, 2006, from http://www.asha.org/about/publications/leader-online/b-line/bl030527.htm

Individuals with Disabilities Education Act (IDEA) of 1990, PL 101-476, 20 U.S.C. §§ 1400 *et seq.*

Individuals with Disabilities Education Improvement Act of 2004, PL 108-446, 20 U.S.C. §§ 1400 *et seq.*

Lieurance, E. (1993 October). Speak up! Get involved in public policy. *The University of Missouri Extension.* Retrieved May 1, 2006, from http://muextension.missouri.edu/xplor/hesguide/famecon/gh3970.htm

Medicare Prescription Drug Modernization Act of 2003, PL 108-173.

Metcalf, S. (2002 January 28). Reading between the lines. *The Nation.* Retrieved May 1, 2006, from http://www.thenation.com/doc.mhtml?i=20020128&s=metcalf

Meyer, L. (2004 May 27). No Child Left Behind fails to pass fairness test. *Albuquerque Journal*. Retrieved May 1, 2006, from http://ourworld.compuserve.com/homepages/JWCRAWFORD/AJ2.htm

Moore, M. (2000). '99 victories in Congress spur 2000 strategies. *The ASHA Leader, 5*(2), 1.

Moore-Brown, B.J., & Montgomery, J.K. (2005). *Making a difference: In the era of accountability*. Eau Claire, WI: Thinking Publications.

Moore-Brown, B.J., Montgomery, J.K., Bielinski, J., & Shubin, J. (2005). Responsiveness to intervention: Teaching before testing helps avoid labeling. *Topics in Language Disorders, 25*(2), 148–167.

National Dissemination Center for Children and Youth with Disabilities (1996). *The education of children and youth with special needs: What do the laws say?* Retrieved May 1, 2006, from http://www.nichcy.org/pubs/outprint/nd15txt.htm#introduction

Nelson, N.W. (1998). *Childhood language disorders in context: Infancy through adolescence*. Boston: Allyn & Bacon.

Newborn and Infant Hearing Screening and Intervention Act, PL 93-406, 88 Stat. 829.

No Child Left Behind Act of 2001, PL 107-110, 115 Stat. 1425, 20 U.S.C. §§ 6301 *et seq.*

Office of Special Education and Rehabilitative Service's rehabilitation services administration legislation page. (2005). Retrieved July 1, 2006, from http://www.ed.gov/print/policy/speced/reg/index.html

Older American Act Amendments, PL 106-501, Stat. 2226, 42 U.S.C §§ 3001 *et seq.*

Older Americans Act of 1965, PL 89-73, 42 U.S.C. §§ 3001 *et seq.*

Rigby, S., & Kipping, P. (2000). *The speech-language pathologist's guide to managing the new Medicare*. Austin, TX: PRO-ED.

Social Security Act of 1935, PL 74-271, 42 U.S.C. §§ 301 *et seq.*

Staskowski, M., & Rivera, E.A. (2005). Speech-language pathologists' involvement in responsiveness to intervention activities: A complement to curriculum-relevant practice. *Topics in Language Disorders, 25*(2), 132-147.

U. S. Department of Education (2002). *No Child Left Behind: Overview*. Retrieved June 22, 2005, from http://www.ed.gov/nclb/landing.jhtml?src=pb

U.S. Department of Education. (2005). *Spellings announces new special education guidelines, details, workable "common-sense" policy to help states implement No Child Left Behind*. Retrieved July 1, 2006, from http://www.ed.gov/news/pressreleases/2005/05/05102005.html

STUDY QUESTIONS

1. What is a public policy? Why is it important for SLPs and audiologists to know about public policies?

2. What are the key elements guaranteed by NCLB and IDEA'04? How do these laws influence audiologists and SLPs who work in school settings?

3. Contrast the important aspects of the Section 504 of the Rehabilitation Act and the ADA.

4. Explain the influence of Medicare, Medicaid, and managed care organizations on speech-language pathology and audiology service provision in medical settings.

5. Describe the term *advocacy*. Why is it important for audiologists and SLPs to take on advocacy roles?

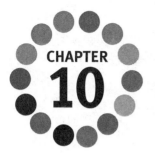

CHAPTER 10

Clinical Service Delivery and Work Settings

PAUL W. CASCELLA, MARY H. PURDY, AND JAMES J. DEMPSEY

Speech-language pathologists (SLPs) and audiologists provide a broad range of professional services aimed at assessing, treating, and preventing speech, language, voice, hearing, swallowing, and related communication disabilities. Estimates suggest one out of every six Americans has a communication disorder and nearly 29 million Americans have a hearing impairment (American Speech-Language-Hearing Association [ASHA], 2004c). We, as audiologists and SLPs, strive to create service delivery models that can accommodate the broad range of communication disabilities faced by our patients, while matching the particular needs of each individual. **Service delivery models** are the systems that are used to organize speech-language and hearing programs within employment settings. These models define our roles in the rehabilitation of persons with communication disorders.

This chapter introduces contemporary service delivery models and work settings within the field of communication disorders. Service delivery includes the formats by which services are rendered, including where, when, and with whom services are provided. To illustrate service delivery, this chapter highlights the typical and unique work settings that are included in professional preparation programs for audiologists and SLPs. A list of common service delivery terms and their acronyms is included in Table 10.1.

SERVICE DELIVERY FEATURES

It is important to become familiar with the core vocabulary that distinguishes one service delivery model from another. In service provision, particular features characterize each approach.

Direct and Indirect Services

Direct services occur when a clinician works in a face-to-face format with an individual patient or a group of patients. In the hospital setting, an SLP might

Table 10.1. Common acronyms related to service delivery

American Academy of Audiology (AAA)
Augmentative and alternative communication (AAC)
Auditory brainstem response (ABR)
Americans with Disabilities Act (ADA)
American Federation of Teachers (AFT)
American Occupational Therapy Association (AOTA)
American Physical Therapy Association (APTA)
American Speech-Language-Hearing Association (ASHA)
Birth-to-three services (B-3)
Commission of the Accreditation of Rehabilitation Facilities (CARF)
Certificate of Clinical Competence (CCC)
Continuum of care (COC)
Certified occupational therapy assistant (COTA)
Committee on Special Education (CSE)
Comprehensive System of Personnel Development (CSPD)
Electronystagmography (ENG)
Ear, nose, and throat doctor (ENT; otolaryngologist)
Extended school year (ESY)
Free and appropriate education (FAPE)
Home health care (HHC)
Health maintenance organization (HMO)
Hard of hearing (HOH)
Health care financing administration (HCFA)
Intermediate care facility/mental retardation (ICF/MR)
Intensive care unit (ICU)
Individualized education plan (IEP)
Individualized family service plan (IFSP)
Individuals with Disabilities Education Act (IDEA)
Joint Commission on the Accreditation of Health Care Organizations (JCAHCO)
Local education agency (LEA)
Least restrictive environment (LRE)
National Education Association (NEA)
National Association for the Education of Young Children (NAEYC)
Neonatal intensive care unit (NICU)
Otoacoustic emissions (OAE)
Occupational therapy (OT)
Occupational therapist, registered (OTR)
Office of Special Education Programs (OSEP)
Office of Special Education and Rehabilitative Services (OSERS)
Planning and placement team (PPT)
Physical therapist (PT)
Physical therapy (PT)
Physical therapy assistant (PTA)
Residential care facility (RCF)
Registered nurse (RN)
State Education Agency (SEA)
Speech-language pathologist (SLP)
Speech-Language pathology assistant (SLPA)
Skilled nursing facility (SNF)
Transitional living center (TLC)
University affiliated program (UAP)
World Health Organization (WHO)
World Health Organization International Classification of Functioning, Disability and Health (WHO-ICF)

provide direct swallowing rehabilitation with a patient at bedside. In an elementary school, a clinician might work directly with a small group of students with language-delays who are learning the vocabulary associated with their first-grade math curriculum. **Indirect services** occur when the clinician does not have hands-on contact with the client but instead is likely to consult with the client's family members, teachers, and/or medical personnel about the client's communication needs. An example of this occurs when a classroom teacher follows the suggestion of a clinician and deliberately emphasizes the way particular sounds are pronounced by the students during a "letter of the week" activity in a kindergarten class. Another example is when the staff of a group home follows a clinician's suggestion and develops a picture board that helps an adult with a developmental disability communicate during community outings.

Clinical and Consultative Services

Direct services can include both clinical and consultative/collaborative services. In a **clinical model,** a school SLP typically takes children out of their classroom so as to provide intensive one-to-one or small group instruction in a separate location. A clinical model is advantageous when trying to initially teach children particular speech-language skills and when standardized testing needs to be completed. A clinical model can also be utilized when a child needs a less distracting environment and when the intervention protocol warrants privacy. This may be necessary, for example, among children who stutter and need a safe place in which to talk about their feelings. The clinical model is also utilized within medical speech-language pathology, when, for example, an adult who has had a stroke leaves his or her home and comes to a university clinic to practice communication skills.

Consultative/collaborative services occur when members of an intervention team work together and share responsibility for client outcomes. In a school setting, the classroom teacher and the SLP can support each other's efforts to enhance students' academic success and communication skills. In one example, an SLP might work directly in a classroom and embed language objectives into small-group learning activities using materials from the academic curriculum. In another example, an SLP might work on literacy by leading phonological awareness activities during class reading time. By engaging in collaborative/consultative services, the SLP becomes better aware of the language demands within the academic curriculum and the social communication demands within the children's peer groups.

Another format for the consultative/collaborative approach is when an SLP works indirectly with a client by providing guidance to the client's family members and professional colleagues (i.e., general and special education teachers, preschool teachers, skilled nursing facility staff, birth-to-3 professionals, **psychologists,**) who work more directly with the patient. This can occur, when we teach parents how to provide home-based language models, or when we help birth-to-3 professionals facilitate early feeding skills among infants with Down syndrome. Also, after a speech-language evaluation, we might make recommendations to home health care staff about communication strategies for people with Alzheimer disease.

Collaborative partnerships require that professionals from different disciplines work together in an effort to integrate patient goals, objectives, and intervention strategies. In these partnerships, participants bring their own field of expertise to their professional colleagues when they mutually design instructions, solve problems, and share teaching responsibilities. In both clinical and consultative/collaborative therapy services, there needs to be considerable scheduling coordination among team members. For example, in a clinical model, classroom teachers may become concerned about the amount of instruction the child misses when absent from the classroom, and in consultative/collaborative model, classroom curricula and activities must be scheduled flexibly to accommodate the future incorporation of speech-language goals. School personnel must also have scheduling flexibility to meet and discuss the integration of speech-language goals into academic curricula. Often, a client's speech-language intervention plan calls for both clinical and collaborative/consultation services.

Individual and Group Services

Sometimes, the SLP will vary the number of clients in a therapy session. *Individual services* are intense and one-to-one in nature and are typically aimed at teaching the client a specific communication skill. An example of individual services occurs when Tom, an adult with apraxia of speech, works on speech production strategies during an individual intervention session at a rehabilitation center. *Group services* include two or more patients who are apt to be working on similar speech-language skills or who need to practice the generalization of learned skills to additional communication partners. For example, after Tom learns speech production strategies during individual services, he might participate in a group session where he is expected to converse with other adults. Although individual services might focus on skill practice and strategies, a group session enables Tom to receive natural feedback from his peers. Another example of group services occurs in a **self-contained classroom** when the SLP is the primary educator providing both academic instruction and intensive speech-language remediation. This can occur when we run a class for preschoolers who need focused stimulation because they have severe speech sound disorders.

Multidisciplinary, Interdisciplinary, and Transdisciplinary Models

SLPs are often asked to work with their professional colleagues from the education, medical, and allied health (i.e., physical therapy, occupational therapy) fields so as to conjointly develop intervention plans which are unified and coordinated by content, objectives, and strategies (see Table 10.2). There are currently three models that identify the relationships shared by team members in the facilitation of patient progress. The first two, multidisciplinary and interdisciplinary, are often interchanged depending on the work setting, and both are popular in medical settings and schools. In a multidisciplinary model, each individual discipline conducts its own assessment and develops discipline specific goals with minimal integration of these goals across disciplines. Each discipline has its own plan for the patient, with goals reflecting only its own field of expertise.

In an interdisciplinary model, each discipline conducts its own particular assessment but also communicates with other disciplines about the results of these assessments. This communication fosters complementary goal development so that as each discipline creates its plan for the client, all disciplines

Table 10.2. Service delivery professionals

	Birth-to-3	School settings	Medical settings
Audiologist	X	X	X
Chaplain			X
Childcare worker	X		
Dietician			X
Neuropsychologist			X
Nurse	X	X	X
Nurse's aide			X
Occupational therapist	X	X	X
Pediatric developmental specialist	X	X	
Physical therapist	X	X	X
Physician	X	X	X
Psychologist	X	X	X
Recreational therapist			X
Rehabilitation paraprofessional	X	X	X
School counselor		X	
Social worker	X	X	X
Special education teacher	X	X	
Speech-language pathologist	X	X	X
Teacher (general education)	X	X	X

incorporate elements of the goals and objectives of related fields into the plan. For example, when working with a patient with TBI, language sequencing may be one objective for the SLP. As part of the program, the SLP might have the patient write down the steps associated with daily tasks (e.g., turn off alarm, get out of bed, go to the bathroom, brush teeth). While writing, the patient can be given instructions about holding the pencil correctly and using eye-hand co-ordination, strategies that had been suggested to the SLP by the patient's occupational therapist (OT). Conversely, during an occupational therapy session, the OT can include verbal sequencing as part of therapeutic activities.

A transdisciplinary model means that team members have an ongoing dialogue in which they share information, knowledge, and skills in order to develop and implement a single integrated service plan for the client. In this model, there is a single assessment of the client that is completed in unison by professionals from several disciplines. Together, they review the assessment data and weave together objectives reflective of all the disciplines. The team typically authorizes one person who, along with the client's family members or caregivers, becomes responsible for carrying out the client's intervention plan. For example, a 17-year-old client with developmental disabilities who is making the transition to living and working independently is likely to have a job coach. This job coach is responsible for teaching vocational skills by integrating several educational domains (i.e., academic, social, speech-language, activities of daily living) as the client learns job and communication skills and how to dress and socialize appropriately in the job setting. In this situation, the job coach can link together the educational plan, and the SLP can teach the job coach strategies to facilitate workplace communication skills.

Table 10.3. Service delivery guidelines from the American Speech-Language Hearing Association (ASHA) and the American Academy of Audiology (AAA)

ASHA and AAA codes of Ethics	Provides an ethical code governing clinician behaviors and actions
ASHA and AAA scope of practice guidelines	Describes the broad range of services and supports offered by these professions
ASHA preferred practice guidelines	Outlines acceptable client care, clinical processes, and anticipated outcomes
ASHA practice guidelines and technical reports	Recommends clinical practice parameters in specific work settings
ASHA position statements	Describes policies in matters of professional practice

PROFESSIONAL GUIDELINES FOR SERVICE DELIVERY

In both speech-language pathology and audiology, there are guidelines from ASHA and the American Academy of Audiology (AAA) that provide direction about clinical activities within service delivery and work settings. These guidelines (see Table 10.3) establish professional practice parameters for ethical practice, specific speech-language-hearing disorders, and typical clinical activities. For example, an ASHA technical report outlines the role of an audiologist in occupational hearing conservation and hearing loss prevention (ASHA, 2004a) and the role of an SLP in school-based preferred practice (ASHA, 2000) and an ASHA position statement identifies the role of an SLP who provides clinical services via telepractice (ASHA, 2005a). Two examples of guidelines from AAA are 1) AAA's scope of practice guidelines (AAA, 2004) and 2) the position statement on the audiologist's role in the diagnosis of vestibular disorders (AAA, 2005).

CONTEMPORARY ISSUES IN SERVICE DELIVERY

Historically, speech-language service delivery has concentrated on the one-to-one or small group intervention approach in which skills are strengthened through a hierarchy of task demands and prompts. Service delivery has seen vast changes since the 1970s and current service delivery models reflect evolving government agencies, health care management, educational philosophy, and human service principles. As service providers, we need to be aware of the many issues that influence service delivery approaches. Table 10.4 provides examples of contemporary issues that affect service delivery. An extensive review of public policies that affect clinical practice is presented in Chapter 9.

EDUCATION WORK SETTINGS FOR THE SPEECH-LANGUAGE PATHOLOGIST

SLPs work in a variety of educational settings for children from birth to age 21. Some of the programs you are likely to participate in as part of your graduate clinical practica are introduced.

Early Intervention Programs

Chapter 9 discusses the public policies that affect clinical practice, including public laws that govern early intervention services. Early intervention applies to

Table 10.4. Contemporary issues that influence service delivery

Issue	Speech-language pathologists are challenged to:
Functional communication	Develop protocols that relate to classroom curricula, independent living and vocational skills, and the natural situations in which their clients communicate.
Assistive and instrumental technology	Increase their technical competence with alternative and augmentative communication (AAC), assistive technology, and medical technology (i.e., ventilators, tracheotomy tubes, nasendoscopy, videofluoroscopy).
Evidence-based practice	Investigate and verify that their assessment and treatment approaches are supported by clinical expertise, research evidence, and client values.
Managed care	Develop effective and efficient service delivery programs.
Accountability	Justify the worth of their clinical services in terms of client progress, cost, and time.
Inclusion	Ensure that communication supports assist children with special needs as they access the regular education curriculum.
Collaboration	Coordinate speech-language services with other education and medical personnel.
Educational standards	Support and document how speech-language intervention can enhance the academic achievement outcomes of students in public schools.
Multicultural issues	Provide services that are culturally sensitive and applicable.
Transition services	Help clients make life transition decisions (e.g., high school to work and reintegration to employment after adult onset disorders).
Regulations and accreditation	Stay familiar with the regulatory and accreditation guidelines governing service delivery.
Self advocacy, family involvement, and client rights	Respect clients and family members as integral participants in designing, implementing, and evaluating the effectiveness of treatment programs.
Eligibility and exit criteria	Balance the opinions of clients, families, and regulatory bodies that may have different opinions about when services are warranted and/or when services are no longer needed.
Speech-language pathology assistants and para-professionals	Understand the issues and guidelines surrounding the use of support personnel.

children from birth to kindergarten. Two systems of early intervention exist, one for children age birth to 3 years, and the second for preschoolers age 3 to kindergarten.

Birth-to-3 services emphasize that the family of the child with a disability is the recipient of services. This means that the SLP must understand family-guided practice that is both culturally sensitive and specific to each family's circumstance. In this model, family members are integral to the design, implementation, and evaluation of services, and they are considered partners with education and rehabilitation professionals in their child's developmental growth (Rini & Whitney, 1999). Birth-to-3 service provision most often operates using a transdisciplinary model by designing a single integrated individualized family service plan (IFSP). When speech-language objectives are recommended for the child, these are designed to coincide with objectives being addressed across other areas of development. The primary interventionist represents every discipline, and, for example, when we assume that role, we facilitate not only communication skills, but also any other goals on the child's IFSP (e.g., fine and gross motor skills, cognition, socialization, adaptive behavior, transition). In this model, service provision occurs in a variety of settings (e.g.., the child's home, a childcare center, a clinic, a segregated or inclusive playgroup) and our role may be direct or indirect, individual or group, and consultative or clinical.

A primary goal of many birth-to-3 programs is to mainstream young children with disabilities so as to provide rich peer language models and promote social development. In doing so, the interventionist becomes responsible for creating educational activities that adapt typical routines by training child care providers and promoting social skills with peers. The topic of service provision in the birth-to-3 model is discussed further in Chapter 13.

Preschool and School-Based Services

The 2003 ASHA omnibus survey indicated that a majority of SLPs work in educational settings (i.e., preschool and school-age). ASHA estimates that nearly 1.1 million school children ages 6–21 have a primary diagnosis of "speech-language impairment" (ASHA, 2004b), and school-based clinicians also provide services to children who have other educational disabilities that affect communication processes. Table 10.5 highlights some of the most frequent communication and educational diagnoses of school-age children and the percentage of school-based SLPs who report serving these children.

Among school-based SLPs, particular service delivery models seem to occur for particular communication disorders. A traditional clinical model is common, either alone or in conjunction with other approaches, for children with disorders of articulation/phonology, fluency, voice, and language. Classroom-based models are often utilized for children with augmentative and alternative communication (AAC) needs, as well as for children with language disorders, cognitive-communication needs, and auditory processing disorders. Collaborative/consultation models occur most frequently for children with language concerns and cognitive-communication needs. Children with related educational diagnoses often receive collaborative/consultation services.

As noted in Chapter 9, school-age children are eligible for speech-language services through the Individuals with Disabilities Education Improvement Act of

Table 10.5. Percentage of school-based clinicians serving communication and related educational disorders

Communication disorders	Percentage of school-based clinicians
Articulation/phonology disorders	91.8%
Fluency disorder	67.5%
Specific language impairment	61.1%
Childhood apraxia	59.4%
Augmentative and alternative communication	50.8%
Hearing disorders	45.8%
Cognitive communicative disorders	43.6%
Voice/resonance disorders	33.8%
Dysphagia	13.8%
Related education disorders	
Autism spectrum disorders	77.4%
Learning disability	72.4%
Intellectual/developmental disability	70.9%
Reading/writing disability	35.7%

Table 10.6. Individuals with Disabilities Education Improvement Act of 2004 requirements for school-based speech-language services

Identification	Students must be screened to determine whether they have speech-language concerns in need of further assessment.
Assessment	Students who are potentially eligible for speech-language services must participate in nonbiased assessment of their strengths, weaknesses, disorders, and/or delays.
Intervention	Students deemed eligible for services are entitled to receive free and appropriate speech-language intervention services in the least restrictive environment.
Consultation/counseling	Family members and educators who are primarily responsible for students with disabilities are entitled to ongoing discussion about the students' problems and remediation plans.
Referral	Students with communication disorders are entitled to the professional advice of related education and rehabilitation disciplines.

2004 (IDEA; PL 108-446), the planning and placement team (PPT) process, and the individual education plan (IEP). IDEA is the most often used mechanism for providing special services to students with disabilities. Table 10.6 outlines IDEA mandated school speech-language pathology services. Preschool and school-based speech-language services require the child to have the label "speech-language impairment" or another educational diagnosis that will affect speech-language development and use (i.e., specific learning disability, autism spectrum disorder, intellectual disability, hearing impairment, and attention-deficit/hyperactivity disorder).

Although school-based clinicians spend a majority of their time in direct intervention, they are likely to have other clinical tasks, including conducting diagnostic evaluations, screenings, and report writing; attending parent and staff meetings; completing paperwork; and supervising student clinicians and/or colleagues. School clinicians are also often asked to take part in tasks shared by the entire teaching staff. These might include performing lunch and bus supervision duties, assisting with kindergarten registration, creating hallway bulletin boards, and helping with school plays and concerts. These additional duties may seem time consuming, given our large caseloads, travel between schools, and lack of planning time. Yet, these tasks provide opportunities to interact cooperatively with the other faculty members and enable us to observe and stimulate children out of the typical classroom and therapy context.

MEDICAL WORK SETTINGS FOR THE SPEECH-LANGUAGE PATHOLOGIST

There are numerous medical conditions that may result in communication or swallowing disorders (see Table 10.7). Consequently, approximately 30% of SLPs work in medical settings (Rosenfield, 2002). The most common work settings are general medical hospitals and skilled nursing facilities. Other medical settings include rehabilitation hospitals, outpatient clinics, home health agencies, or pediatric hospitals. In general hospitals and skilled nursing facilities, a large portion of your time may be spent treating individuals with dysphagia. In both inpatient and outpatient rehabilitation centers, however, more time may be spent with remediation of aphasia or **cognitive communication disorder** (see Table 10.8). In each of these settings, our role typically includes assessment, development of

Table 10.7. Medical conditions resulting in communication and/or swallowing disorders

Medical conditions	Communication and swallowing disorders
Stroke	Aphasia
Traumatic brain injury	Dysarthria
Progressive disease	Apraxia
Spinal cord injury	Cognitive-linguistic disorder
Head and neck tumors	Dysphonia
Brain tumors	Aphonia
Dementia	Speech-language delay/disorder
Vocal fold abnormalities	Dysphagia
Acquired immune deficiency syndrome	
Respiratory disorders	
Congenital and genetic disorders	
Premature birth	

an intervention plan, and patient/family education, although the proportion of these duties may vary depending on the setting.

ASHA has adopted the **World Health Organization's (WHO)** International Classification of Functioning, Disability, and Health (ICF) framework (WHO, 2001) for guiding assessment and intervention services to people with communication disorders (ASHA, 2004d). This framework considers the influence of body structure and function on the performance of daily activities and an individual's ability to participate in life functions. Participation may be further influenced by a variety of personal or environmental variables. For example, Tina has had a stroke (health condition) and a resulting aphasia (impairment in body function), and she is not able to speak intelligibly to a conversation partner (activity limitation) or return to work (participation restriction). Tina is, however, exceptionally motivated to return to work and therefore regularly practices her speech exercises (positive personal variable). In addition, Tina's employer may adapt Tina's work environment and encourage Tina to use her AAC strategies during interactions (positive environmental factor; see Figure 10.1). Knowing the impact of the communication disorder on daily life functioning helps the SLP manage patients' care and facilitate transitions from one medical setting to another as the patients recover and the goals of rehabilitation change.

The transition through various settings is referred to as the **continuum of care (COC)** (see Figure 10.2). As part of the intervention team, SLPs participate in the decision to move patients through the continuum. Various regulatory bodies, however, also influence the placement of a patient in a specific type of facility. One of the major issues related to service delivery in medical settings is the concept of **managed care.** This is the collective term for approaches to the

Table 10.8. Percentage of time spent by medically-based clinicians

Dysphagia	42%
Aphasia	20%
Cognitive communication	20%
Motor speech	10%
Voice	6%
Other	2%

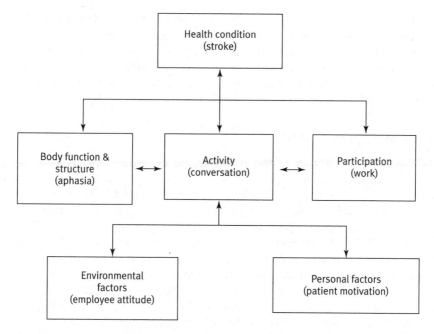

Figure 10.1. World Health Organization international classification of disease.

delivery of health care that attempt to control quality while containing costs. Third-party payers that cover the costs of rehabilitation (e.g., Medicare, private insurance) now have a great influence in determining the number of sessions a patient may receive and may even influence how a patient progresses through the COC.

Other regulatory bodies that may influence service delivery are the accreditation commissions. The **Joint Commission on the Accreditation of Health**

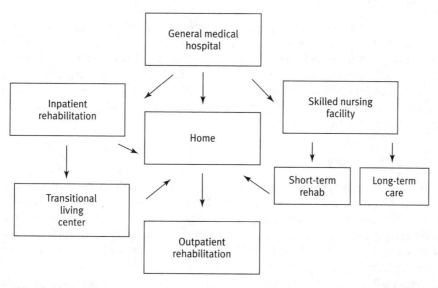

Figure 10.2. Continuum of care.

Care Organizations (JCAHCO) and the **Commission of the Accreditation of Rehabilitation Facilities (CARF)** both have regulations that must be met regarding documentation, amount of therapy provided, communication among team members, goal setting, and inclusion of the patient in the plan for his or her intervention. SLPs must adhere to the guidelines imposed by both the insurance companies and the accrediting bodies.

General Medical Hospitals

Individuals are admitted to a general medical hospital due to needs for immediate medical management. As a result, these individuals are often medically unstable and may be admitted to the **intensive care unit (ICU)** where they receive continuous medical monitoring. Once stabilized, they are moved to the main hospital floor. Because hospital stays are often brief, our role is typically that of a consultant. We are responsible for evaluating the patient in order to determine the presence, type, and severity of the communication or swallowing disorder, and educating the patient, family, and staff regarding the findings and recommendations of the evaluation. For example, we may receive a referral from a **neurologist** to evaluate a patient, Marie, who had a stroke. Marie is having difficulty speaking and swallowing. We evaluate her and determine she has a severe dysarthria. Her speech is difficult to understand due to severe weakness in the oral musculature. The weakness extends from the mouth to the pharynx, resulting in a severe dysphagia, and Marie cannot eat or drink safely. Due to her immediate need to receive adequate nutrition, you recommend a **videoflouroscopic swallowing study (VFSS)** to determine the specific swallowing problem and possible management approaches. The procedure is carried out in the Radiology Department by a **radiologist.** Following the study, a **nasogastric tube** is recommended as an alternative method of feeding. In addition, you also recommend speech therapy to work on Marie's speech and swallowing. You also collaborate with medical and rehabilitation staff such as the physical therapist (PT) and OT regarding the continued needs and the most appropriate discharge destination.

Within many hospitals, premature infants or other infants with severe medical problems immediately after birth may be transferred to the **neonatal intensive care unit (NICU).** Many of these infants have feeding and swallowing problems. For example, an infant delivered at 32 weeks' gestation has numerous respiratory problems and an uncoordinated suck/swallow. The SLP may observe and evaluate the baby during feedings and provide suggestions to parents and nursing staff.

Children's Hospitals

Some SLPs may work in a hospital that provides medical care specifically to children from infancy through late adolescence. Some of these children may have communication or swallowing difficulties as a result of a birth defect such as **Möbius syndrome.** Other children may have an acquired communication or swallowing disorder resulting from a medical condition such as a brain tumor or traumatic brain injury (TBI). The role of the SLP is largely the same as in the general medical setting. We are responsible for evaluation, intervention, education, and discharge planning as part of the interdisciplinary team. In addition, the SLP in a children's hospital may act as a consultant once a child is discharged. For example, we may meet with the birth-to-3 team to provide swallowing recommendations for an infant with a **cleft palate.** Or, we may meet with a child's elementary school teachers and school-based SLP following the child's discharge from the hospital following a TBI. Our goal is to provide as smooth a transition as possible from the hospital to the school.

Rehabilitation Units and Hospitals

Some hospitals have a dedicated rehabilitation unit, while other intensive rehabilitation programs are housed in specialized rehabilitation hospitals. Rehabilitation hospitals often have specific programs for acquired brain injury (ABI) (e.g. stroke, traumatic brain injury), spinal cord injuries, or respiratory dysfunction. The SLP may be assigned to a single unit, or required to work in all programs. Patients admitted to these programs are generally medically stable and are able to participate in several hours of therapy each day, which can be a combination of speech, occupational, physical, recreational, and/or psychosocial therapies. The SLP's first role is to assess the patient. At this stage, patients can tolerate longer sessions and the assessment can be more in depth than in the general hospital. When testing is completed, an appropriate intervention plan is developed given the specific diagnosis and needs of the patient. The SLP also functions as a member of a team. Depending on the philosophy of the rehabilitation program, the type of team may vary (multi-, inter-, transdisciplinary). In this setting, the SLP will likely provide a combination of individual and group therapy. In addition, the SLP may cotreat patients with professionals from other disciplines. For example, if a patient has **cognitive impairments** that interfere with **executive function,** the SLP might conduct an intervention session with the OT in a kitchen and focus on assisting the patient with organization and sequencing skills required for the patient to prepare a meal, while the OT addresses the patient's hand and arm control and trains the patient in the use of adaptive equipment. The primary goal of therapy is to enhance communicative and cognitive functioning and prepare the patient for discharge home. Regular team meetings are held to discuss the patient's progress, and, prior to discharge, a meeting is held with the patient and family to assist with the transition home.

Outpatient Rehabilitation Centers

Outpatient rehabilitation centers may be affiliated with a general medical hospital or a rehabilitation hospital or may be an independent center. Individuals participating in outpatient rehabilitation programs are transported from their homes to the center. Similar to our responsibilities within inpatient programs, we evaluate the patient and set up an individualized intervention plan. The patient and his or her family are likely to have significant input into the goals of intervention. For example, a patient with a mild dysarthria due to Parkinson's disease may state, "I want to talk better so I can be understood on the telephone and get back to work." Or, an elementary school teacher with dysphonia due to vocal nodules may state, "I want to learn to use my voice so I don't get hoarse at the end of the day." Goals typically are geared toward maximizing communicative functioning in the home and the community as well as those communication skills necessary for return to work or school. The intensity of intervention may vary from daily to once a week. Individual and group interventions are typically provided, and multiple interventions may occur at the same time. Some intervention may even occur in the community. For example, you may take a patient to a fast food restaurant to practice using his or her verbal skills or AAC system to order a meal.

Transitional Living Centers

Transitional living centers are geared toward those individuals who need to return to an independent lifestyle. Most residents of this type of program are young and have sustained a traumatic brain injury (e.g., as a result of a vehicular accident). The SLP works very closely with other rehabilitation staff and directs intervention toward self-management and community reentry skills. For example, we may help the nursing staff develop a plan to teach the patient his or her medication schedule and compensate for memory problems, or we may address managing the patient's finances. Therapy is often provided in a group setting led by the SLP or cofacilitated by the SLP and another team member, depending on the focus of the group.

Skilled Nursing Facilities

Individuals are admitted to a skilled nursing facility if they need ongoing nursing and medical care which cannot be managed by family members in the home. These facilities often have two distinct units: short-term (or subacute) care and long-term care. Individuals on the short-term units typically have the goal of returning home. They may be slower to recover from an illness or injury and therefore do not qualify for intensive rehabilitation programs. For example, we may see a patient on the short-term unit with swallowing problems due to **multiple sclerosis** who was admitted to regulate his or her medications and to improve his or her endurance, self-care, and safety while swallowing. The goal for intervention may be to train the patient and his or her family members and caregivers to use some strategies to make swallowing easier and to recognize any signs of difficulty when the patient returns home. Individuals in long-term care are likely to remain in the facility for the rest of their lives. These patients may have a progressive neurological disease such as **Alzheimer disease.** These individuals may be seen in a group setting for general cognitive stimulation. In addition, education and training may be provided to caregivers regarding supportive communication techniques. Because Alzheimer disease is progressive, the goal of intervention would not be to improve the patients' memory and communication but to facilitate and maintain communication as long as possible to improve quality of life. Medicare regulations have greatly influenced the provision of speech therapy and other rehabilitation services within these facilities. Strict guidelines must be followed regarding the amount and type of therapy provided.

Home Health Care

Individuals may be eligible to receive therapy in the home if they are considered "homebound"; that is, they are unable to leave their home. They may be transported by family members or other caregivers to their doctor appointments, but they do not leave the home for any other purpose. These individuals often require the services of a registered nurse and a home health aide. The SLP may be seeing an **oncology** patient who had his or her larynx removed and can no longer speak. The patient is still very weak and cannot drive. The patient has had difficulty maintaining weight due to side effects of medications and needs supplemental tube feeds. A nurse may help the patient manage the tube feeds, and a home health aide may assist the patient with bathing, dressing, and household chores. The SLP's role is to help the patient learn to communicate with an **electrolarynx** and to educate the patient and the caregivers regarding techniques that help facilitate communication.

CASE EXAMPLE 1

Bob is a 58-year-old man admitted to a general medical hospital with the diagnosis of a stroke. The SLP completes an evaluation and diagnoses a moderate aphasia. The PT and the OT determine Bob has a paralysis of his right side and is unable to complete basic activities of daily living (ADLs; e.g., dressing, bathing, cooking). Given his age, motivation, and potential for good progress, the rehabilitation team recommends that he be discharged to an inpatient rehabilitation program.

At the **inpatient rehabilitation** program, the SLP begins intensive intervention. Bob is scheduled for 1 hour of individual speech therapy per day. He starts to make progress in his ability to understand directions and questions, express some basic thoughts and ideas, and read sentences. Progress is also made in his physical therapy and occupational therapy, though Bob continues to need moderate assistance to complete his ADLs. After 3 weeks, the rehabilitation team determines that Bob's wife could manage him at home. After some education and training for his family members, Bob was discharged.

Once at home, Bob receives occupational, physical, and speech therapy through **home care services.** Rapid progress is made with his mobility and ability to perform his ADLs. The SLP continues to work with him on his language skills. After 4 weeks, Bob makes significant progress in all language areas. Physically, he can now get around the house and in and out of the car, so PT discharges him. A referral to outpatient therapy is recommended for continued speech therapy.

Bob begins therapy at an **outpatient facility.** His speech and language program is geared toward return to work. He participates in individual and group therapy, as well as some activities in the community. After 8 weeks, Bob is ready to return to work on a part-time basis.

Private Practices and Other Work Settings for Speech-Language Pathologists

Running an independent private practice is similar to running any other small business. The challenges and risks, both financial and emotional, of such an endeavor are greater than in other professional settings. The rewards of a successful private practice, however, are equally great. SLPs who work in a private practice have a lot of flexibility in choosing the setting in which they may work. Some may see individuals in a private office; some may contract with various facilities such as hospitals, rehabilitation agencies, schools, or group homes; and some may act primarily as consultants. In private practice, the SLP can specify the types of communication disorders he or she may treat and accept only those referrals. Depending on the setting and type of client seen in a private practice, we may work completely independently or be part of a team. For example, one SLP may specialize in management of communication disorders in children with autism spectrum disorders. She may contract with several school systems and be called upon to evaluate a child, provide specific intervention recommendations, and train the teachers in management of the child's intervention. Another SLP may be hired by parents of children with communication disorders and provide therapy outside of school. Or, an SLP may have contracts with several nursing homes or hospitals, which would contact the SLP when a client needs to be evaluated and have an intervention plan set up. This SLP may also be hired privately by a family to provide therapy in the home.

Colleges and Universities

Some SLPs may function as a professor or clinical supervisor in a college or university setting. Here, we may provide direct services to the clients, but our main role is to provide undergraduate and graduate education and supervise graduate student clinicians who are training to become SLPs themselves. Services may be provided at a university-based clinic or in a variety of educational or medical settings with whom the university has a contract. When we function as a clinical instructor, our role is to provide a foundation in the principles of diagnosis and intervention and expose our students to a wide variety of communication disorders encountered in children and adults. In this college or university setting, an SLP may act as a consultant and provide a second opinion to school or hospital-based SLPs.

Psychiatric Centers

Some SLPs work in a psychiatric facility among individuals who present with severe behavioral disabilities secondary to psychiatric illness, mental health concerns, and/or social-emotional maladjustment. For this population, the SLP needs an understanding of behavioral management and the potential communicative function of aberrant or challenging behavior. In psychiatric centers, we work with **psychiatrists, behavior modification specialists,** and psychiatric **social workers.**

Group Home and Employment Settings
for People with Developmental Disabilities

Since the mid-1970s, small, local community group homes have gradually replaced large state institutions for people with developmental disabilities and/or intellectual disability (ID; i.e., mental retardation). Service provision to these individuals is often indirect and consultative. Assessment includes documenting the skills of the individual, and determining whether the individual is provided opportunities to actualize communication skills during daily routines. Intervention strategies focus on functional communication within everyday routines and community recreational events (Cascella & McNamara, 2004; ASHA, 2005b).

WORK SETTINGS FOR AUDIOLOGISTS

Audiologists practice their profession in a variety of settings. The majority of audiologists practice in some type of health care setting. As smaller number of audiologists practice in school systems, universities, and industrial environments.

Scope of Practice

In defining the scope of practice for the field of audiology it is important to realize that audiologists are autonomous professionals. This means that we have earned the right to function independently. Patients who seek the services of an audiologist can do so directly, without the referral of a physician. In order to maintain this autonomy, it is important that the audiologist provide services that fall under the true mission of the profession.

Audiologists are involved in activities that identify; assess; diagnose; manage in a nonmedical fashion; and interpret test results related to disorders of human hearing, balance, and other neural systems (AAA, 2004; ASHA, 2004e). These activities would include traditional **behavioral audiologic tests** of hearing sensitivity (i.e., air and bone conduction thresholds) as well as **electrophysiological tests** (i.e., auditory brainstem response). Audiologists are uniquely qualified to assess the hearing sensitivity of children and adults. In addition to assessing peripheral hearing sensitivity, audiologists are also involved in evaluation and management of children and adults with **auditory processing disorders.**

Audiologists often serve in a consultative capacity. When dealing with school-age children, audiologists may be called upon to consult with an educational team regarding educational implications of a hearing loss, educational programming, classroom acoustics, and large-area amplification systems for children with hearing impairments. Audiologists may also serve as consultants with regard to compliance with the *Americans with Disabilities Act (ADA) of 1990* (PL 101-336). In this capacity, the audiologist may be called on to determine accessibility for persons with hearing loss in public and private buildings and facilities. Many audiologists serve as expert witnesses for legal interpretations of audiological findings and the general effects of hearing loss. Consulting with industrial businesses regarding prevention of noise-induced hearing loss and implementing **hearing conservation** techniques has been a staple of the audiological profession for many years. More recently, many audiologists have gotten involved in consultation and provision of rehabilitation to persons with balance disorders through habituation, exercise therapy, and balance retraining.

The scope of practice for the audiologist has been rapidly expanding in recent years. One area in which audiologists have become involved is in the use of **otoscopic** examination and external ear canal management for removal of **cerumen.** In the past, cerumen management was a function performed exclusively by physicians or nurses. An ear canal that is clear of excessive cerumen is critical to obtaining an accurate audiological evaluation and impression of the external ear. In an attempt to expedite the diagnostic evaluation process, many audiologists have become involved in cerumen management.

Technological advances have led to additional activities becoming part of the audiological scope of practice. Many audiologists who are familiar with electrophysiological equipment now find themselves working in the operating room side by side with surgeons. In these instances, the audiologist is providing neuro-physiologic **intraoperative monitoring** and cranial nerve assessment. The purpose of intraoperative monitoring is to try to alert the surgeon to possible nerve damage during surgery in an attempt to maintain complete nerve function.

Another technological advancement that has broadened the scope of practice of the audiologist is the **cochlear implant.** Audiologists are involved in determining candidacy for cochlear implants as well as fitting, programming or mapping the device. Audiologists also provide rehabilitative services to optimize the benefits derived from the cochlear implant.

Although audiologists have been involved in newborn hearing screening programs for many years, legislation in many states during the 1990s has increased the need for involvement in this area. Many states now have mandated universal hearing screening for all newborns. The development of the otoacoustic emission (OAE) test battery has provided one tool by which these universal screening programs can be carried out. The **auditory brainstem response (ABR)** also continues to be used for this purpose.

Audiologists are also involved in **tinnitus** assessment and management. New developments in nonmedical management of tinnitus using biofeedback, masking, hearing aids, education, and counseling have led to an increase in this area by many audiologists.

The reduction of communication disorders is a primary theme that runs through the activities of the audiologist. Audiologists screen for obvious speech-language disorders, are involved in use of sign language, and provide rehabilitative services including speechreading and communication management strategies.

Practice Settings

Audiologists work in a wide variety of settings (ASHA, 2003). Figure 10.3 contains a breakdown of the primary settings in which audiologists practice.

Schools Those individuals who work in the school systems are referred to as educational audiologists. Their role will be mainly rehabilitative in nature. Educational audiologists work in a collaborative fashion with educators as a member of an interdisciplinary team. Educational audiologists provide input about amplification issues as well as communication management, educational implications of hearing loss, educational programming and classroom acoustics.

An example of a common scenario faced by an educational audiologist would be the case of a 10-year-old girl with a moderate to severe hearing loss who has recently moved into the school district. The educational audiologist in this setting would be called upon to provide input to the child's educational team regarding use of an **frequency modulation (FM) amplification system** in the classroom. The audiologist would also provide information regarding the expected influence of the hearing loss on educational performance for this child.

Hospitals or Medical Centers Approximately 20% of audiologists work in a hospital or medical center. In this setting the audiologist is almost always an employee of the hospital. The hospital setting provides a broad array of duties for audiologists. Diagnostic procedures will include in depth electrophysiological and behavioral assessments of inpatients and outpatients of all ages. If the hospital is a birthing hospital, audiologists will likely be involved in a universal

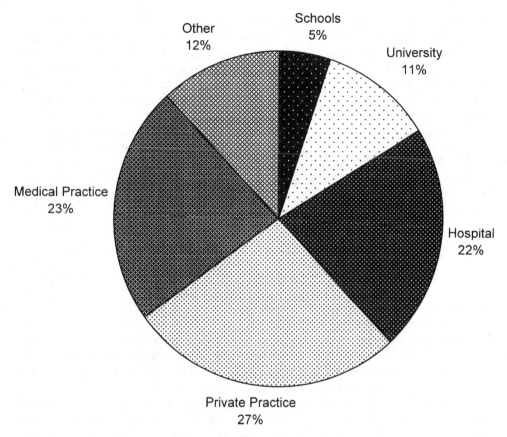

Figure 10.3. Primary settings in which audiologists practice. (From Stach, B. [1998]. *Clinical audiology: An introduction* [p. 11]. San Diego: Singular Publishing Group; reprinted with permission.)

neonatal hearing screening program. Audiologists may also be involved in hearing screenings and diagnostic evaluations of babies who spend time in the NICU. In many hospital settings, audiologists will have the opportunity to be involved in intraoperative monitoring in order to measure the integrity of various nerves during surgical procedures. The hospital setting is the environment in which audiologists are most likely to be involved in working with cochlear implants. It is also in the hospital or medical center where audiologists are most likely to be called upon to assess the possible **ototoxic** effects of various types of drug therapies.

One example of a clinical scenario in the hospital setting would be the case of the 20-year-old man with **cystic fibrosis.** This patient's team of doctors has recently prescribed the drug *Amikin* to help him with his breathing. This particular drug is known to have possible ototoxic side effects. The other team members have asked the hospital audiologist to perform repeated serial audiograms in order to monitor the patient's hearing sensitivity very closely. Ototoxic effects are usually first evident as shifts in hearing sensitivity in the very high frequencies. Under these circumstances, audiologists may choose to perform a combination of repeated high frequency audiograms as well as repeated OAEs.

Medical Practices Approximately 25% of audiologists work in a medical practice. In this setting, audiologists are most often an employee of the corporation that is usually managed by a physician or a group of physicians. The medical specialty of the physicians who hire audiologists is almost always **otolaryngology.**

The duties of audiologists in this setting will usually have a diagnostic emphasis. In addition to routine behavioral diagnostic measures of hearing sensitivity, audiologists will often be called upon to perform electrophysiological tests such as the ABR and **electronystagmography (ENG)** to assist the physician in making diagnoses regarding hearing and balance disorders.

An example of a common clinical scenario in a medical private practice could be seen in the case of a 62-year-old man who has been seen by the otolaryngologist with a complaint of episodes of dizziness. The physician has referred the patient to the audiologist for an audiological evaluation to measure hearing sensitivity and an ENG to evaluate the vestibular (balance) system. The audiologists' responsibility is to perform the requested tests and provide the results to the physician. The audiologist's role in this case is primarily diagnostic in nature and interpretation of test results will usually be left up to the otolaryngologist.

Private Practices   The practice setting that has grown most dramatically in the past few years and is most likely to continue to grow is the independent private practice. Almost 30% of audiologists currently work in this setting. One obvious reason for the growth in this area is related to a change in the official scope of practice guidelines for the profession (AAA, 2004; ASHA, 2004d). In the 1970s, dispensing hearing aids was not considered to be in the audiologist's scope of practice. In 2007, dispensing hearing aids is an integral part of the audiologist's duties and has provided the main source of income for many who are maintaining an independent private practice. Although diagnostic evaluations are an important part of most private practices, the emphasis is usually on the rehabilitative services of dispensing and fitting hearing aids. Most private practitioners state that they experience a tremendous feeling of satisfaction in running their own business. In addition, the potential for financial benefit is great as well. Median earnings for a successful independent private practice are estimated to be between 33% and 100% higher than the salary of other audiologists (Stach, 1998).

An example of a common clinical scenario in an independent private practice would be illustrated by the case of a 72-year-old woman who has recently noticed a decrease in her hearing sensitivity. This client has sought the advice of her family physician regarding her increase in communication difficulties. The physician has provided medical clearance for amplification to her and has referred her to the audiologist's private practice. Audiologists in private practice are responsible for assessment of the client's hearing sensitivity as well as the selection and fitting of appropriate hearing aids. In addition to the formal test protocols that may be used, a good deal of the audiologist's efforts will be rehabilitative in nature. The audiologist will spend significant time counseling the client regarding proper use of the instruments and establishing realistic expectations concerning aided performance.

Industry   Audiologists who work in industry are referred to as industrial audiologists or as environmental audiologists. Industrial audiologists are involved in the prevention of hearing loss to a greater extent than audiologists in other professional settings. A primary role of industrial audiologists is to be a manager of an effective hearing conservation program.

An industrial hearing conservation program includes assessing the levels of noise exposure experienced by workers, performing baseline and annual audiometric evaluations, and providing recommendations for utilizing hearing protection devices. An important part of an effective hearing conservation program is providing education to workers and supervisory personnel regarding noise-induced hearing loss. In addition, many industrial audiologists will be called on to make suggestions for engineering and administrative controls that will reduce the levels of noise exposure to employees.

Colleges and Universities   Some audiologists work at colleges and universities as professors or clinical instructors. Although these professionals may be involved in clinical activities, their main role is to provide graduate-level education and training to audiology students. It is common for audiologists in these settings to divide their time between lecturing to graduate students regarding diagnostic and rehabilitative procedures and providing actual services to a clinical population.

Hearing Aid Manufacturers   Companies that manufacture hearing aids employ some audiologists. In this setting, the audiologist will be responsible for bringing ideas to the company regarding design of instruments and communicative needs of hearing-impaired individuals. Audiologists working for hearing aid companies will often serve as in-house consultants to practicing audiologists regarding specific instruments produced by their company. These audiologists are available to provide hearing aid fitting suggestions over the telephone to other audiologists. On occasion, audiologists working in this capacity will travel to various facilities as a product representative for their particular company.

CONCLUSION

In conclusion, SLPs and audiologists have a myriad of opportunities to match their personal interests and styles to a work setting. All settings in which we practice make high levels of demand in terms of productivity, accountability, and technical competence. All settings also provide the personal satisfaction that is unique to our profession, knowing that we are helping clients to engage in one of the most important human functions: communication.

REFERENCES

American Academy of Audiology. (2004). *Scope of practice*. McLean, VA: Author.

American Academy of Audiology. (2005). *Position statement on the audiologist's role in the diagnosis and treatment of vestibular disorders*. Retrieved June 1, 2006, from http://www.audiology.org/professional/positions/vestibular.pdf

American Speech-Language-Hearing Association. (2000). *Guidelines for the roles and responsibilities of school-based speech-language pathologist*. Rockville, MD: Author.

American Speech-Language-Hearing Association. (2003). *2003 omnibus survey: Practice trends in audiology*. Rockville, MD: Author.

American Speech-Language-Hearing Association. (2004a). The audiologist's role in occupational hearing conservation and hearing loss prevention programs: Technical report. *ASHA Supplement 24*. Rockville, MD: Author.

American Speech-language-Hearing Association. (2004b). *Communication facts: Incidence and prevalence of communication disorders and hearing loss in children, 2004 edition*. Retrieved October 1, 2005, from http://www.asha.org/members/research/reports/children.htm

American Speech-Language-Hearing Association. (2004c). *Incidence and prevalence of hearing loss and hearing aid use in the United States, 2004 edition.* Retrieved October 1, 2005, from http://asha.org/members/research/reports/hearing.htm

American Speech-Language-Hearing Association. (2004d). *Preferred practice patterns for the profession of speech-language pathology.* Rockville, MD: Author.

American Speech-Language-Hearing Association. (2004e). *Scope of practice in audiology. ASHA Supplement 24.* Rockville, MD: Author.

American Speech-Language-Hearing Association. (2005a). *Roles and responsibilities of speech-language pathologists serving persons with mental retardation/developmental disabilities.* Retrieved December 1, 2005, from http://www.asha.org/members/deskref-journals/deskref/default

American Speech-Language-Hearing Association. (2005b). Speech-language pathologists providing clinical services via telepractice: Position statement. *ASHA Supplement 25.*

Americans with Disabilities Act (ADA) of 1990, PL 101-336, 42 U.S.C. §§ 12101 *et seq.*

Cascella, P.W., & McNamara, K.M. (2004). Practical communication services for high school students with severe disabilities: Collaboration during the transition to adult services. *The ASHA Leader, 9*(9), 6–7, 18–19.

Individuals with Disabilities Education Improvement Act of 2004, PL 108-446, 20 U.S.C. §§ 1400 *et seq.*

Rini, D.L., & Whitney, G.C. (1999). Family centered practice for children with communication disorders. *Child and Adolescent Psychiatric Clinics of North America, 8,* 1, 153–174.

Rosenfield, M. (2002). *Report on the ASHA speech-language pathology health care survey.* Retrieved October 1, 2005, from http://www.asha.org/members/slp/healthcare/healthcare_survey.htm

Stach, B. (1998). *Clinical audiology: An introduction.* San Diego: Singular Publishing Group.

World Health Organization. (2001). *International classification of functioning, disability and health (ICF).* Geneva: Author.

STUDY QUESTIONS

1. Describe some of the service delivery features that influence the role of the SLP. What are the relative strengths and weaknesses of these service delivery features?

2. Contrast multi- inter-, and transdisciplinary service provision.

3. Describe some of the contemporary factors affecting speech-language service provision in birth-to-3, public schools, and medical settings.

4. How is the work setting of the SLP in birth-to-3 services uniquely different than that of the school-based clinician?

5. Describe the parameters that contribute to a patient's progression through the continuum of care.

6. Compare and contrast the role of a SLP in a medical setting versus a school setting.

7. Describe three different settings in which audiologists may practice. Which one of these appeals to you the most and why?

8. How have recent technological developments broadened the scope of practice of the audiologist?

CHAPTER 11

Issues of Cultural and Linguistic Diversity

BRIAN GOLDSTEIN AND AQUILES IGLESIAS

A personal story from Brian Goldstein

As a speech-language pathologist (SLP) at Massachusetts General Hospital in Boston, I was asked to evaluate a 4-year-old Vietnamese-speaking child suspected of having a speech and language delay. At the time, I was perplexed about how I, as a speaker of English and Spanish, would assess the speech and language skills of a child who did not speak the languages I did. Moreover, I knew little about the cultural characteristics of the Vietnamese people. To prepare for this evaluation, I read material on Vietnam and the Vietnamese people, culture, and language. I also consulted with an individual from the local Vietnamese community center about the culture, language, and dialect of the region from which this child emigrated. After I provided some training, that individual served as my interpreter during this assessment. The knowledge I obtained from the individual at the community center and my training in a bilingual-bicultural emphasis graduate program allowed me to provide this child an appropriate assessment.

Not every SLP will have access to individuals who can provide cultural and linguistic information about clients or will have been enrolled in a training program with a major focus on providing appropriate clinical management skills to individuals from culturally and linguistically diverse populations. It should be noted, however, that the American Speech-Language-Hearing Association (ASHA) mandates academic and clinical education that prepares students in accredited programs to practice in a multicultural society (ASHA, 2004). This chapter provides a road map to the linguistic and cultural differences found in the United States of America today and shows how those differences influence the field of speech-language pathology. The overarching goal of this chapter is to better prepare and equip you for situations in which you provide clinical services to individuals who do not share your cultural and/or linguistic experiences.

CULTURALLY AND LINGUISTICALLY DIVERSE DEFINED

What individuals are considered *culturally and linguistically diverse*? For the most part, normative information about speech and language development and disorders comes from European American, middle-class individuals. That is, clinicians have tended to base their diagnostic and intervention approaches on one group. In a sense, everyone except those who make up that group would fall into the category of *culturally and linguistically diverse*. For the purposes of this chapter, we are concerning ourselves with individuals who diverge from the traditional group.

DEMOGRAPHICS

Historically, the United States of America has been called a "melting pot" because individuals from diverse countries came representing diverse races, ethnic groups, religions, languages, and so forth and then were thought to assimilate into mainstream American (however *mainstream* is defined) culture. The obvious disadvantage to assimilation was the loss of cultural and linguistic identities. In the early 21st century, the term *mosaic* is more commonly used to represent how individuals new to the United States help form the fabric of the country. Individuals retain some or all of their historical identities while creating a new and different picture of the United States. In the future, that picture will continue to change. Table 11.1 represents United States population statistics from 2000 and projected for the year 2050 (U.S. Bureau of the Census, 2000).

By the year 2050, it is predicted that the percentage of culturally and linguistically diverse individuals will increase as the percentage of individuals of European decent declines. The percentage of individuals of Asian descent will double, and the percentage of individuals of Hispanic descent will almost double. The percentage of African Americans/Blacks[1] in the U.S. population will increase by 2%; the percentage of Native Americans will increase to 1%. The percentage of Whites (i.e., European Americans) will decrease, forming slightly over half of the population.

There is a misperception that individuals from culturally and linguistically diverse populations exist mainly in large, urban areas such as Chicago, New

Table 11.1. United States population statistics: 2000 & 2050

Group	Number[a] (2000)	Percent[b] (2000)	Percent[b] (2050)
African American/Black	33.0	12.1	14.6
Asian American	10.1	3.6	8.0
Hispanic	35.0	12.6	24.4
Native American	2.1	0.7	1.0
White	195.0	69.1	50.1
Total	275.2	98.1[c]	98.1[c]

Source: U.S. Bureau of the Census, 2000.
[a]In millions.
[b]Represents percent of total US population.
[c]2% "other"/not specified.

---

[1]Terms are those used by the U.S. Department of Commerce, Bureau of the Census.

York, Philadelphia, and Los Angeles; however, that is clearly not the case. For example, there are large Spanish-speaking communities in Arkansas, Georgia, Nebraska, and Oregon. There are Native Americans in North Carolina and Minnesota. There are sizeable Hmong (Southeast Asian) communities in Massachusetts, Minnesota, and California. This linguistic diversity extends to speakers of English dialects as well. For example, Washington and Craig (1994) indicated that the number of children speaking African American English (AAE) is increasing and will continue to do so in the foreseeable future. Thus, children from culturally and linguistically diverse populations are well-represented in U.S. school systems. In 2001, approximately 48 million children were enrolled in elementary and secondary schools in the United States, 19.2 million (40%) of whom were from culturally and linguistically diverse populations (U.S. Department of Education, 2003a). In addition, there were more than 3 million (6.7% of all students) English language learners (ELLs; i.e., individuals acquiring a language in addition to English) in public schools during the 1999–2000 academic year, an increase from 2.1 million students (5.1% of all students) in 1993–1994 (U.S. Department of Education, 2003b). This diversity influences school-based SLPs directly. Roseberry-McKibbin, Brice, and O'Hanlon (2005) surveyed school-based SLPs on a number of issues concerning students from culturally and linguistically diverse backgrounds, particularly ELLs. The authors found that 11.3% of all the children on SLPs' caseloads were ELLs. The most commonly reported issues that SLPs faced in working with ELLs included: 1) the inability to speak the language of the child, 2) the lack of least-biased assessments, 3) the lack of support personnel who speak the child's language, and 4) the lack of information on developmental norms in the student's home language. In a national survey of SLPs, Roseberry-McKibbin, and Eicholtz (1994) found that 78% of SLPs had 0–3 students with limited English proficiency on their caseloads; 11% had 4–7 students; 4% had 7–10 students; and 6% had more than 10 students. The majority of SLPs were working with children of Latino descent although they were also working with children of Chinese, Filipino, Hmong, Korean, European, Middle Eastern, Portuguese, and Vietnamese descent. Peters-Johnson (1998) conducted a national survey of school-based SLPs and found that 35% of the 1,718 SLPs who responded to the survey indicated that a percentage of their caseload spoke a language other than English although only 10% of 1,718 respondents were proficient in languages other than English. If you are a SLP working almost anywhere in the United States, you are almost certain to encounter individuals from culturally and linguistically diverse backgrounds.

COMMUNICATION AND CULTURE

The way in which we communicate reflects, among many things, the culture in which we were raised. Parents socialize their children to be "good" communicators within their own community. Given the diversity that exists in the United States, SLPs may find that the ways in which parents interact with their children vary greatly. That variation may be reflected in the responses to the tasks we ask families to perform during the clinical management process. For example, during an evaluation of Nina, 4-year-old child of Latino descent, a student clinician asked Sra. Flores, Nina's mother, to go into the diagnostic room and "play with your child as you do at home." Nina and Sra. Flores entered the playroom, which was full of toys and games appropriate for Nina's age. After entering the room, Nina promptly went to the kitchen area and began playing with the pots and pans. Sra. Flores sat nearby and observed Nina as she played. Every once in a while, Sra. Flores would ask Nina in Spanish to bring her something to drink or eat. Nina complied with all requests that were repeated more than twice. Nina's verbal utterances were limited in quantity and quality. The student clinicians in the observation room were dismayed because they felt Nina and Sra. Flores's interaction was stilted and the language sample was not rich. They wondered why Sra. Flores did not ask questions, make comments or statements, or engage with her daughter in play. The student clinicians began to wonder whether Nina's low verbal output and possible language delay was due in part to Sra. Flores's interaction style.

The clinical supervisor then asked one of the student clinicians to go into the playroom with a rather complex puzzle. The student was instructed to ask Sra. Flores to explain to Nina how to put the puzzle together. After hearing the instructions, Sra. Flores asked Nina to sit in a chair next to her. She began asking Nina questions and making commands using a large number of nonspecific words (e.g., "Where do you put this one?" "Put that one next to that thing") Nina's expressive language was more complex and receptively she appeared to understand all of Sra. Flores's utterances. The language output, however, was still less than one would expect of a 4-year-old child, and the student clinicians were almost positive that Nina had a language delay. Finally, Nina's 6-year-old sister, Pilar, was brought into the room, and the two were allowed to play together. Pilar informed Nina that they were going to play school, pulled out a book, and proceeded to play the role of the teacher. She asked such questions as, "What is the girl's name?" "What happened when she sat in the Papa Bear chair?" and "What happened next?" Nina's verbal output in this situation amazed the evaluation participants. She used language for a variety of purposes, her sentences were complex, and her vocabulary was diverse. The student clinicians were not prepared for the fact that there are cross-cultural differences in parent-child interaction and communication that vary by context (Iglesias & Quinn, 1997). For example, parents do not necessarily engage in cooperative play with their children. Parents may see their role as being that of a caregiver, and, in a situation in which language is contextualized, parents may use a high degree of nonspecific vocabulary (Scheffner Hammer, Miccio, & Rodriguez, 2004).

It is necessary to gather cultural and linguistic information to provide appropriate services to individuals who come from cultures other than your own or speak languages other than yours. You might read and study about various cultural groups, talk to and work with individuals from a variety of cultures, participate in the life of someone from another culture, and/or learn another language (Lynch, 2004). There are a number of specific **sociolinguistic factors** (both verbal and nonverbal) that might influence your interaction with a client and his or her family (Damico & Hamayan, 1992; Kayser, 1993; Lynch, 2004; Roseberry-McKibbin, 1994; 2002; Terrell & Terrell, 1993; Wyatt, 2002). First, child socialization practices and children's play characteristics should be considered. For example, children who typically utilize peers as conversational partners might be less comfortable interacting in play situations with adults. In terms of the assessment process, the SLP would want to use peers (or perhaps siblings) to interact with the client in order to obtain a language sample. Second, family characteristics also need to be taken into account (e.g., Westby, 2000). These include factors such as country of birth, degree of acculturation into American society, knowledge of the U.S. education system, family attitude toward English and English speakers, family attitude toward disabilities, family structure, geographic location (e.g., urban, rural), religious beliefs, social status, and socioeconomic status. For example, adults from some cultures may be more comfortable interacting with female clinicians rather than male clinicians (Roseberry-McKibbin, 2002). Third, in assessing clients from culturally and linguistically diverse populations, SLPs must also consider individual differences. For example, not all African Americans speak AAE, and speakers of AAE are all not African Americans (Wolfram & Schilling-Estes, 1998).

BILINGUALISM AND DIALECTS

In providing assessment and intervention services to individuals from culturally and linguistically diverse populations, you undoubtedly will encounter individuals who either speak more than one language (e.g., are bilingual) or speak a dialect of English (we focus on dialects of English in this book although there are dialects of all languages). We will first discuss bilingualism and then turn our attention to dialects.

Bilingualism

Speaking only one language is the exception to the norm if we take a world perspective. According to the Linguistic Society of America (1996), the majority of the world's countries are at least bilingual and many are multilingual. For example, the European Union has more official languages than the United Nations, and nearly 60% of Europeans have learned a second language (Sollors, 1998). The United States, although officially not bilingual, is home to almost 34 million speakers of languages other than English (U.S Bureau of the Census, 2000). In addition, of those 34 million, 11 million do not speak English "well" or "at all." According to the U.S. Bureau of Census (2000), there are 30 languages spoken in the United States and more than 100,000 speakers, ranging from Hungarian with 117,000 speakers to Spanish, with more than 28 million speakers. In addition to Spanish, French, German, and Italian, more than one million individuals speak Chinese, Vietnamese, and Tagalog.

Historically, bilinguals have been placed in one of two categories, simultaneous or sequential. Traditionally defined, simultaneous learners were individuals who acquired both languages from birth, and sequential learners were those who acquired one language after the other (e.g., the second language being acquired on entrance into the school system). As Baker (1996) said, however, "Defining who is or is not bilingual is essentially elusive and ultimately impossible. Some categorization is often necessary and helpful to make sense of the world" (p. 13). Thus, bilingualism should be viewed on a continuum with changing levels of input, output, use, and proficiency over time. At the two extremes of the continuum are monolingual individuals raised and living in monolingual environments (e.g. Spanish-speaking children raised and living in remote areas of Mexico). Bilingual individuals fall between those ends of the continuum and will differ from monolingual speakers of each language across phonological, semantic, morphosyntactic, and pragmatics areas (see Goldstein, 2004 for specifics in each of these areas for Spanish-English bilinguals). The degree of bilingualism achieved by an individual will be dependent on linguistic, social, emotional, political, demographic, and cultural factors (e.g., Baker, 1996; Hakuta, 1986; Pease-Alvarez, 1993). In addition, studies in bilingualism suggest that the degree of bilingualism depends on such factors as generational level, age, occupation, opportunity for contact with speakers of English, exposure to English media, and the nature of interactions with members of their community (Romaine, 1995, 1999).

Bilingual speakers demonstrate various degrees of proficiency in either language depending on the situation, topic, interactants, and context. Impressionistically, many bilingual individuals appear indistinguishable in normal social interactions, what Cummins (1984) refers to as possessing *Basic Interpersonal Communication Skills (BICS)*. Differences, however, are evident in cognitively demanding, decontextualized interactions—what Cummins refers to as having *Cognitive Academic Language Proficiency (CALP)*.

For an illustration of that difference, we return to the example of Nina's evaluation for a possible language delay. In the first interaction between Sra. Flores and Nina, they both were speaking in Spanish, although in the second interaction Sra. Flores used English and Spanish. The interaction between Nina and Pilar was all in English. The first interaction could be classified as one in which Nina was relying heavily on her BICS to communicate with her mother. The second interaction was more demanding and required Nina to understand and use more cognitively demanding language. To facilitate the linguistic experience in this interaction, Sra. Flores used contextual cues (using modeling behaviors) and also used both languages to facilitate the conversation. Sra. Flores's use of both languages is typical of that seen when both speakers are bilingual. The interaction of Nina and Pilar was all in English and required Nina to further use more cognitively and academically demanding language. As a result of the situations, the speakers, and the topics, Nina demonstrated different proficiencies in the two languages.

Although there are many specific definitions of bilingualism, most people accept Grosjean's "holistic" view of bilingualism (Grosjean, 1989, 1992, 1997). This view posits that the languages of bilinguals are an integrated whole that cannot be easily separated into the component languages. According to Grosjean, bilinguals have one linguistic system that results in different surface structures. This interdependence between the two languages allows for the transfer of skills across languages. From the standpoint of an SLP, adopting this view of bilingualism means that the communication assessment of bilinguals, both children and adults, will necessitate 1) studying bilinguals as a whole without comparison to monolinguals, 2) examining both of the bilingual's languages, and 3) investigating how bilinguals organize and use both languages.

Dialects

There are many dialects spoken in the United States, including those such as Southern White Standard, Appalachian English, Caribbean English, African American English, and General American English. A **dialect** is a rule-governed variety of a language characterized by social, ethnic, and geographical differences in its speakers. Dialects are mutually intelligible forms of a language associated with a particular region, social class, or ethnic group. Dialects may differ across all areas of language-phonology, syntax, morphology, lexicon, and pragmatics. In fact, every person has his or her own unique way of speaking, termed an

idiolect. Varieties of a language that depend on the context and conversational participants are called **registers,** which change depending on the participants, setting, and topic. For example, an individual would usually use one register when talking to a potential employer and another variety when speaking to friends. The terms *dialect* and **accent** are often (erroneously) used interchangeably. The term *dialect* refers to all aspects of a language, and *accent* refers only to the pronunciation of a language variety. Accent does not take into account lexical, syntactic, morphological, and pragmatic aspects of the language variety.

No dialect of any language is superior to any other dialect. This is not to say that all varieties of a language are equally prestigious. Some varieties of a language, specifically those used by the "dominant" groups in any socially stratified society, will be considered to have higher prestige (Wolfram, 1986), to be preferred in the educational system (Adler, 1984), and to be valued by the private sector of the society (Terrell & Terrell, 1983). General American English is considered the prestige dialect in the United States and is preferred in the educational system. Because of mass media saturation, there have been some decreased differences between dialects and greater acceptance of others. There has also been, however, increasing difference between dialects because of the isolation of some groups, especially those in the lower socioeconomic status in society (Wolfram & Schilling-Estes, 1998). The increased immigration and ethnic isolation that has occurred among some subgroups has further increased the number of ethnic dialects. At least in terms of dialects, the "melting pot" hypothesis appears to be a myth for certain segments of our society.

COMPLETING MOST APPROPRIATE ASSESSMENTS

SLPs will need to use information on communication and culture, bilingualism, and dialects to complete reliable and valid assessments. The goal of an assessment with an individual from a culturally and linguistically diverse population is to conduct a **least-biased assessment.** This means that you understand the individual's culture and language (and/or dialect) and understand how the factors cited previously might influence the diagnostic process. The result of a least-biased assessment is to differentiate individuals developing typically who may have a **language difference** (i.e., expected community variations in syntax, semantics, phonology, pragmatics, and lexicon) from those with **language disorders** (i.e., communication that deviates significantly from the norms of the community; Taylor & Payne, 1994). So why is it necessary to make adjustments in the way that individuals from culturally and linguistically diverse populations are assessed? Historically, individuals from culturally and linguistically diverse populations have not been assessed appropriately. For example, bilingual adults with aphasia have only been assessed in one language (i.e., English) because of the lack of a bilingual SLP or trained support personnel. In the case of school-age children, this has resulted in an overreferral to and enrollment in special education for children from culturally and linguistically diverse populations despite recognition of cultural differences and their influence on linguistic development. That is, many children from culturally and linguistically diverse backgrounds were placed in special education because of a language difference, not a language disorder. It has also meant, in some cases, an underidentification of language disorders due to the assumption that any variation from what is expected is due to cultural and linguistic differences.

Many laws have been passed and lawsuits have been brought to help ensure that children are placed appropriately into special education. For example, public laws such as Individuals with Disabilities Education Improvement Act (IDEA) of 2004 (PL108-446) mandate that a child's native language must be used in all direct contact with the child. Thus, SLPs must find means to conduct assessments employing the language the child uses in the home or learning environment. Lawsuits such as *Larry P. v. Riles* (1979) nullified the use of standardized IQ tests in California to place African American children in special education. Thus, society at large and the courts have acknowledged the rights of linguistic minority populations. This acceptance has resulted in greater acceptance of the variety of dialects that are spoken in the United States. Although General American English is the most common and dominant language variety spoken in the United States, there has been a realization that other varieties have a right to exist in the linguistically pluralistic society. These laws have a definite influence on conducting least-biased assessments.

To diagnose individuals who truly have a communication disorder, communicative standards of one group cannot be imposed on another. Operationally, a communication disorder is defined as communication that differs from the norm. It is imperative that the norm be, among other things, culturally based (Taylor & Clarke, 1994). To be certain that least-biased assessments take place, you should take into account factors that may influence the assessment process (e.g., Goldstein, 2000; Iglesias, 2001; Kayser, 1993, 1995a; Roseberry-McKibbin, 2002; Seymour & Pearson, 2004; Terrell & Terrell, 1993).

Clinician Factors

Prior to conducting an assessment, clinicians must assess their cultural and linguistic competence. Our attitudes, knowledge, and actions have an influence on the quality of the services we provide. To respond optimally to the individuals we serve, we must have 1) a positive attitude towards the families' values and beliefs, even if they are significantly different from our own; and 2) an understanding of typical and atypical language development, including an understanding of what is considered to be a disorder. As we gain a better understanding and an appreciation of the families we serve, our intervention goals and approaches will be congruent with those of the families.

We must also assess the extent to which our linguistic skills in a language other than English are sufficient to evaluate our assessment tools and carry out an assessment. Although some working knowledge of a language is helpful, clinicians should be aware that less-than-native or near-native proficiency in a language is not be sufficient to carry out a proper assessment. In the case of a bilingual child, the clinician must not only be proficient in both languages but also should able to create an environment where the child can freely code-switch or mix, thus using his or her full linguistic repertoire. In preparing to complete a least-biased assessment, you should conduct a self-assessment (i.e., know your own culture and world view), have a solid understanding of variations across and within cultural-linguistic groups, and determine whether you have the language skills and training to provide assessment and intervention for bilingual individuals. According to ASHA (1989), an SLP or audiologist may be considered bilingual if he or she speaks one native language and speaks a second language with native or near-native proficiency in lexicon, semantics, phonology, morphology, and pragmatics. To provide bilingual clinical services in the child's language, the bilingual SLP should

- Be able to describe typical speech and language development using contemporary data and theory

- Possess knowledge of dialects in the child's home language

- Use least-biased evaluation tools to gauge speech and language skills

- Administer and interpret formal and informal evaluation tools

- Apply intervention strategies in the child's language

- Recognize cultural factors that affect assessment and intervention

- Be able to aid parents and other professionals in understanding the diagnosis, assessment results, and intervention options and approaches

General Assessment Factors

During the assessment process, there are ways in which you can increase the likelihood of an appropriate diagnosis. First, use an assessment framework, such as the one outlined by Gillam and Hoffman (2001). Although the framework was designed for children, it has implications for adults as well and can be adapted for that purpose, especially as it relates to assessing the client across multiple contexts with multiple interlocutors. They suggest that assessment should take place in four domains: 1) functions and activities (e.g., interviews, language samples, dynamic assessment), 2) participation (e.g., portfolios with homework, class assignments, tests, writing samples) and naturalistic observation in the home and at school, 3) contextual (e.g., curriculum measures, reading miscues; see Laing, 2002), and 4) decontextual (e.g., standardized tests). Using such a framework will increase the likelihood of a least-biased assessment. Second, administer several formal (i.e., standardized) and informal (i.e., nonstandardized) measures. Using both types of measures will allow for a more representative sample of the individual's abilities. Third, assess skills in all languages/dialects. It is quite common for individuals to exhibit some skills in one language/dialect and other skills in the other language/dialect. For example, some bilingual, Latino children first learn the names of colors in preschool, when their English-speaking teacher produces the names of colors in English. Thus, the children will know the names of colors in English only and not in Spanish. If bilingual children were tested in Spanish only, they might not label colors in Spanish leading the clinician to mistakenly believe that the children did not know color names. Bilingual adults with aphasia may recover some language skills in the one language but other skills in the other language (Paradis, 2001). Clinicians should also observe whether the language disorder exists in all languages/dialects; it should. Fourth, recognize that different modes of communication may be in effect and that performance may vary because of those factors rather than the clients' abilities. A mismatch of communicative styles between the family and SLP is always possible.

Assessment Tool Factors

Most SLPs administer formal (i.e., standardized) assessment tools to their clients. Not all formal assessments, however, will be appropriate for all clients.

In administering formal assessments to your clients, you should take into account the following issues (e.g., Goldstein, 2000; Kayser, 1993, 1995a; Roseberry-McKibbin, 2002; Wyatt, 2002):

- Examine each item before administering the test to determine whether the client may have had prior access to the information and if failure should be considered indicative of a disorder.

- Determine whether modification of specific test items can reduce bias.

- Consider first administering a child's test to an adult in order to get information on the appropriateness of test items and the likely responses from a child.

- Have families complete case history information, permission forms, and release of information documents in person.

- Make an effort to identify those measures that include individuals from culturally and linguistically diverse populations in the normative sample.

- Observe code switching (i.e., alternations between languages at the word, phrase, or sentence levels; e.g., an individual may start a sentence in one language and finish it in another; Mattes & Omark, 1991) and **language interference** (i.e., the influence of one language on another; e.g., a native speaker of Japanese may pronounce English with a Japanese accent; Roseberry-McKibbin, 2002).

- Report all modifications of standardized administration procedures.

- Report norms only if they are valid for the population being assessed.

- Select a test that examines those aspects of language that need to be assessed.

- Use a variety of elicitation procedures.

ALTERNATIVE METHODS OF ASSESSMENT

Just as you would alter the assessment process for evaluating someone with a language disorder versus someone with a voice disorder, you also need to tailor the assessment of individuals from culturally and linguistically diverse populations to their specific language and culture. That is, you design your assessment to fit the specific needs of the client. Alternative methods of assessment also need to be used in order to make a proper differential diagnosis. Without using such modifications, there is a chance for either **overdiagnosis** or **underdiagnosis.** Overdiagnosis may occur when an individual is labeled with a communication disorder because his or her abilities were assessed using a test standardized based on a sample from which the client does not come. Underdiagnosis may occur because the assessment does not take into account the individual's linguistic features or because the SLP may not understand how the individual's language or dialect differs from General American English. For example, in the assessment of a 5-year-old child who speaks AAE, the SLP may find a language sample and note some anomalies in form (e.g., "He eated the doughnut") that were initially, erroneously labeled as a dialect feature (i.e., "eated" is not grammatically correct in AAE).

A number of suggestions in completing alternative methods of assessment have been suggested by many researchers (compiled from Cheng, 1993; Erickson

& Iglesias, 1986; Goldstein, 2000; Kayser, 1989, 1993, 1995a; Langdon, 1992; Norris, Juarez, & Perkins, 1989; Roseberry-McKibbin, 1994, 2002; Taylor & Payne, 1983; Terrell & Terrell, 1993; Toliver Weddington, 1981; Van Keulen, Weddington, & DeBose, 1998; Vaughn-Cooke, 1986; Wyatt, 2002). These suggestions include solutions such as developing new tests, standardizing existing tests on individuals from culturally and linguistically diverse backgrounds, and administering standardized tests in nonstandardized ways. No matter which route you choose, if a standardized test does not include individuals from culturally and linguistically diverse populations in the standardization sample, you should question the test's validity. Because many standardized assessments must still be developed with these populations in mind, clinicians frequently use tests already in existence and administer them to their clients in alternative ways. If you use an alternative format when assessing a client, your assessment report must detail how the test was modified and the report must indicate the underlying motivation of the modifications. For example, you might alter a test by allowing an individual to go back and revise his or her test responses, repeating and/or rewording instructions, providing additional time for an individual to respond, testing beyond the ceiling of the assessment, adding practice items, and asking an individual to explain his or her answers. If modifying existing tests will not yield helpful information, another option is to restandarize the existing tests by developing **local norms.** You can do this by administering the test to individuals without language disorders in the community in which you are working, note the scores they receive and the quality of their responses, and use their test results as the "standard" to which the client's test scores can be compared.

Because it can be difficult and time-consuming to restandardize existing tests or develop new tests, it is also recommended that clinicians use alternative testing formats (i.e., measures other than standardized tests). Alternative testing formats might include

- *Criterion-referenced tests:* These are tests that specify the linguistic behaviors to be tested, establish criteria for acceptable responses, and do not compare the client's responses against some other standard. One disadvantage is that the criteria used to develop these tests often come from standardized assessments.

- *Dynamic assessment* (e.g., Peña, 1996; Peña, Iglesias, & Lidz, 2001): Performance is gauged by examining **modifiability** (i.e., change through mediation or teaching). Examiners can determine how a client learns, what is needed for a client to learn, and how a client generalizes a task to new situations. Modifiability is composed of three factors: 1) client responsiveness (i.e., how a client responds to and uses new information), 2) examiner effort (i.e., the quantity and quality of effort needed to make a change), and 3) transfer (i.e., the generalization of new skills).

- *Portfolio assessment:* This is a procedure in which you collect a client's work over time representing a variety of tasks and assignments; assignments might include writing samples, observations from teachers, parents, and so forth; language samples; and tapes of performance.

- *Ethnographic assessment* (Heath, 1982, 1983; Westby, 2000): This is a procedure in which you observe the client in many contexts with many conversational partners. Ask family members about their own culture, their attitudes about the host culture (i.e., the new culture in which they are living), and their communication in the home. Interact with clients, being sensitive to their culture, their frame of reference, and what they see as important. Describe clients' communicative abilities during genuine communication in a naturalistic environment.

- *Probe techniques:* This assessment technique assesses a small amount of information over a short period of time (e.g., weekly, biweekly) to gauge rate and amount of learning.

If a school-age child is being evaluated, the SLP might obtain academic information from teachers and school records in addition to utilizing the alternative testing formats described above. Damico (1993) and Gillam and Hoffman (2001) suggested that clinicians obtain information by observing in the classroom, analyzing academic tasks and the curriculum, and assessing the child's test-taking abilities during structured activities.

You should also follow some testing guidelines to decrease the possibility of misdiagnosis (Kayser, 1993; Roseberry-McKibbin, 1995).

1. Do not use norm-referenced tests only.

2. Do not use only a language sample to qualify someone for services.

3. Do not use multiple assessments in order to get low scores so that someone will be qualified for services.

4. Do not use translations of tests (Roseberry-McKibbin, 1994). First, there are differences in structure and content in each language. The same translated item may differ in structure and difficulty across the two languages. Second, using such tests mistakenly implies that children acquiring English proficiency and English-speaking children receive similar socialization, life experiences, language input, academic instruction, and so forth. Third, differences in the frequency of target words vary from one language to the next. Fourth, grammatical forms may not be equivalent between the languages. Fifth, translated tests do not tap an individual's ability to acquire language.

5. Do not use only one elicitation technique.

6. Do not use tests administered in English-only if the individual is bilingual.

7. Do not assume that features of a second language or a dialect of English are characteristics of a disorder.

8. Do not assume that support personnel are automatically trained to aid in the diagnostic process.

RESPONSIBILITIES AND ROLES OF THE MONOLINGUAL SPEECH LANGUAGE PATHOLOGIST

Given the demographic changes occurring in the United States and the fact that most SLPs are monolingual and English speaking, ASHA has developed guidelines regarding the responsibilities of monolingual SLPs to individuals who are bilingual. According to ASHA (1985; see also ASHA, 2004), monolingual SLPs may test in English, perform the oral-peripheral exam, conduct hearing screenings, complete nonverbal assessments, and conduct the family interview (with appropriate support personnel) in English. In preparing to assess an individual whose language they do not speak, monolingual SLPs should research the culture, language, and dialect of the person they are going to assess and use least-biased assessment tools. They should also be prepared to ask for help if necessary, be an advocate for the individual, and be willing to refer the individual to another clinician if necessary.

Monolingual SLPs might also consider some other alternatives (ASHA, 1985):

1. Establishing contacts and hiring bilingual SLPs as consultants or diagnosticians to provide clinical services

2. Establishing cooperative groups in which group of school districts or programs might hire an itinerant bilingual SLP

3. Establishing networks such as forging links between university settings and work settings to help recruit bilingual speakers into the workforce

4. Establishing Clinical Fellowship Year and graduate student practica sites

5. Establishing interdisciplinary teams in which monolingual SLPs are teamed with bilingual professionals from other fields

6. Training support personnel such as bilingual aides, students, family members, or members of the community

You should be aware that there is a limit as to the types of tasks that support personnel can complete (ASHA, 1996). Support personnel can conduct speech-language screenings, follow intervention plans or protocols, document client progress, and assist during assessment, but there are also other tasks that support personnel should not complete. These tasks include performing standardized or nonstandardized diagnostic tests; interpreting test results; participating in parent conferences, case conferences, or any interdisciplinary team without the supervising SLP present; and writing, developing, or modifying a client's individualized intervention plan.

INTERVENTION

Intervention is a process by which a clinician deliberately sets out to systematically change the course of an ongoing behavior. This process always involves an expert who has an awareness of what is appropriate behavior (i.e., intervention goal) and what to do to achieve this goal (i.e., intervention approach). The specific goals and approaches selected are driven by the clinician's values, beliefs, and knowledge. As clinicians, it is our ethical responsibility to examine how our own biases and the limits of our knowledge base influence the direction and outcome of our intervention. To achieve this, we must identify and overcome our biases and engage in activities that expand our conceptual perspective of sociocultural and linguistic factors that have an influence on intervention. We must be aware that in many cases we will be implementing interventions based on limited empirical research. The majority of our intervention programs will be based on this limited knowledge coupled with logic and experience. Ongoing evaluation of our goals, intervention approaches, and outcomes should be a source for our ongoing decision-making process.

Let us return to our example of Nina being evaluated for a language disorder. Based on the results of the evaluation, the supervising clinician decided that

Nina needed to receive intervention to facilitate her language acquisition and that one of the goals of the intervention should be to increase Nina's use of questions, commands, and statements. The SLP reasoned that greater use of these communicative functions would increase Nina's academic communication skills. Unfortunately, Nina's parents were excluded from the decision-making process. Although on the surface the goal appears to be appropriate, the clinician should have noted that this goal required a shift in Sra. Flores's child-rearing practices—Nina is to view her parent as an equal partner instead of as a caregiver. The clinician did not consider if this shift would create new adjustment problems for the family. Sra. Flores returned to the clinician 3 weeks later to complain about the Nina's new, disrespectful behavior towards adults. Another intervention strategy may have worked better while still assuming the same goals. For example, the clinician could have discussed with the Sra. Flores the need to achieve these goals and asked Sra. Flores' advice on optional ways to attain them. Perhaps Sra. Flores would have suggested that the SLP explicitly state that this type of communication is only to be used in Nina's classroom or that the intervention should be carried out in a group situation where Nina would be interacting with her peers. There is even the possibility that Sra. Flores would have agreed to change her own rules regarding what behaviors of Nina are appropriate once the SLP thoroughly explained the intervention strategy. Any or all of these strategies could have avoided the negative side effects of Nina's intervention.

Providing appropriate intervention services to individuals from culturally and linguistically diverse populations has often proved to be difficult. There is a severe lack of research into effective intervention strategies. We have, however, provided you with general intervention guidelines to apply when treating individuals from culturally and linguistically diverse populations with communication disorders (compiled from Beaumont, 1992; Cheng, 1989, 1996; Damico & Hamayan, 1992; Damico, Smith, & Augustine, 1996; Goldstein, 2000; Kayser, 1995b; Seymour, 1986).

General Considerations

There are a number of general guidelines you should follow when providing intervention services to individuals from culturally and linguistically diverse populations. First, assess the individual continuously. Each session should be a mini-assessment that will help you plan for the next session. Complete comprehensive reevaluations of the individual's intervention needs periodically (e.g., every 3–6 months). Second, set up opportunities for language to be used in natural interactions, utilize natural language learning activities, and interrelate activities. The activities, and the materials used in them, should be meaningful and interesting. We acquire new knowledge in situations that require us to use multiple bases of knowledge. Third, consider a holistic strategies approach by encouraging clients to 1) explain new information in their own words, 2) abstract information, 3) generalize information to new contexts, and 4) analyze new information (Roseberry-McKibbin, 2002). SLPs should focus on language meaning as well as language structure; have clients relate new information to previously learned information; teach strategies for learning and remembering new content; and use an intervention strategy that teaches the "whole" of a concept, breaks the concept down into its "parts," and then reconstructs it into a "whole" again (Roseberry-McKibbin, 2002). Fourth, allow clients to think, discuss options, make decisions, establish accountability, and show knowledge both verbally and nonverbally. If the use of printed material is emphasized during the intervention, SLPs will need to build a literacy-rich environment for clients, which will help empower individuals as learners. Fifth, use a variety of social organizations (e.g., large group projects, small group projects, peer-peer projects) and use individual, peer-peer, and group work. Sixth, if appropriate, use a bidialectal/bilingual approach. That is, incorporate clients' home language and/or dialect into the intervention process. Research has shown that language skills in the second language can be predicted, in part, by skills in the first language (e.g., Cobo-Lewis, Eilers, Pearson, & Umbel, 2002; Lopez & Greenfield, 2004; Perozzi & Sanchez, 1992). Finally, use all resources available to you (e.g., if you are working in a school, get help from English as a second language teachers, general classroom teachers, and so forth; if you are employed in a health care setting, utilize a cross-disciplinary approach).

Family-Centered Intervention

It is likely that the people who will know your client best are his or her family members. Therefore, it is imperative to involve your client's family in the intervention process (Lynch & Hanson, 2004). Family members' involvement, however, must be at a level at which they are most comfortable. Some families may be comfortable actually participating in the intervention by being in the room with you although other families may wish to observe the intervention sessions and ask questions following the intervention.

There are some specific ways in which you ought to work with families in the intervention process. First, educate the family about the purpose of the sessions and who will be present in them. Second, attempt to involve the family in the decision making, if appropriate. Third, match your client's goals to the family's concerns and needs. Fourth, allow time for the family to ask questions but also be prepared to answer the same question posed by different members. Fifth, utilize practices that are culturally appropriate. These strategies include checking often for comprehension, emphasizing key words continually, reviewing previously learned material on a daily basis, including literacy activities, rephrasing information, teaching concepts in naturalistic situations, teaching the client to monitor his or her own learning activities, using all modalities, and using stories and narratives. These strategies have been shown to be effective for individuals from culturally and linguistically diverse populations (Roseberry-McKibbin, 2002).

CONCLUSION

Providing appropriate assessment and intervention services to individuals from culturally and linguistically diverse populations is challenging. Before the assessment even takes place, you will probably have to gather information on your client's language, dialectal variety, verbal and nonverbal communication styles, and so forth. This information will have to be applied to the specific person you are evaluating. It may be necessary for you to employ support personnel to aid in the clinical management process, particularly if you do not speak the client's language. You may also have to alter your typical assessment protocol in order to ensure that you are making a valid diagnosis. Accurate diagnosis will lead to intervention approaches and techniques that are suited to your particular client.

REFERENCES

Adler, S. (1984). *Cultural language differences: Their educational and clinical-professional implications.* Springfield, IL: Charles C. Thomas.

American Speech-Language-Hearing Association. (2004). *Accreditation manual: Council on academic accreditation in audiology and speech-language pathology.* Rockville, MD: Author.

American Speech-Language-Hearing Association. (1996, Spring). Guidelines for the training, credentialing, use, and supervision of speech-language pathology assistants. *ASHA, 38*(Suppl. 16), 21–34.

American Speech-Language-Hearing Association. (1989). Definition: Bilingual speech-language pathologists and audiologists. *ASHA, 31,* 93.

American Speech-Language-Hearing Association. (1985). Clinical management of communicatively handicapped minority language populations. *ASHA, 27*(6), 29–32.

Baker, I. (1996). *Foundations of bilingual education and bilingualism* (2nd ed.). Clevedon, England: Multilingual Matters.

Beaumont, C. (1992). Language intervention strategies for Hispanic LLD students. In H. Langdon (Ed.), *Hispanic children and adults with communication disorders: Assessment and intervention* (pp. 272–333). New York: Aspen Publishers.

Cheng, L.R.L. (1989). Intervention strategies: A multicultural approach. *Topics in Language Disorders, 9,* 84–91.

Cheng, L.R.L. (1993). Asian-American cultures. In D. Battle (Ed.), *Communication disorders in multicultural populations* (pp. 38–77). Boston: Andover Medical Publishers.

Cheng, L.R.L. (1996). Enhancing communication: Toward optimal language learning for limited English proficient students. *Language, Speech, and Hearing Services in the Schools, 27,* 347–354.

Cobo-Lewis, A., Eilers, R., Pearson, B., & Umbel, V. (2002). Interdependence of Spanish and English knowledge in language and literacy among bilingual children. In D.K. Oller & R.E. Eilers (Eds.), *Language and literacy in bilingual children* (pp. 118–134). Clevedon, England: Multilingual Matters.

Cummins, J. (1984). *Bilingualism and special education: Issues in assessment and pedagogy.* San Diego: College-Hill Press.

Damico, J. (1993, October). Appropriate speech and language assessment for bilingual children. Seminar presented at *Bilingualism: What every clinician needs to know.* Symposium sponsored by the American Speech-Language-Hearing Association, Alexandria, VA.

Damico, J., & Hamayan, E. (1992). *Multicultural language intervention.* Buffalo, NY: Educom Associates.

Damico, J., Smith, M., & Augustine, L. (1996). Multicultural populations and language disorders. In M. Smith & J. Damico (Eds.), *Childhood language disorders* (pp. 272–299). New York: Thieme New York.

Erickson, J., & Iglesias, A. (1986). Assessment of communication disorders in non-English proficient children. In O. Taylor (Ed.), *Nature of communication disorders in culturally and linguistically diverse populations* (pp. 181–217). San Diego: College-Hill Press.

Gillam, R., & Hoffman, L. (2001). Language assessment during childhood. In D. Ruscello (Ed.), *Tests and measurements in speech-language pathology* (pp. 77–117). Boston: Butterworth-Heinemann.

Goldstein, B. (2000). *Cultural and linguistic diversity resource guide for speech-language pathology.* San Diego: Singular Publishing Group.

Goldstein, B.A. (Ed.). (2004). *Bilingual language development and disorders in Spanish-English speakers.* Baltimore: Paul H. Brookes Publishing Co.

Grosjean, F. (1989). Neurolinguists, beware! The bilingual is not two monolinguals in one person. *Brain and Language, 36,* 3–15.

Grosjean, F. (1992). Another view of bilingualism. In R. Harris (Ed.), *Cognitive processing in bilinguals* (pp. 51–62). New York: Elsevier.

Grosjean, F. (1997). Processing mixed languages: Issues, findings, and models. In A. de Groot & J. Kroll (Eds.), *Tutorials in bilingualism: Psycholinguistic perspectives* (pp. 225–254). Mahwah, NJ: Lawrence Erlbaum Associates.

Hakuta, K. (1986). *Mirror of language: The debate on bilingualism.* New York: Basic Books.

Heath, S. (1982). What no bedtime story means: Narrative skills at home and school. *Language in Society, 11,* 49–76.

Heath, S. (1983). *Ways with words: Life and work in communities and classrooms.* New York: Cambridge University Press.

Iglesias, A. (2001). What test should I use? *Seminars in Speech and Language, 22*, 3–16.

Iglesias, A., & Quinn, R. (1997). Culture as a context for early intervention. In S.K. Thurman, J.R. Cornwell, & S.R. Gottwald (Eds.), *Contexts for early intervention: Systems and settings* (pp. 55–71). Baltimore: Paul H. Brookes Publishing Co.

Individuals with Disabilities Education Improvement Act of 2004. PL 108-446, 20 USC 1400 *et seq.*

Kayser, H. (1995a). Assessment of speech and language impairments in bilingual children. In H. Kayser (Ed.), *Bilingual speech-language pathology: An Hispanic focus* (pp. 243–264). San Diego: Singular Publishing Group.

Kayser, H. (1995b). Intervention with children from linguistically and culturally diverse backgrounds. In M.E. Fey, J. Windsor, & S.F. Warren (Eds.), *Communication and language intervention series: Vol. 5. Language intervention: Preschool through the elementary years* (pp. 315–331). Baltimore: Paul H. Brookes Publishing Co.

Kayser, H. (1989). Speech and language assessment of Spanish-English speaking children. *Language, Speech, and Hearing Services in the Schools, 20*, 226–244.

Kayser, H. (1993). Hispanic cultures. In D. Battle (Ed.), *Communication disorders in multicultural populations* (pp. 114–157). Boston: Andover Medical Publishers.

Laing, S. (2002). Reading miscues in school-age children. *American Journal of Speech-Language Pathology, 11*, 407–416.

Langdon, H. (1992). Speech and language assessment of LEP/bilingual Hispanic students. In H. Langdon (Ed.), *Hispanic children and adults with communication disorders: Assessment and intervention* (pp. 201–271). New York: Aspen Publishers.

Linguistic Society of America. (1996). *Statement on language rights.* Washington, DC: Author.

Lopez, L., & Greenfield, D. (2004). The cross-linguistic transfer of phonological skills of Hispanic Head Start children. *Bilingual Research Journal, 28*, 1–18.

Lynch, E.W. (2004). Developing cross-cultural competence. In E.W. Lynch & M.J. Hanson (Eds.), *Developing cross-cultural competence: A guide for working with children and their families* (3rd ed., pp. 41–77). Baltimore: Paul H. Brookes Publishing Co.

Lynch, E.W, & Hanson, M.J. (2004). Steps in the right direction: Implications for service providers. In E.W. Lynch & M.J. Hanson (Eds.), *Developing cross-cultural competence: A guide for working with children and their families* (3rd ed., pp. 449–466). Baltimore: Paul H. Brookes Publishing Co.

Mattes, L., & Omark, D. (1991). *Speech and language assessment for the bilingual handicapped* (2nd edition). Oceanside, CA: Academic Communication Associates.

Norris, M., Juarez, M., & Perkins, M. (1989). Adaptation of a screening test for bilingual and bidialectal populations. *Language, Speech, and Hearing Services in the Schools, 20*, 381–389.

Paradis, M. (2001) Bilingual and polyglot aphasia. In H. Goodglass & A.R. Damasio (Eds.), *Handbook of neuropsychology* (2nd ed., pp. 69–91). New York: Elsevier Science.

Pease-Alvarez, L. (1993). *Moving in and out of bilingualism: Investigating native language maintenance and shift in Mexican-descent children.* Santa Cruz, CA: National Center for Research on Cultural Diversity and Second Language Learning.

Peña, E.D. (1996). Dynamic assessment: The model and its language applications. In K.N. Cole, P.S. Dale, & D.J. Thal (Eds.), *Communication and language intervention series: Vol. 6. Assessment of communication and language* (pp. 281–307). Baltimore: Paul H. Brookes Publishing Co.

Peña, E., Iglesias, A., Lidz, C.S. (2001) Reducing test bias through dynamic assessment of children's word learning ability. *American Journal of Speech-Language Pathology, 10*, 138–154.

Perozzi, J., & Sanchez, M. (1992). The effect of instruction in L1 on receptive acquisition of L2 for bilingual students with language delay. *Language, Speech, and Hearing Services in the Schools, 23*, 348–352.

Peters-Johnson, C. (1998). Action: School services. *Language, Speech, and Hearing Services in the Schools, 29*, 120–126.

Romaine, S. (1999). Bilingual language development. In M. Barrett (Ed.), *The development of language* (pp. 251–275). East Essex, England: Psychology Press.

Romaine, S. (1995). *Bilingualism* (2nd edition). Oxford, England: Blackwell Publishing.

Roseberry-McKibbin, C. (1994). Assessment and Intervention for children with limited English proficiency and language disorders. *American Journal of Speech-Language Pathology, 3*, 77–88.

Roseberry-McKibbin, C. (1995). *Multicultural students with special language needs.* Oceanside, CA: Academic Communication Associates.

Roseberry-McKibbin, C. (2002). *Multicultural students with special language needs* (2nd ed.). Oceanside, CA: Academic Communication Associates.

Roseberry-McKibbin, C., Brice, A., & O'Hanlon, L. (2005). Serving English language learners in public school settings: A national survey. *Language, Speech, and Hearing Services in the Schools, 36,* 48–61.

Roseberry-McKibbin, C., & Eicholtz, G. (1994). Serving children with limited English proficiency in the schools: A national survey. *Language, Speech, and Hearing Services in the Schools, 25,* 156–164.

Scheffner Hammer, C., Miccio, A.W., & Rodriguez, B.L. (2004). Bilingual language acquisition and the child socialization process. In B.A. Goldstein (Ed.), *Bilingual language development and disorders in Spanish-English speakers* (pp. 21–50). Baltimore: Paul H. Brookes Publishing Co.

Seymour, H. (1986). Clinical principles for language intervention among nonstandard speakers of English. In O. Taylor (Ed.), *Treatment of communication disorders in culturally and linguistically diverse populations* (pp. 115–133). San Diego: College-Hill Press.

Seymour, H.N., & Pearson, B.Z. (Eds.). (2004). Steps in designing and implementing an innovative assessment instrument. *Seminars in Speech and Language, 25,* 27–32.

Sollors, W. (1998). Introduction: After the culture wars; or, from "English only" to "English plus." In W. Sollors (Ed.), *Multilingual America: Transitionalism, ethnicity, and the languages of American literature* (pp. 1–13). New York: New York University Press.

Taylor, O., & Clarke, M. (1994). Communication disorders and cultural diversity: A theoretical framework. *Seminars in Speech and Language, 15,* 103–113.

Taylor, O. & Payne, K. (1983). Culturally valid testing: A proactive approach. *Topics in Language Disorders, 3,* 8–20.

Taylor, O., & Payne, K. (1994). Language and communication differences. In G. Shames, E. Wiig, & W. Secord (Eds.), *Human communication disorders: An introduction.* (4th ed., pp. 136–173). New York: Merrill.

Terrell, S., & Terrell, F. (1983). Effects of speaking Black English upon employment opportunities. *ASHA, 25,* 27–29.

Terrell, S., & Terrell, F. (1993). African-American cultures. In D. Battle (Ed.), *Communication disorders in multicultural populations* (pp. 3–37). Boston: Andover Medical Publishers.

Toliver Weddington, G. (1981). *Valid assessment of children.* San Jose, CA: San Jose State University.

U.S. Bureau of the Census. (2000). *Statistical abstract of the United States: 2000* (120th ed.). Washington, DC: U.S. Department of Commerce.

U.S. Department of Education. (2003a). *Percentage distribution of enrollment in public elementary and secondary schools, by race/ethnicity and state or jurisdiction: Fall 1991 and fall 2000.* Retrieved February 10, 2005, from http://nces.ed.gov/programs/digest/d03/tables/dt042.asp

U.S. Department of Education. (2003b). *English language learner students in U.S. public schools: 1994 and 2000.* Washington DC: National Center for Education Statistics. Retrieved May 24, 2005, from http://nces.ed.gov/pubs2004/2004035.pdf

Van Keulen, J., Weddington, G., & DeBose, C. (1998). *Speech, language, learning and the African American child.* Boston: Allyn & Bacon.

Vaughn-Cooke, F. (1986). The challenge of assessing the language of nonmainstream speakers. In O. Taylor (Ed.), *Treatment of communication disorders in culturally and linguistically diverse populations* (pp. 23–48). San Diego: College-Hill Press.

Washington, J., & Craig, H. (1994). Dialect forms during discourse of poor, urban African American preschoolers. *Journal of Speech and Hearing Research, 37,* 816–823.

Westby, C. (2000). Multicultural issues in speech and language assessment. In. J.B. Tomblin, H. Morris, & D.C. Spriestersbach (Eds.), *Diagnosis in speech-language pathology* (2nd ed., pp. 35–62) San Diego: Singular Publishing Group.

Wolfram, W. (1986). Language Variation in the United States. In O. Taylor (Ed.), *Treatment of communication disorders in culturally and linguistically diverse populations* (pp. 73–116). San Diego: College-Hill Press.

Wolfram, W., & Schilling-Estes, N. (1998). *American English: Dialects and variation.* Oxford, England: Blackwell Publishing.

Wyatt, T. (2002). Assessing the communicative abilities of clients from diverse cultural and language backgrounds. In D. Battle (Ed.), *Communication disorders in multicultural populations* (pp. 415–459). Boston: Butterworth-Heinneman.

STUDY QUESTIONS

1. Describe your own culture, language, and dialect. How have aspects of each one changed since high school? How does your culture, language, and dialect compare to the group you think is most different from you? How might your culture, language, and dialect influence assessment and intervention of an individual from a different cultural and/or linguistic group?

2. How do culture and communication relate? Consider three ways in your own experience that culture and communication are interrelated.

3. Describe four alternative methods of assessment in the diagnosis of communication disorders of individuals from culturally and linguistically diverse populations.

4. What is the relationship between child socialization practices and language development? In an assessment, how might you determine that a child's linguistic performance was due to socialization and not the result of a communication disorder?

5. Gather different definitions of bilingualism. How might monolingual SLPs assess and treat bilingual individuals?

6. Do you think immigrants to the United States should maintain their home language? Provide a rationale for your response. How would their maintenance or loss of their home language influence your selection of an intervention approach and intervention goals?

7. Using data from the U.S. Census Bureau (http://www.census.gov), determine the racial or ethnical composition of your community.

8. Go to the grocery store, department store, or airport (or anywhere diverse groups of individuals congregate) and describe the different ways that individuals interact with one another. You might compare how adults interact with other adults, how adults interact with children, and how children interact with other children.

CHAPTER 12

Assistive Technology in Communication Disorders

MELANIE FRIED-OKEN

Consider your typical morning routine. You wake up to the sound of an alarm clock, and you realize that you forgot to reset to an earlier time! You quickly call a classmate on your cellular telephone and have a message passed along to your professor to say that you will be late for class. You dress for the day, heat up old coffee in the microwave, and run out of the apartment. You take the elevator to the garage, use the keyless remote to unlock your car door automatically, jump in your car, turn on your favorite radio station, open the garage door with the remote control, and zoom to class. You have already used eight **assistive technology (AT)** devices within 10 minutes.

Consider Steve's typical morning routine. He wakes up to the sound of a ventilator that moves air in and out of his lungs for respiration. He moves his head to the left and hits a pillow switch that is attached to an alerting system that let his caregivers know that he is ready to get out of bed. A Hoyer lift helps the caregivers move Steve's body from the bed into his electric wheelchair. He then uses the five switches in his headrest to activate his communication device, which he uses to thank his caregivers, and drives the wheelchair into his bathroom. The bathroom has been redesigned for universal access. Steve has amyotrophic lateral sclerosis (ALS) and is quadriplegic. He used six AT devices within an hour to get from his bed to his bathroom.

There are thousands of items that can be called AT, and there are many ways to categorize them. According to the Technology-Related Assistance for Persons with Disabilities Act of 1988 (the Tech Act), AT is "any item, piece of equipment, or product system, whether acquired commercially off the shelf, modified, or customized, that is used to increase, maintain, or improve functional capabilities of people with disabilities" (PL 100-407).

AT includes tools that help people overcome limitations related to a disability by either enhancing the skills the person has or by compensating for absent or nonfunctional skills. It can be a commercial product or something that someone made for a personal use. It can be a simple low-technology ("low-tech") device such as a magnifying glass to read small text or an expensive high-technology ("high-tech") device such as screen-reading computer software. AT is powerful enough to influence an individual's potential to learn, to be independent, to have a good quality of life, and to have a healthy self-esteem (http://www.atstar.org). Think, for example, of the power of a telecommunication device for the deaf (TDD) which functions as a telephone for people who cannot hear or produce speech. A young man who is deaf can use the AT to call his parents and tell them that he just got engaged. Likewise, if skill enhancement is not possible, AT provides alternative ways to accomplish a task. Reciting the calendar during morning circle time, for example, is important to Kayla, a preschooler with autism. When she is called upon during circle time, she can simply press a speech-generating device that has a peer's prerecorded voice with that day's information. It results in the same outcome, and Kayla can participate verbally. *Every person needs AT devices and every person's AT needs are unique.* Individual needs are matched with necessary technology in a functional environment, rather than matching available equipment to individual needs.

The writers of the Tech Act knew that people could not just be given devices, because people need training to learn how to use equipment. Rick Creech, an AT user and vocational rehabilitation counselor in Pennsylvania, believes that, "assistive technology without training is not assistive" (Creech, personal communication, 1992). The Tech Act defines AT services as "any service that directly assists an individual with a disability in the selection, acquisition, or use of an assistive technology device." Within the field of communication disorders, AT devices and services are becoming standard intervention options for children and adults with complex communication impairments for expressive and receptive language, reading, writing, learning, and hearing.

The Rehabilitation Engineering & Assistive Technology Society of North America (RESNA; www.resna.org), is an interdisciplinary association of people with a common interest in AT and disability. RESNA's goal is to help people with disabilities achieve their goals through the use of technology. They have divided AT according to special interest groups (SIGs). The organization has 21 SIGs that address the diverse needs of consumers, physicians, engineers, service providers, therapists, and industry around each AT specialty area. These SIGs include, augmentative and alternative communication (AAC), special education, service delivery and public policy, rural rehabilitation, job accommodation, and international appropriate technology.

ASSISTIVE TECHNOLOGY LEGISLATION

The benefits of AT have become so important in the United States of America that AT has been legislated by Congress into a number of acts. Legislation for AT mimics the societal changes that have occurred within the U.S. disabilities community since 1980. As disability policy moves from a caregiver and institutional perspective to one of community inclusion and self-determination, so does the development of AT (Wallace, Flippo, Barcus, & Behrmann, 1995). The four important pieces of legislation that affect the delivery of AT devices and services by professionals in the fields of communication disorders are: the Tech Act, the Americans with Disabilities Act (ADA) of 1990 (PL 101-336), the Rehabilitation Act Amendments of 1992 (the Rehab Act; PL 102-569), and the Individuals with Disabilities Education Act Amendments of 1997 (IDEA'97; PL 101-476) with its 2004 reauthorization (IDEA'04, PL 108-337).

The Tech Act stated that

> Provision of assistive technology devices and services enables some individuals with disabilities to:
> A. Have greater control over their own lives;
> B. Participate in and contribute more fully to activities in their home, school, work environments, and in their communities;
> C. Interact to a greater extent with non-disabled individuals; and
> D. Otherwise benefit from opportunities that are taken for granted by individuals who do not have disabilities. (PL 100-407, p. 1044)

The ADA provided direct references to AT. It protects individuals against discrimination in the workplace and provides them with equal access to public services and accommodations, transportation, and telecommunications. The availability of TDDs in public buildings and the use of adapted computers for writing in the workplace are both examples of reasonable accommodations under the ADA.

The Rehab Act addressed the requirements of state vocational rehabilitation agencies for adults who are seeking to find or continue employment or independence. It calls for "a range of services and devices which can supplement and enhance individual functions" (p. 4) and describes eligibility for rehabilitation engineering services. The Rehabilitation Act Amendments of 1992 further empowered individuals and families through the provision of AT and training.

IDEA'97 clearly included AT devices and services. Section 300.308 stated that "each public agency shall ensure that assistive technology devices are assistive technology services, or both, as those terms are defined in 300.5–300.6, are made available to a child with a disability if required as a part of the child's Individualized Education Plan (IEP)." IDEA'97 also ensured that every IEP team for a child with a disability must consider the child's need for assistive technology (IDEA'97, 300.346 (a)(2)(v)). This simple statement has a powerful effect on the lives of many students with disabilities. The law makes it very clear that every child with a disability might need assistive technology and that school has a responsibility to provide it when it is needed. IDEA's revision, the Individuals with Disabilities Education Improvement Act of 2004 (PL 108-779), at the time of this writing, have not yet been specified for enactment. It is, however, encouraging to read an introductory statement in IDEA'04: "Almost 30 years of research and experience has demonstrated that the education of children with disabilities can be made more effective by ....(Section H) including assistive technology devices and assistive technology services, to maximize accessibility for children with disabilities."

ASSISTIVE TECHNOLOGY FOR COMMUNICATION

Larry is a retired linguistics professor who has had a stroke and was subsequently diagnosed with global aphasia. He now uses an AAC system. Terry, Larry's wife, described the system in her own words:

> The AAC device is only part of his communication. It's a smaller piece of the pie than sometimes we wish it would be, but the reality is that it's a very useful piece. It has its place, but it is only a part of his system. His system is saying 'yes' and 'no' and looking over to me and all the other ways to express himself. There's a whole system that you use and that you go back and forth among. If somebody doesn't get it, you go to a backup. The AAC device is only one of the tools in the toolbox (Thompson & Thompson, 2000).

AT for communication is called AAC. It is based on a robust human communication model (Denes & Pinson, 1993) that is composed of three processes: 1) a means to represent an idea, 2) a means to select the representation of that idea, and 3) a means to transmit that idea (Lloyd, Fuller, & Arvidson, 1997). The primary role of AAC systems is to facilitate individuals' participation and engagement in meaningful events in their daily lives. AAC focuses on the role of current and prospective communication partners and settings in which interactions occur (American Speech-Language-Hearing Association [ASHA], 2004). *AAC is defined as*

> An area of research, clinical and educational practice, AAC involves an attempt to study and when necessary compensate for temporary or permanent impairments, activity limitations, and participation restrictions of persons with severe disorders of speech-language production and/or comprehension, including spoken and written modes of communication. (ASHA, 2005, p. 1)

In 2004, ASHA described the multimodal AAC system with four critical terms: *symbols, aids, strategies,* and *techniques.* A *symbol* is a method for visual, auditory, and/or tactile representation of conventional concepts (e.g., a word, vocalization, gesture, photograph, manual sign, printed word, object, Braille word). An *aid* refers to "a device, either electronic or nonelectronic, that is used to transmit or receive messages" (ASHA, 2004, p. 2). The electronic aid is called a **speech-generating device (SGD)** and will be discussed in detail later in this chapter. A *strategy* refers to "the way in which symbols can be conveyed most effectively and efficiently" (ASHA, 2004, p. 2). Some people with dysarthria, for example, point to the first letter of a word on an alphabet board while speaking. This strategy helps their communication partners understand their speech and slows down the speaker so that there is a pause between each word. A *technique* is "a way in which messages can be transmitted" (ASHA, 2004, p.2). Techniques include, but are not limited to, speaking, signing, natural gestures, selecting with one's eyes, selecting with a mouse, scanning with a computer, or using Morse code. Examples of these terms are explored within the following discussion of AT functions for children and adults.

Speech-Generating Devices

Many professionals consider AAC to be speech generating devices. This is not the case, but an SGD may be an integral part of an AAC system. SGDs are grouped according to whether they are dedicated devices (i.e., individual devices that are customized to function only as communication aids) or integrated systems (i.e., standard computers that have been adapted to serve the function of communication devices with specialized software and hardware components). Both dedicated and integrated SGDs are selected based on three categories of features: 1) language representation (the symbols used to form a message), 2) selection technique (the technique used to select the symbols), and 3) output (the product that is formed upon selection) (Fishman, 1987).

Language Representation *Symbols* are publicly used representations of meaning (Lloyd et al., 1997). For example, an image of a tree could be a 2-dimensional symbol for the concrete concept *tree,* or the abstract concept *spring, nature,* or *shade.* A 3-dimensional object, such as a small twig or a plastic leaf, also could represent these concepts. Written words (i.e., print), 2-dimensional drawings, and 3-dimensional objects are all symbols. The most common symbol used by adults to represent language is orthography, a very structured, abstract set of characters used to transcribe a specific linguistic system. In fact, letters only form one orthographic system. Braille, an alphabet formed by a series of six embossed dots, is considered a tactile orthographic system.

Every symbol system implies a certain level of representation, a specific degree or type of relatedness between symbol and referent. Written words illustrate a completely abstract level of representation. The letters themselves have no relationship to the concept they describe. There are a number of alternative symbol systems that depict meaning with various degree of concreteness (Lloyd et al., 1997). Nonorthographic symbol sets often are used by children before and during the development of literacy skills, by children who will never learn to read, and by adults who are not literate. Table 12.1 shows examples of the word *sister* represented by commonly used AAC symbol sets.

Selection Technique   Because many of the individuals who use AAC have physical disabilities that can affect the use of their hands for pointing, writing, or typing, the technique for selecting communication symbols for each SGD must be considered. Two different ways to access or select symbols on an SGD are *direction selection* and *scanning* (Fishman, 1987).

Table 12.1.   Examples of the word *sister*, represented by common used augmentative and alternative communication (AAC) symbol sets

Symbol	Description	Example
Tangible symbols	An object, piece of an object, or item that represents the concept, as in a *doll* for the word *sister*.	
Photograph	Color or black and white photographs to represent actual objects, activities, locations, actions, and people.	
Picture communication symbols	Simple line drawings that represent an object.	
Rebus symbols	A representation of words or syllables by pictures of objects.	
Blissymbols	Pictographic, ideographic, and arbitrary symbols with abstract representations of concepts.	
Orthography	A set of characters that represent a linguistic code.	*sister*
Morse Code	A system of dits and dots that represent orthography.	... . - . .-.

Direct selection refers to the user's ability to point directly to a desired symbol. People usually isolate their dominant index fingers to press a box on a device or picture board, but there are ways to point without using hands. People can point with eyes, feet, or any anatomical pointer. Aids, such as a headpointer, chinpointer, or laser attached to a headband, can also be used. Technology is available to allow individuals to directly select a symbol without touching anything. A headmouse, for example, permits the user to select items simply by moving his or her head. A small camera attached to a computer and a reflective dot worn on the forehead provides the necessary contact. The camera follows the movement of the dot and projects it on the screen as a mouse selection. Technology beginning to appear in the AT marketplace permits direct selection with brainwaves, which allows the user to place electrodes on his or her forehead and "think" the mouse location.

Scanning refers to the user depending upon a tool (i.e., switch) to select from presented items. Scanning can be electronic or nonelectronic. A familiar example of nonelectronic scanning is the game 20 Questions, in which a number of choices are presented to the user, and a yes or no response is required until the preferred information is selected. Another example is the auditory alphabet scan, where letters of the alphabet are orally presented to a user. When the correct letter is spoken, the user makes a visible gesture (e.g., closes the eyes, moves a finger). There are many examples of electronic scanning communication systems in AT. Stephen Hawking, the famous physicist with ALS, uses a single switch to write his books (Hawking, 1988). While viewing an alphabet grid on a computer screen, he closes a switch when the letter or word that he wants is visibly before him. Hawking also uses a more advanced method of scanning, called *encoding*. He can choose a code to represent a large string of words or letters (e.g., BH could stand for "black hole," UI could represent "present universe"). This technique reduces keystroke selections and increases scanning speed. Scanning is a very slow way to communicate, but it remains an important option for individuals with severe physical impairments.

Output The output parameters of SGDs are changing rapidly as advances in speech synthesis, computer screens, printers, and wireless options appear. Despite changes in the quality, size, shape, and cost of output devices, the basic types of output for SGDs remains the same (Fishman, 1987). There are four types of output: 1) attention getters (i.e., sound generated by a device that causes attention by communication partners), 2) speech (i.e., digitized and synthesized speech), 3) visual display (i.e., computer screen), and 4) print (i.e., hard copy). The presence of different output parameters is determined by the needs of the user. For example, if a user converses with someone who is not literate (e.g., a young child), then speech output would be desired over printed output. If a user needs to complete homework with the SGD, then printed output might be preferred. Most SGDs have multiple output methods. It is the responsibility of an individual's AAC team to determine what outputs are needed for the user and to make sure that the selected SGD has the necessary options.

Who Can Use Augmentative and Alternative Communication?

Everyone is a candidate for AAC. We all rely on a multimodal communication system. If you need to speak to a friend in a noisy bar, you might use gestures, eye gaze, exaggerated speech, or writing (e.g., on a napkin or hand). If you need to speak to a friend during a class seminar, you might send a written note and follow the note with a gesture (e.g., a wink, raised eyebrows). Mirenda (1993) wrote

> Communication has only one prerequisite: and it has nothing to do with mental age, chronological age, prerequisite skills, mathematical formulae, or any of the other models that have been developed to decide who is an AAC candidate and who is not. That is because *breathing is the only prerequisite* that is relevant to communication. Breathing equals life, and life equals communication. It is that simple. (p. 4)

The National Joint Committee (NJC) for the Communication Needs of Persons with Severe Disabilities (1992) prepared a bill of rights that proclaims that all people with a disability of any extent or severity have a basic right to affect, through communication, the conditions of their existence. NJC emphasized that communication services and supports may not be denied on the basis of discrepancies between cognitive and communication functioning, chronological age, diagnosis, or absence of cognitive or other skills believed to be prerequisites (see http://www.asha.org/NJC).

Models of Augmentative and Alternative Communication Service Delivery

AAC services may be offered in all practice settings. Because of the complexity of the communication impairments and the multimodal nature of AAC, the unidisciplinary model of one professional providing all service is not recommended (Lloyd et al., 1997). Instead, professional members of an AAC team most often work together in one of three models: multidisciplinary, interdisciplinary, or transdisciplinary approach (Locke & Mirenda, 1992). Table 12.2 lists an example of possible team members. The models of delivery apply to all settings—whether school, intensive care unit, rehabilitation hospital, or home health—and the goal in all settings is the same: to provide the best means to augment, supplement, or replace individuals' impaired speech, language, or writing skills so that they may participate to their best abilities in daily functioning.

Augmentative and Alternative Communication Assessment

The AAC assessment is much broader and eclectic than a typical communication disorders assessment. The participation model (Beukelman & Mirenda, 2005) is the recommended heuristic for AAC evaluation. It is based on the concepts that AAC users should have opportunities to functionally participate on a level commensurate with their chronological peers in activities today, tomorrow, and in

Table 12.2.   Possible members of an augmentative and alternative communication (AAC) team

Person with AAC needs	Family, guardians, and/or parents
Teacher or physician (usually team leader)	Speech-language pathologist
Audiologist	Occupational therapist
Physical therapist	School or rehabilitation psychologist
Nurse or social worker	Rehabilitation engineer
Vendor	

the future. In addition to assessing peoples' skills and identifying their strengths, the participation model assesses opportunity or access barriers that prevent or lessen the AAC users' participation in daily activities. Tony's case is an example of the benefits of the participation model.

Tony, a 10-year-old boy with severe spastic cerebral palsy and dysarthria, is in a fifth-grade class with peers who are typical learners. His school speech-language patholo-gist (SLP) has determined that he has age-appropriate receptive language and read-ing skills, but his severe speech and motor impairments reduce his expressive and physical participation at school. During the AAC assessment, the school team observed the daily class schedule and conducted an ecological inventory of all the opportunities that existed for Tony's communication (Reichle, York, & Sigafoos, 1991). Upon arrival at school, Tony's peers discussed what computer games they had played the night before and what television shows they had watched. Tony's class read silently for 30 minutes every morning before instruction started. Later, the class moved into history groups where they usually worked on art projects that corresponded to their history units (e.g., making relief maps of the country they were studying with paper-mâché and paint). The AT team determined that Tony could use AT to participate in all of these activities. He could direct his electric wheelchair into the school (which has accessible doors) and enter his classroom. His SGD could be programmed with greetings and information about computer games. Although Tony could not turn the pages of a book, he could read an electronic book on a computer and turn pages with his adapted joy-stick. The art project during history created some functional barriers for Tony, but his classroom decided that Tony could access the necessary maps on the Internet and print them out to copy for the relief maps.

Tony was very lucky. He did not encounter policy barriers to AT access in this school setting. Not every school has enough funding or room to allow every student with ready access to a computer, let alone provide a student a single, personal computer with specific adaptations. Also, schools frequently assign a specific reading list to each grade. Many of the books typically assigned are not freely available on the Internet, and schools do not always have additional funds to buy electronic books from online providers. Tony, however, had tools that would help him participate in class, and he spent the year learning how to use them for maximal participation.

Evaluation of Individuals for Augmentative and Alternative Communication

For many individuals with complex communication needs, formal assessment with standardized instruments may not be possible. Nonstandardized tools and adapted tests should be considered in these cases. There are many ways to adapt a test so that its content, rather than procedure, is maintained (Allen & Collins, 1955). A child with visual impairments might need the position of the test to be changed or the size of pictures in the manual to be enlarged. A child who cannot hold a pencil easily might do better with an adapted writing implement or a computer mouse to select responses. A child with physical impairments may use eye gaze to point to responses. An example of what an AAC specialist can do to adapt a test for a child who may not be able to isolate a finger for pointing to pictures on a receptive language test would be to cut up each page, separate the pictures, and laminate the pictures onto 16-inch by 20-inch sheets of plastic. The specialist holds up the laminated page in front of the child and says the test stimulus. Now the child can point to the correct answer on the laminated pages with the eyes instead of the fingers. When a clinician considers using an SGD for a child, he or she should make note of all the equipment features needed to meet the child's communication needs and abilities for present and future participation and increased opportunities.

ASSISTIVE TECHNOLGY FOR LEARNING

Tiara, a high school student with muscular dystrophy, emphasized the use of AT for learning when she said, "It should be clear that I would not be able to attend school or carry on a relatively normal life without assistive technology" (Shattuck, 2001, p. 43).

Individuals with learning disabilities, as well as those with motor or sensory impairments, benefit from AT for learning. The equipment enhances academic achievement in written expression, reading, mathematics, and spelling; it improves organization and fosters social acceptance (Quenneville, 2001). AT can include low-tech options, such pressure-sensitive paper (i.e., carbonless paper that allows the user to tear off copies of classroom lecture notes to share with a fellow student who may not be able to take notes easily), and high-tech options, such as sophisticated real-time captioning software for a student with an auditory processing disorder who needs to read, not just hear, information to learn it (for more information, see http://www.atstar.org).

A student with language literacy disabilities can use small electronic talking devices, such as a Franklin Ace, to assist with spelling and grammar. A laptop computer can assist with note taking, reading, or organization of information. Screen reading software can enhance reading rate and comprehension and increase the length of time that reading can be sustained (Elkind, 1998). Indeed, MacArthur (1996) found that a word processor that provides speech synthesis and a personalized word bank benefits the student with learning disabilities who often finds the writing process frustrating because the processor helps facilitate writing. When these students have the opportunity to accommodate writing challenges, they are more successful in the general education classroom. Hetzroni and Schrieber (2004) showed that the use of a word processor for text generation enhanced the academic outcomes of three students with writing disabilities in a junior high school. They found a clear difference between handwritten and computer generated prose. In traditional handwritten phases, the students produced more spelling mistakes, more reading errors, and lower overall quality of organization and structure in comparison with tasks in which a computer equipped with a word processor was used.

Evaluation with Assistive Technology for Learning

Zabala (1993) introduced an AT framework that has proved the test of time in school settings. The **SETT** framework helps individuals with disabilities, their family members, and the professional team that supports them to identify appropriate AT devices and services. It was developed to help the AT team with decision making at all stages of AT service delivery, from consideration through evaluation of effectiveness. The SETT framework gets its name by considering the **S**tudent, the **E**nvironment(s), and the **T**asks a student needs to accomplish before attempting to determine what **T**ools will be required. The SETT framework assists the team in goal setting and maintenance and is an excellent guide for school-based professionals. The SETT framework is part of the recommendations that Bowser and Reed (2002) offered to educators who are implementing AT into the curriculum. In their *Tech Points* manual, the authors stressed examining all aspects of the child's curriculum in a team environment, making a plan that addresses the role of each member, and creating quality indicators that can be measured for AT success. In addition, the Council for Exceptional Children has published several monographs to help implement AT in the classroom (for a list of monographs available for purchase, see http://www.tamcec.org).

ASSISTIVE TECHNOLOGY TO SUPPORT COGNITION

AT to support individuals with cognitive impairments is generally discussed with three groups in mind: 1) individuals with traumatic brain injuries, 2) children and adults with developmental disabilities, and 3) adults with dementia. One example of AT in the functional domain of support cognition is the Picture Planner software (Keating & Ames, 2004; see Figure 12.1). This software sits on a laptop computer, is completely graphically driven, and provides an easy-to-use life skills application suite for a range of users with cognitive disabilities. The user simply manipulates pictures to build and manage daily, weekly, and monthly schedules or to get assistance for task planning and prompting. The Picture Planner can be used by individuals with developmental disabilities, such as autism spectrum disorders, as well as individuals with traumatic brain injuries and individuals with dementia.

Consider, for example, an adult with developmental disabilities who lives independently in a supported apartment and uses public transportation to get to work and visit friends. AT is available to help this person with organizational

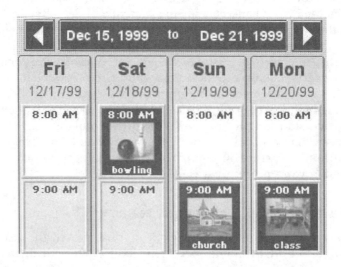

Figure 12.1. Example of a Picture Planner screen. (Courtesy of Picture Planning, http://www.eugeneresearch.org)

skills, memory, managing personal calendars and activities, and time management. A personal digital assistant (PDA) with specialized software can be used to personalize picture, audio, and visual-based prompts. The Think and Link e-mail interface, which has been designed to support the basic functions for receiving, composing, and sending e-mail, can help keep contact with friends and family (Sohlberg, Ehlhart, Fickas, & Sutcliffe, 2003). Companies such as Ablelink Technologies (http://www.ablelinktech.com) have been developed to address research and development of AT for individuals with intellectual and cognitive disabilities. Low-tech solutions are also available, especially for youth with cognitive impairments in schools. Hart, Hawkey, and Whyte (2002) found that a simple portable voice organizer can help school-age children with traumatic brain injuries recall therapy goals and plans. Students rely on a full range of AT for learning in the school setting, including highlighters, index cards, color-coding stickers, graph paper, beepers and buzzers, digital clocks, digital watches, talking watches, headphones or earplugs, tape recorders, pocket recorders, voice-activated day planners, and software programs (e.g., personal data managers, free-form data bases). The future of AT to support persons with cognitive impairments lies in telerehabilitation and virtual cognitive prostheses. The concept is simple: Customized prompts and coaching through real-time, online software in a person's daily environment will help them participate successfully in activities of daily living (Tam et al., 2003).

ASSISTIVE TECHNOLOGY FOR PEOPLE WITH VISUAL IMPAIRMENT OR BLINDNESS

Nicaise Dogbo is the director of employment technology services at the Rose Resnick Lighthouse for the Blind and Visually Impaired in San Francisco. He is also blind. He relies on a scanner, a refreshable Braille display, a synthesized speech output, and a Braillelyte note taker. He stated, "Technology is not just a luxury thing for us, it's for access. Start using technology because it will help you be what you want to be and help you be at the same level as everyone else" (Dogbo, 2002).

For students or adults with visual impairment or blindness, AT is a fundamental work tool, equivalent to pencil and paper for typical students. With AT, students with visual impairments can participate on an equal basis with their peers in the general electronic educational environment. They can have access to literature and writing tools to complete educational tasks such as homework or tests. Table 12.3 describes some AT for reading, but remember that this field is constantly growing new forms of screen readers, note takers, Braille embossers, and other such technologies.

ASSISTIVE TECHNOLOGY FOR WRITING

AT for people who find writing challenging can be categorized into access technologies (i.e., specialized keyboards, built-up pens) and writing generation technologies (i.e., spelling checkers, speech recognition software). Slant boards, pens with enlarged grips, and paper with raised lines are all examples of low-tech

Table 12.3. Assistive technology to support people with visual impairments

Braille embosser: A Braille printer that embosses Braille onto paper

Braille translation software: A program that translates and formats text into appropriate Braille characters for hard copy printout

Braille writing equipment: Devices for creating paper Braille materials

Closed-circuit television: A device that magnifies a printed page through a special television camera with a zoom lens and displays the image on a monitor

Portable note taker: Portable units that use Braille or standard keyboards to allow the user to enter, store, and edit information

Refreshable Braille display: A mechanical display that provides tactile output of text from the computer screen to the user

Screen magnification: Software that focuses on a single portion (e.g., one quarter) of the screen and enlarges it to fill the screen

Screen reader: Software that includes a speech synthesizer to provide verbalization of everything on the screen, including menus, text, and punctuation

access technologies to support the mechanics of writing. MacArthur (1999) found that students who are challenged by writing often struggle with the basic transcription processes, including handwriting or typing, spelling, capitalization, and punctuation. Problems with transcription are important both because they affect written products and because they interfere with students' ability to attend to higher order processes such as planning and evaluation. Computer tools, including word processing, spelling checkers, speech synthesis, word prediction, and speech recognition software, offer support to writers.

Writing generation technologies permit a user to direct writing efforts toward the language-generation task instead of concentrating on the mechanics of writing and error detection. This, in turn, boosts the user's self-confidence and the perception of others about the user's abilities. Often specialized features are added to word processors, such as spelling checkers, dictionaries, thesauruses, grammar checkers, word prediction, abbreviated expansion, and proofreading software programs, to assist the writer. This sort of technology has seen widespread use since 1990. Voice recognition software in particular is frequently used in telephone menus where the listener is prompted to give an oral command or response (e.g., "Yes," "No," "Help"), but consider the value of voice recognition software for a student with severe physical impairments who can speak but cannot write or use his or her hands.

ASSISTIVE TECHNOLOGY FOR HEARING IMPAIRMENT OR DEAFNESS

Children and adults who are hearing impaired rely heavily on AT to meet their communicative, social, vocational, and educational needs in many settings. The **Telecommunication Access Program** dictates that every state will have a procedure in place to ensure that citizens have access to telecommunications (Act 501 of 1995 and Act 530 of 2001). This important legislation for people who are deaf and blind and have speech or motor impairments has made equipment available free of charge and stressed the importance of AT for hearing. **Telecommunications for the Deaf, Inc.** is an active national advocacy organization focusing its energies and resources to address equal access issues in telecommunications and media for people who are deaf, hard of hearing, late-deafened, or deaf-blind (http://www.tdi-online.org/tdi/orgnization.asp). AT for people who are deaf or hard of hearing can be divided into the following three categories: 1) **assistive listening devices,** 2) **devices for telecommunications** (e.g., telecaption decoders), 3) and **alerting devices.**

Assistive Listening Devices

Assistive listening devices include both personal listening devices (i.e., hearing aids) and group listening enhancement systems (i.e., audio loops or frequency modulation [FM] transmission systems). The hearing aid is the most commonly used assistive listening device. Conventional hearing aids rely on analog components, amplifying all environmental sounds (e.g., speech, water running, keyboard typing, automobile and pedestrian traffic) equally. In response, digital technology has been incorporated into hearing aids. Digital hearing aids block out background noise and are customized to the necessary amplification for the user's hearing loss profile. Cochlear implants, the newest and most exciting listening device, are best characterized as technology that provides those who are deaf with access to the sound environment. The single channel or multiple channel cochlear implant provides prosthetic activation of auditory nerve afferent fibers so that auditory centers of the brain can process information for speech and other sounds (Niparko & Blankenhorn, 2003). Listening enhancement systems for communication access in groups and large rooms is accomplished with audio loops systems, amplitude modulation (AM) systems, FM systems, and infrared systems. These systems are used to direct sounds into the listener's ears and block background noise. Since the ADA was passed, audio loops can be found in many public places. They range in size from room-based systems to accommodate large number of listeners to portable, individualized systems for the single user.

Telecommunication Devices

Telecommunication devices are the second type of popular AT for hearing. Assistive devices to improve public communication include text captions, text and digital telephones, and relay systems. TDDs available in public places and private homes help make the telephone accessible. Amplifier headsets are also available in many public telephones. Portable amplifiers can be carried by users and simply placed on telephones to make them functional for the person with hearing impairment. In fact, cellular telephones with text messaging capabilities are an AT that is widely used by people with hearing impairments and deafness. Interface devices for computers are used by people with partial hearing loss and allow a computer to pair visual cues simultaneously with auditory cues. There are a number of multimodal presentation platforms that convert speech to real time, on-screen text or sign language for users with different hearing profiles (e.g., see http://www.myicommunicator.com).

Alerting Devices

Alerting devices are available so that important sounds are converted into sight, different auditory signals, or vibration for users with different needs. A vibrating pad attached to the home smoke alarm can wake a sleeping person with hearing impairment. An alarm clock with flashing lights can arouse the night shift nurse who is deaf. Alerting devices have been designed for many daily functions.

ASSISTIVE TECHNOLOGY FOR PLAY

Play is the work of children and their vehicle for gaining basic knowledge about the world around them. When typically developing children are learning that their actions have an effect on their environment, however, children with significant physical, sensory, and cognitive disabilities are limited in their ability to produce action from and interact with the environment. The early use of adaptive toys and switches can change this. AT is a tool to enhance play and learning (Lesar Judge & Lahm, 1998). For children in the sensorimotor stage of play, battery-operated toys controlled by switches can be used to establish cause and effect (e.g., when a switch is pressed, the toy dog barks and wages its tail). There is a wide range of switches available (http://www.tashinc.com) that fit the motor and sensory needs of young children. The switches can turn on popcorn poppers, swirl art machines, and machines that blow bubbles. Homemade switches work well also and "make it yourself" directions can be found via the Internet (see Burkhart, 2001).

AT for symbolic or pretend play requires a bit more imagination. Certainly, switch-operated computer games are now accessible for all children (e.g., see http://www.rjcooper.com). If a child is pretending to be the teacher at school, for example, a switch can be attached to battery powered scissors, a lamp, a television, and an electric stapler (see, http://www.ablenetinc.com). The highest level of play is game play. Materials for rule-governed board games are very adaptable. Spinners are easily made with switches. Commercial software, video game consoles, and other electronic options are available in the educational tool market. Many low-tech adapted toys and high-tech computers are available for children with disabilities (see http://cosmos.ot.buffalo.edu/letsplay/AT/at.html for more information).

ASSISTIVE TECHNOLOGY AND CULTURAL DIVERSITY

Of course, a person's cultural, ethnic, and/or socioeconomic background will influence his or her decisions about the use of AT. Parette, VanBiervliet, and Hourcade (2000), for example, found that AT devices that draw considerable attention to a person's disability in public places might not be acceptable to African American families, because these families tend to value fitting into their community by not appearing different. Hourcade, Parette, and Huer (1997) also noted that for many Asian and Native American families, there is a value and expectation on a certain degree of dependence within a family, and AT for independence is not considered important. Additionally, families from low socioeconomic backgrounds often must consider basic needs such as health care, food, employment, and transportation, which can leave little time, energy, or funds for participation in AT evaluation and training sessions (Kemp & Parette, 2000). The priorities of these families may be very different than those of the professionals working with them. These kinds of considerations obviously have important implications for the AT decision-making process.

MEASURING ASSISTIVE TECHNOLOGY OUTCOMES

Rick Creech stated

> We have the technology to improve the quality of life for people with disabilities. Having this technology, we are accountable for its use. Who would forgive

this generation if we use this technology destructively and selfishly? A hammer can be used to build or to tear down or, even, to kill. The choice is in the hand that holds the hammer. We hold technology. What will we choose to do with it? How will we know if it's right?" (1992, p. 66)

How do we know if AT works? How do we know if it is important, effective, or timely? How do we know if a school team is adequately using the SETT framework, or buying the appropriate equipment for students? What indicators do we have that quality AT services are offered? These questions become even more important as we enter an era when evidence-based practice is expected for evaluation and intervention programs (Schlosser, 2003; see also Chapter 7). The questions lead us to examine *assistive technology outcomes,* questions of whether AT works or what happens as a result of using an AT device or service (DeRuyter, 1995, 1997). The outcome from the use of AT can cover a wide range of issues. They include whether AT, 1) was used or abandoned, 2) led to efficient completion of specific tasks/activities, 3) played a role in productive employment, 4) realized cost savings, 5) decreased family or caregiver support, 6) increased independence, or 7) enhanced an individual's quality of life.

AT outcomes may have somewhat specific measures depending on the various AT service areas and reimbursement models. The Consortium on Assistive Technology Outcomes Research (CATOR) has developed a taxonomic framework for AT device outcomes that is driven by *health related outcomes.* CATOR divides the assessment into three areas: effectiveness, social significance, and subjective well-being (Jutai, Fuhrer, Demers, Scherer, & DeRuyter, 2005). Conversely, the educational model emphasizes achievement of *educational goals for a free and appropriate public education.* The vocational rehabilitation model emphasizes achievement of *vocational goals and enhancing productivity.* These distinctions have a tremendous influence on the types of services and equipment that are funded.

CONCLUSION

It is apparent that *assistive technology* is, indeed, a broad term that has been assimilated into every area of communication disorders, education, and rehabilitation. The descriptions in this chapter merely skim the surface of applications and outcomes that AT can have on children, families, and society as a whole. If we, as professionals in the communication disorder field, can use AT to start changing attitudes about functional limitations caused by communication impairments, then we have made an important change. Parette and Brotherson reminded us that "it is difficult to overstate the contributions AT is making in the quality of life for people with disabilities" (2004) Bob Williams, former commissioner of the U.S. Administration on Developmental Disabilities and an AT user, said it best:

> You know, we all talk a good game about the power and the potential of assistive technology. And, it is all very true. But I am increasingly seeing, both as an individual and a federal officer, that where the real rubber meets the information highway is in transforming that power and potential into everyday realities in people's lives! . . . Access to assistive technology . . . is vital. Having the power to speak one's heart and mind changes the disability equation dramatically. In fact, it is the only thing that I know that can take a sledgehammer to the age-old walls of myths and stereotypes and begin to shatter the silence that looms so large in many disabled people's lives (2000, pp. 251–252, 249).

It is the role and, indeed, the ethical responsibility of every professional in the field of communication disorders to provide AT options to people with disabilities so that they can maintain or begin their independent, expressive contributions to society.

REFERENCES

Allen, R.M., & Collins, M.G. (1955). Suggestions for the adaptive administration of intelligence tests for those with cerebral palsy. *Cerebral Palsy Review, 16,* 11–14.

American Speech-Language-Hearing Association. (2004). Roles and responsibilities of the speech-language pathologist with respect to alternative communication: Technical report. *ASHA Supplement 24.*

American Speech-Language-Hearing Association. (2005). *Roles and responsibilities of the speech-language pathologists with respect to alternative communication: Position statement.* Retrieved June 20, 2006, from http://www.asha.org/about/continuing-ed/ASHA-courses/JSS/jss7420.htm

Americans with Disabilities Act (ADA) of 1990, PL 101-336, 42 U.S.C. §§ 12101 *et seq.*

Beukelman, D.R., & Mirenda, P. (2005). *Augmentative and alternative communication: Supporting children and adults with complex communication needs* (3rd ed.). Baltimore: Paul H. Brookes Publishing Co.

Bowser, G., & Reed, P. (2002). *Education tech points: A framework for assistive technology planning.* Winchester, OR: CATO.

Burkhart, L. (2001). *"Make it yourself" directions and workshop handouts.* Available from the Technology Integration web site, http://www.lindaburkhart.com/handouts

Castelanni, J., Zabala, J., & Reed, P. (2004). *Considering the need for AT within the individual education plan.* Arlington, VA: Council for Exceptional Children.

Church, G., & Glennen, S. (1992). *The handbook of assistive technology.* San Diego: Singular Publishing Group.

Creech, R. (1992). *Reflections from a unicorn.* Greenville, NC: RC Publications.

Denes, P., & Pinson, E. (1993). *The speech chain: The physics and biology of spoken language.* Fort Worth, TX: Worth Publishers.

DeRuyter, F. (1995). Evaluating outcomes in assistive technology: Do we understand the commitment? *Assistive Technology, 7*(3), 3–16.

DeRuyter, F. (1997). The importance of outcome measures for assistive technology service delivery systems. *Technology and Disability, 6,* 89–104.

Dogbo, N. (2002). Ethnic minorities and assistive technology. In T.M. Doe (Ed.). *A review of AT successes and barriers: Is it working?* San Francisco: California Foundation for Independent Living Centers.

Elkind, J. (1998). Computer reading machines for poor readers. *Special Education Perspectives, 24*(2), 9–14.

Fishman, I. (1987). *Electronic communication aids: Selection and use.* San Diego: College-Hill Press.

Hart, T., Hawkey, K., & Whyte, J. (2002). Use of a portable voice organizer to remember therapy goals in traumatic brain injury rehabilitation: A within-subjects trial. *Journal of Head Trauma Rehabilitation, 17*(6), 556–570.

Hawking, S. (1988). *A brief history of time.* New York: Bantam Books.

Hetrzroni, O.E., & Shrieber, B. (2004). Word processing as an assistive technology tool for enhancing academic outcomes of students with writing disabilities in the general classroom. *Journal of Learning Disabilities, 37*(2), 143–54.

Hourcade, J.J., Parette, H.P., & Huer, M.B. (1997). Family and cultural alert! Considerations in assistive technology assessment. *Exceptional Children, 30*(1), 40–44.

Individuals with Disabilities Education Act (IDEA) of 1990, PL 101-146. 20 U.S.C. §§ 1400 *et seq.*

Jutai, J.W., Fuhrer, M.J., Demers, L., Scherer, M.J., & DeRuyter, F. (2005). Toward a taxonomy of assistive technology device outcomes. *American Journal of Physical Medicine and Rehabilitation. 84*(4), 294–302.

Keating, T.J. & Ames, J. (2004, March). *Cognitive accessibility for individuals with disabilities: Picture Planner graphic activity planning software.* Presentation at the Center On Disabilities Technology and Persons with Disabilities Conference. Los Angeles.

Kemp, C.E., & Parette, H.P. (2000). Barriers to minority family involvement in assistive technology decision-making processes. *Education and Training in Mental Retardation and Developmental Disabilities, 35*(4), 384–92.

Lesar Judge, S., & Lamn, E.A. (1998). Assistive technology applications for play, mobility, communication, and learning for young children with disabilities. In S. Lesar Judge & H.P. Parette. (Eds.). *Assistive technology for young children with disabilities: A guide to family-centered services* (pp. 16–44). Brookline, MA: Brookline Books

Lloyd, L.L., Fuller, D.R., & Arvidson, H. H. (1997). *Augmentative and alternative communication: A handbook of principles and practices.* Boston: Allyn & Bacon.

Locke, P.A., & Mirenda, P. (1992). Roles and responsibilities of special education teachers serving on teams delivering AAC services. *Augmentative and Alternative Communication, 8,* 200–214.

MacArthur, C.A. (1999). Overcoming barriers to writing: Computer support for basic writing skills. *Reading & Writing Quarterly, 15*(2), 169–192.

MacArthur, C.A. (1996). Using technology to enhance the writing processes of students with learning disabilities. *Journal of Learning Disabilities. 29*(4), 344–354.

Maschkau, M. (2001). Get the job done. In H. Bersani, T. Anctil, & M. Fried-Oken (Eds.). *Me and my AT.* Eugene, OR: Northwest Media.

Meyer, A. (2001). Hear it, feel it, do it. In H. Bersani, T. Anctil, & M. Fried-Oken (Eds.). *Me and my AT.* Eugene, OR: Northwest Media.

Mirenda, P. (1993). AAC: Bonding the uncertain mosaics. *Augmentative and Alternative Communication, 9,* 3–9.

National Joint Committee for the Communicative Needs of Persons with Severe Disabilities. (1992). Guidelines for meeting the communication needs of persons with severe disabilities. *ASHA, 34*(Suppl. 7), 2–3.

Niparko, J.K., & Blankenhorn, R. (2003). Cochlear implants in young children. *Mental Retardation and Developmental Disabilities Research Reviews, 9*(4), 267–275.

Quenneville, J. (2001). Tech tools for students with learning disabilities: Infusion into inclusive classrooms. *Preventing School Failure, 45*(4), 167–170.

Parette, H., & Brotherson, M.J. (2004). Family-centered and culturally responsive assistive technology decision making. *Infants & Young Children, 17*(4) 355–367.

Parette, H.P., VanBiervliet, A., Hourcade, J.J. (2000). Family-centered decision making in assistive technology. *Journal of Special Education Technology, 15*(1), 15–55.

Rehabilitation Act of 1973, PL 93-112. (September 26, 1973). 93rd Congress, 1st session. §§ 504 *et seq.*

Reichle, J., York, J., & Sigafoos, J. (1991). *Implementing augmentative and alternative communication: Strategies for learners with severe disabilities.* Baltimore: Paul H. Brookes Publishing Co.

Scherer, M., & Galvin, J. (1994). Matching people with technology. *Rehabilitation Management, 7*(2) 128–130.

Schlosser, R. (2003). *The efficacy of augmentative and alternative communication.* Boston: Academic Press.

Shattuck, T. (2001). A shining star. In H. Bersani, T. Anctil & M. Fried-Oken (Eds.). *Me and my AT.* Eugene, OR: Northwest Media.

Sohlberg, M.M., Ehlhardt, L.A., Fickas, S., & Sutcliffe, A. (2003) A pilot study exploring electronic mail in users with acquired cognitive-linguistic impairments. *Brain Injury, 17*(7), 609–629.

Tam,S., Man, W.K., Hui-Chan, C.W.Y., Lau, A., Yip, B., & Cheung, W. (2003). Evaluating the efficacy of tele-cognitive rehabilitation for functional performance in three case studies. *Occupational Therapy International, 10*(1), 20–38.

Technology-Related Assistance for Individuals with Disabilities Act of 1988, PL 100-407, 29 U.S.C. §§ 2201 *et seq.*

Thompson, L.C., & Thompson, M.T. (2000). Partners with a view. In M. Fried-Oken & H.A. Bersani, Jr. (Eds.). *Speaking up and spelling it out* (pp. 135–145). Baltimore: Paul H. Brookes Publishing Co.

Wallace, J.F., Flippo, K.F., Barcus, J.M., & Behrmann, M.M. (1995). Legislative foundation of assistive technology policy in the United States. In Flippo, K.F., Inge, K.J., & Marcus, J.M. (Eds.) (1995). *Assistive technology: A resource for school, work, and community* (pp. 3–21). Baltimore: Paul H. Brookes Publishing Co.

Williams, B. (2000). More than an exception to the rule. In M. Fried-Oken & H.A. Bersani, Jr. (Eds.). *Speaking up and spelling it out* (pp. 245–255). Baltimore: Paul H. Brookes Publishing Co.

Zabala, J. (1993, October). *The SETT framework: Critical issues to consider when choosing and using assistive technology.* Presentation at the Closing the Gap Conference, Minneapolis, MN.

STUDY QUESTIONS

1. Define and state the purpose of *AT*.

2. Cite three examples of federal legislation that influenced the provision of AT services.

3. Why is it important to consider the language representation level associated with different types of symbols?

4. Describe the participation model of AAC assessment. How would you assess communication opportunities and barriers?

5. What are some ways you could adapt a standardized test for a student with a physical disability?

6. Describe examples of AT applications for people who are blind or have visual impairments, are deaf or hard of hearing, or have cognitive impairments.

7. Why is it important to consider cultural differences in AAC assessment and intervention?

8. Describe why it is important to assess client-specific outcomes after the introduction of AT.

13

Family-Centered Practice

DENISE LAPRADE RINI AND JANE HINDENLANG

Family: It is the genesis of our being: the primary and most powerful context for development of our values, beliefs, human interactions, rules, roles, and responsibilities; daughters and sons, brothers and sisters, mothers and fathers, aunts and uncles, nieces and nephews, cousins.

Every person is a member of a family and assumes many different family roles throughout his or her lifetime. Yet, many clinicians who are first entering home- and family-based clinical situations experience some trepidation. Although they feel prepared to provide treatment and have been trained in a wide range of techniques, they often feel overwhelmed when faced with the multiple and personal demands of the family context. Traditional service delivery methods have centered on the needs of the client as an individual. According to those methods, the professional has assumed responsibility for decision making and is seen as the "expert." While clinicians typically work with an individual or a small group within a clinical setting, such as a speech center, a hospital, or a school, services are increasingly being provided within the contexts natural to clients, such as their homes, vocational settings, or recreational settings. While we are expected to use **family-centered practice** in our work with very young children, it is applicable throughout the client's lifespan and across the various communication disorders we encounter.

A number of federal and state legislative provisions, as well as certain insurers, mandate that services be provided through a family-centered, natural environment framework while recognizing the important role of clients and families in the assessment and intervention process. It is important to obtain input from clients and their families about their needs and desires and to ultimately strive to make therapy more meaningful. In the current health care climate, there is a demand to demonstrate functional changes in everyday environments. Occasionally our roles shift to that of a consultant in educating family members and others, rather than a direct service provider. The increasing rate of an aging population predicts that the incidence and prevalence of communication disorders will rise, as will the need to provide services through a family-centered framework.

It is likely that, in the near future, the family milieu will be second only to school settings, in terms of frequency, as a site for practice in communication disorders. As clinicians, we must ask ourselves to what extent can we draw upon our own experiences as family members in order to deliver services successfully in a family-centered context? What roles do family members assume when one of them is involved in treatment for a communication disorder? Who constitutes family? How does this influence the manner in which the clinician provides the intervention? In order to answer these questions and to effectively implement family-centered practice, we need to know something about family systems and available clinical tools and resources for assessment and intervention according to this service delivery model.

FAMILY SYSTEMS THEORY

When we work with clients and their families, we need to understand what families are and how they function. The shift from the individual to the family as a focus of study, and the concept of family as a functioning transactional system and as an entity in itself through which individuals are viewed and understood, was considered a revolution in psychotherapy when the concept of *family therapy* began in the 1950s (Goldenberg & Goldenberg, 2004). Rosin and colleagues (1996) discussed the diversity of contemporary American families and the impact that this diversity has on professionals and educators who interact with them. They listed four sources of diversity that present particular challenges for clinicians:

1. The growing number of families whose ethnic and cultural backgrounds are different than those of service providers

2. The differences in family structure (e.g., decrease in traditional two-parent homes)

3. The impact of poverty on disability

4. The increase in the number of families that have parents or adults with disabilities

In addition, it is important to be aware that the family unit is not a static entity but rather a dynamic and complex system. The family may include primary relatives and secondary persons, such as more distant relatives (e.g., grandparents, aunts, uncles), significant partners and/or friends and neighbors who fulfill family roles. *Family* refers to those individuals who provide care giving, emotional, physical, and/or financial support, and who affect the client's quality of life and well-being. Families change and develop over time. Major life experiences, such as new partnerships, the birth of a child, children leaving home, aging, illness, and death create changes. Many situations can challenge families, such as a change in an economic situation, a change in employment, a household move, an acute or chronic illness, or an accident.

Often, the clinician does not enter the family system during the system's typical functioning but during one of these challenging stages. It is important to be aware that the family may be in flux and that family member roles and responses to illness, disability, and developmental delay may be different than typically expected. Specific reactions related to the age and role of the affected family member may also occur. A family with an infant or young child recently diagnosed with a disability may react to the loss of their dreams for the child and their loss of hope regarding future experiences that they believe the child may never have. There may also be an awareness of the demands of lifelong care if the disability is serious. When an adult family member experiences illness or a condition resulting in communication disorder, the effect is different because that person has held certain roles in the family that may no longer be possible to carry out. The economic status of the family may be directly and significantly affected, and there may be a reversal in caregiver roles due to the disability. The concomitant communication disorder itself further creates frustration and difficulty coping, negotiating, and exchanging important information.

THE KEY CONCEPTS OF A
FAMILY SYSTEMS PERSPECTIVE (BEGUN, 1996)

The family as a whole is greater than the sum of its parts. This concept reflects that each family has its own patterns, rules, behaviors, and boundaries. The family as a whole has meaning and its preservation may transcend the goals and interests of any one member.

Change in one part of the family affects the whole family system. The interdependence among family members will cause any change or experience that occurs to any one member to affect the entire family (e.g., member illness and concomitant communication disruption).

Subsystems are embedded within the larger family system. Different family members have their own particular relationships/systems (e.g., siblings, spouses, parent-child).

The family system exists within a larger social and environmental context. The family is a component of larger systems, such as extended families, neighborhoods, religious communities, and political and economic communities.

Families are multigenerational. Most family systems of multiple generations are also interwoven with members and ideas of past generations, along with future anticipated generations.

What implications do these concepts have for professionals in the field of communication disorders? If we acknowledge and act on these concepts, our approach to the family will be different than if we hold a more traditional client-centered approach. For example, in a traditional approach, the clinician might consider how a specific therapeutic intervention will affect the client. In a family systems approach, however, the clinician will also consider how therapy approaches affect the other members of the family and their relationships to one another. In a traditional approach, a clinician might make assumptions about a family member's role based on his or her position (e.g., parent, sibling), but in a systems approach, each family member's true role would be deduced through interview and observation of how members interact and how that interaction may change over time with new experiences (Begun, 1996).

Each clinician brings to the experience his or her own beliefs about what families are and how they "should" function, as well as the roles that the clinician and all family members should assume. Within a family-centered approach, the clinician needs to place these beliefs aside in order to be effective and clear-sighted in the service delivery process. As professionals, it is important to recognize not only what we have to offer but also what we can learn from our clients and their families or significant partners to establish more ecologically valid management paradigms.

DEFINING FAMILY-CENTERED PRACTICE

Family-centered practice has its roots in the consumer-led movements of the 1960s; consumers of health care and other human services were granted the rights to safety, to be informed, to choose, and to be heard (Goldenberg & Goldenberg, 2004). Head Start, created in 1965, mandated parent involvement and control of local programs (Johnson, 2000). One definition of family-centered practice, generated by the Beach Center on Disability (formerly the Beach Center on Families and Disability, 1997), states, "Family-centered service delivery, across disciplines and settings, recognizes the centrality of the family in the lives of individuals. It is guided by fully informed choices made by the family and focuses upon the strengths and capabilities of these families" (p. 1).

The family support movement acknowledges and builds on the many strengths and resources of families and communities (Rini & Whitney, 1999). The Beach Center lists key components of family-centered service delivery (Table 13.1). In addition, core concepts indicated by the Institute for Family-Centered Care (1998) include respect, support, choice, flexibility, collaboration, information, and identification of family strengths. *Family empowerment* extends beyond support by systematically assisting family members to direct their strengths and resources toward meeting the present and future needs of their members, themselves, and their communities. Thus, it is accepted as best practice that the client's relations to both family and community should be explored when formulating and implementing an intervention plan. Even though every family-centered intervention cannot address the full range of a complex set of systems, an acceptance of the family context as part of the individual's treatment has become a standard of clinical practice. For example, Gadow offers a response to the typical roles assumed by professionals when developing decision-making procedures. In her 1981 study, she proposed an advocacy model in "an effort to

Table 13.1. Principles of family support

Staff and families work together in relationships based on equality and respect.

Staff embrace families' capacity to support the growth and development of all family members—adults, youth, and children.

Families are resources to their own members, to other families, to programs, and to communities.

Programs affirm and strengthen families' cultural, racial, and linguistic identities and enhance their ability to function in a multicultural society.

Programs are embedded in their communities and contribute to the community-building process.

Programs advocate with families for services and systems that are fair, responsive, and accountable to the families served.

Practitioners work with families to mobilize formal and informal resources to support family development.

Programs are flexible and continually responsive to emerging family and community issues.

Principles of family support are modeled in all program activities, including planning, governance, and administration.

Source: Beach Center on Families and Disability, 1997.

Table 13.2. Premises of family support

The primary responsibility for the development and well-being of children lies within the family, and all segments of society must support families as they rear their children. The systems and institutions on which families rely must effectively respond to their needs if families are to establish and maintain environments that promote growth and development. Achieving this requires a society that is committed to making the well-being of children and families a priority and to supporting that commitment by allocating and providing necessary resources.

Assuring the well-being of all families is the cornerstone of a healthy society and requires universal access to support programs and services. A national commitment to promoting the healthy development of families acknowledges that every family, regardless of race, ethnic background, or economic status, needs and deserves a support system. Because no family can be self-sufficient, the concept of reaching families before problems arise is not realized unless all families are reached. To do so requires a public mandate to make family support accessible and available, on a voluntary basis, to all.

Children and families exist as part of an ecological system. An ecological approach assumes that child and family development is embedded within broader aspects of the environment, including a community with cultural, ethnic, and socio-economic characteristics that are affected by the values and policies of the larger society. This perspective assumes that children and families are influenced by interactions with people, programs, and agencies, as well as by values and policies that may help or hinder families' ability to promote their members' growth and development. The ecological context in which families operate is a critical consideration in programs' efforts to support families.

Child-rearing patterns are influenced by parents' understanding of child development and of their children's unique characteristics, personal sense of competence, and cultural and community traditions and mores. There are multiple determinants of parents' child-rearing beliefs and practices, and each influence is connected to other influences. For example, a parent's view of his or her child's disposition is related to the parent's cultural background and knowledge of child development and to characteristics of the child. Because the early years set a foundation for the child's development, patterns of parent–child interaction are significant from the start. The unique history of the parent–child relationship is important to consider in programs' efforts.

Enabling families to build on their own strengths and capacities promotes the healthy development of children. Family support programs promote the development of competencies and capacities that enable families and their members to have control over important aspects of their lives and to relate to their children more effectively. By building on strengths rather than treating impairments, programs assist parents in dealing with difficult life circumstances as well as achieving their goals, and in doing so, enhance parents' capacity to promote their children's healthy development.

The developmental processes that make up parenthood and family life create needs that are unique at each stage in the life span. Parents grow and change in response to changing circumstances and the challenges of nurturing a child's development. The tasks of parenthood and family life are ongoing and complex, requiring physical, emotional, and intellectual resources. Many tasks of parenting are unique to the parent's point in her or his life cycle. Parents have been influenced by their own childhood experiences and their own particular psychological characteristics, and are affected by their past and present family interactions.

Families are empowered when they have access to information and other resources and take action to improve the well-being of children, families, and communities. Equitable access to resources in the community—including up-to-date information and high-quality services that address health, educational, and other basic needs—enables families to develop and foster optimal environments for all family members. When families have meaningful experiences, participate in programs, and influence policies it strengthens existing capabilities and promotes the development of new competencies, such as the ability to advocate on their own behalf.

Source: Family Resource Coalition, 1996.

help individuals become clear about what they want in a situation, to assist them in discerning and clarifying their values, and to help them in examining available options in light of their values" (p. 137). Family-centered services means that the full context of the family, assessed with the family, is taken into consideration whenever intervention occurs (Table 13.2).

There are legal provisions that mandate family primacy in communication assessment and intervention. The Individuals with Disabilities Education Improvement Act (IDEA) of 2004 (PL 108-446), with its birth-to-3 component, requires that parents or guardians direct the contents of the Individualized Family Service Plan (IFSP), including outcomes for the child and family, and a statement of family needs and resources around which intervention must be designed. For children ages 3–21, IDEA'04 requires family input for permission to assess and develop the Individualized Education Program (IEP). Although school-based services are less likely to be fully family-centered, many school systems require clinicians to have contact with the family on a regular basis to discuss the course of assessment and intervention, to integrate family goals, and to share ideas for both school- and home-based intervention. For adults in hospitals, rehabilitation centers, or long-term care settings, there is the Patient Bill of Rights, which ensures family notification and patient/family input and/or attendance at all case conferences. A patient and his or her family may also partner with professionals to set short- and long-term plans of care, as well as to formulate statements of family needs. In its standards for care, The Joint Commission on Accreditation of Healthcare Organizations (JCAHO) cites involvement of residents and family in care decisions to maximize the client's functional status. The International Classification of Functioning, Disability and Health (ICF; World Health Organization [WHO], 2001) has challenged our thinking about service delivery by considering how any disability influences an individual's ability to reintegrate into activities at home, at work, and in the community. Audiologists and speech-language pathologists (SLPs) need to consider limitations in communication experienced by clients within daily activities (i.e., activity level) and the emotional, psychological, and social consequences of the impairment for the individual, spouse, caregiver, and family (i.e., participation level).

CULTURAL AND SOCIOECONOMIC CONSIDERATIONS

Contemporary practice also requires the audiologist and SLP to consider the unique ethnic, linguistic, and cultural background of the family. When there is a discrepancy between the culture of the family and client and their service providers, these differences can impede the development of a positive, family-centered intervention program if the clinician imposes his or her own beliefs and values onto the therapeutic situation. It is critically important for the clinician to understand how culture and tradition influence communication behavior, both at the level of clinician-family information exchange and at the level of clinician-client therapy interaction (see Chapter 11).

In her discussion of family-centered services among the chronically impoverished, Humphrey (1995) described issues that affect parents' and clinicians' views of each other and that threaten the effectiveness of the intended partnership. She noted the influences of poverty on parenting and pointed out that the demographics between those of low socioeconomic status and the clinician are often radically different. Rini and Whitney (1999) surveyed a number of studies that illustrate the deleterious effect poverty has on families and children in particular. Poverty is often accompanied by a host of other deficits in family resources, such as inadequate food and housing (which may include toxins such as lead paint and asbestos that are directly dangerous to health); restricted access to medical care, medications, and equipment; lack of transportation; and below-standard education. Chronic illness of family members may be more common than in families of high socioeconomic status. If further complicated by substance abuse (i.e., alcohol, legal and illegal drugs), environmental or domestic violence, and/or mental illness, the family of low socioeconomic status experiences multiple stressors that threaten family function. If different cultural backgrounds are also involved, then the number of obstacles between the members of this intervention team increases greatly. When families are experiencing multiple stressors, additional resources besides those directed at remediating a communication disorder in one family member are needed.

FAMILY-CENTERED PRACTICE IN COMMUNICATION DISORDERS

Traditionally, service delivery in communication disorders has followed a model in which the professional is viewed as the authority who identifies the presence and severity of the communication disorder along with treatment recommendations, if appropriate. Intervention would include educating family members and modeling interactive intervention behaviors that family members would be expected to imitate. Family members of persons with communication disorders were often perceived as being unsophisticated or too subjective to adequately observe or delineate the aspects of the person's communication disorder. Cress (2004) found this perception to be inaccurate. A review of multiple sources "confirmed that parents are accurate and thorough observers of their children, although they may not convey their observations in the same terms as professionals" (p. 51).

During the 1990s, particularly with the initiation of birth-to-3 services across the country (Individuals with Disabilities Education Act Amendments of 1997; PL 105-17) and the expansion of home health care services for adults, there has been an increasing movement toward true inclusion of family members in the decision-making process. Families are now involved in planning and conducting assessment tasks, identifying and prioritizing desired intervention outcomes if delays are diagnosed, developing intervention objectives, and implementing intervention activities. Wahrborg and Bornstein (1989), in investigating family attitudes and rehabilitation outcomes, suggested that an important positive relationship exists between active family support and stroke rehabilitation outcomes and, conversely, a nonsupportive family may interfere with stroke recovery resulting in physical and emotional deterioration of the client.

There are no prescriptive procedures to family-based approaches but the tenets of this practice suggest that both assessment and intervention are dynamic and collaborative, occur over time in several different contexts, and include relevant stakeholders. Functional communication and social relevance are embraced, particularly in our work with persons with complex communication needs. Outcomes and goals focus on improving individuals' quality of life by enabling them to become participating members in their families and communities and to experience a sense of personal competence. Client and family education contributes to achieving improved outcomes, and clients tend to fare better when their families and partners are involved.

The nature, content, and methods of interpersonal communication are critically important in the overall service delivery process. In particular, the ways in which service providers relay information and suggestions may be key to how the clinician's communication is important:

1. Clarity: Information should be provided in language that is familiar and understandable to the family

2. Succinctness: Information needs to be directed at the specific areas being discussed

3. Redundancy: Information should be provided frequently to allow family members to internalize and consider it

4. Respectfulness: Information should be provided in a manner that acknowledges the contribution of the family

5. Genuineness: The clinician must present him- or herself as a sincere human being and be perceived as such in order for necessary trust to develop among the persons involved

---

FAMILY-CENTERED ASSUMPTIONS AND ATTITUDES

1. Any circumstance that affects one family member (the client) affects other members, as well as the family as a whole.
2. The family has a right to establish its own priorities.
3. The family must be accepted as being the experts concerning their family member.
4. The clinician must evidence genuine listening in collaboration with family members to obtain assessment information and in developing intervention goals.
5. The family must be acknowledged as having the right to form their own approach to raising their child or caring for an older family member, as long as health and safety are not at issue.
6. The clinician must acknowledge any personal bias regarding preconceived notions of expected role behavior in approaching a family and must place these notions aside in order to assess the function of the specific family and client.
7. In situations in which a family report appears to differ significantly from a clinician's observation (particularly in situations in which communication behaviors are underreported), it is the responsibility of the clinician to explore with the family the situations in which they may perceive the client differently or to assist them in identifying behaviors that help them become aware that the client may have expanded skills.

FAMILY-CENTERED ASSESSMENT IN COMMUNICATION DISORDERS

Best practice suggests that we view assessment as a dynamic process that should be completed over time and in a variety of contexts in order to sample a representative set of communication behaviors (Lidz & Pena, 1996). Naturalistic contexts are also emphasized (Lund & Duchan, 1993). These contexts include the places where clients are comfortable and familiar, places that contain objects that are salient and immediate for them, and places in which typical social and communication exchanges occur. Linder (1993) discussed the limitations of traditional assessment in communication disorders, which has often required that the client be evaluated out of context (e.g., in an unfamiliar office or clinic setting, separated from family, individually rather than in a setting with peers or siblings) and presented with tasks that are often unrelated to any immediate activity, interest, or communication exchange. For example, federal and state birth-to-3 guidelines ensure that developmental assessment takes place within a natural environment and with family as key team members.

A number of family factors must be included in the assessment process. Knowledge of the cultural and linguistic contexts and characteristics of the family is primary in developing a preliminary understanding of the communication expectations and style of the environment (Halpern, 1993; Lund & Duchan, 1993). Size of the family, educational and socioeconomic backgrounds, and family members' expectations of each other all have an influence on what clinicians will see and what families perceive as areas of competence and need. One of the greatest challenges involves obtaining a representative sample of client and family communication behavior within the constraints of time and materials set by the agencies that govern the provision of services. A clinician must also conduct a comprehensive family assessment in such a way that the family does not feel that its privacy is violated (Donahue-Kilburg, 1992).

Utilizing intensive family interviews and observing family-client interactions are aspects of family-centered assessment. **Ethnographic interviewing** refers to information that is gained from observations made of a family in context and told from a family's perspective (Hammer, 1998). These techniques are applied in such a way that families are not assessed for their adequacy, rather they are valued for engaging in a dialogue to obtain valid information about the client's behavior (Hanson, 2000). Family and/or caregiver interviews are the typical means by which information is obtained, often in the absence of an already established relationship between the clinician and the family. It is obviously important for the clinician to be perceived as trustworthy and responsive to the concerns voiced by the family. At times, these concerns may go beyond communication to include illness, housing, coping issues, education, domestic issues, substance abuse, and so forth. At other times, the family may need to solely focus on communication problems; in which cases, trust revolves around the clinician's ability to hone in on the important communication issue.

FAMILY-CENTERED ASSESSMENT QUESTIONS

1. Is there a communication difference in this client in comparison to peers of his or her chronological and/or mental age and linguistic/cultural community?
2. Is this difference interfering with daily interactions within the family unit?
3. Is the client's communication functional for the purposes of attending to safety issues, expressing needs, negotiations, coping, planning, and developing literacy skills?
4. If the client's communication appears adequate within the immediate family context, is it sufficient for the larger context of the world outside of the family and for purposes that the family and the client intend (school, work, social settings)?
5. Do issues with the client's communication indicate areas of need, such as medical, economic, or mental health, to be addressed by and for the entire family?

Family-Centered Assessment with Infants, Toddlers, and Children

For children younger than 3 years, there are a number of instruments and procedures that enable the clinician to obtain information regarding speech-language development from the parent. The Vineland Adaptive Behavior Scales II (Sparrow, Balla, & Ciccietti, 2005) include a communication scale that provides parent report about receptive and expressive language. The MacArthur-Bates Communicative Development Inventories (CDIs), Second Edition (Fenson et al., in press) assesses receptive and expressive vocabulary size and early grammatical production. These two instruments provide results in terms of standard scores, which are often required to determine eligibility for intervention services. In addition, these scales are also available in Spanish, under the names Vineland-II and the MacArthur Inventarios del Desarrollo de Habilidades Communicativas (Jackson-Maldonado et al., 2003), respectively. Among other available parent-report format instruments are the Receptive-Expressive Emergent Language Scale-3 (Bzoch, League, & Brown, 2003), the Rossetti Infant-Toddler Language Scale (Rossetti, 2005), and the Early Language Milestone Scale, second edition (Coplan, 1993). These scales include areas of specific speech-language milestones rated by parents. Wetherby and Prizant's (2002) Communication and Symbolic Behavior Scales: Developmental Profiles™ (CSBS-DP™) include two tools in which parents provide information about the child's communication status, the Infant-Toddler Checklist and the Caregiver Questionnaire.

Although the assessment of communication disorders among school-age children usually includes background information provided by parents, there are few published assessment tools for older children that rely on parent report. When assessments are completed within the school system, it is easy for the family to become separated from the assessment experience. Yet, special education laws require that parents be notified in writing and give signed consent for assessment, so that presumably parents are aware of an upcoming evaluation and have the opportunity to initiate input into the process. It is incumbent on the clinician to obtain information from family members and to verify assessment results with the family. Clinicians must also recognize that the child's wishes, perceptions, and input are critical components in the assessment process.

Family-Centered Assessment Among Adolescents and Adults

In the case of adults or adolescents with acquired and chronic disabilities, clinicians can gather information through the use of questionnaires and rating scales that rely on client, family, and/or significant others' observations and knowledge. Some of these questionnaires and scales can be administered to the client and family via interviews or the family members can administer or complete them independently. Access to families or partners who know the client well can be helpful in determining the reliability of normative test scores. Family members can provide a window into a client's premorbid functioning that can assist in assessment. For example, the clinician can consider how a person's low score on a reading comprehension test might be interpreted differently once it is revealed the person was illiterate preinjury. Two published tools are available to clinicians, The General Health & History Questionnaire (Kreutzer, Leininger, Doherty, & Waaland, 1987) asks for information on current levels of functioning as well as premorbid status as does the *Pre-interview or Referral Form for Collecting Family and Medical History and Status Information* (Chapey, 2001).

There are several family-needs assessments that provide insight into the relative strengths of the family and its need for information or resources. These tools are useful for developing communication goals, educational programming, and referrals. One example is the Everyday Communicative Needs Assessment (Worrall, 1992). There are also partner skill and attitudinal surveys that assist in providing information for creating comprehensive management plans. The Quality of Communication Life Scale (Paul et al., 2004) is a tool that is used to attain information about the influence of a person's communication disorder on his or her relationships, communication interactions, participation in social, leisure, work and education activities, and overall quality of life. Lubinski's (2001) Communication/Environment Assessment and Planning Guide may be used to identify opportunities for communication, barriers to successful communication, and overall effectiveness of communication interactions. The Communication Effectiveness Index (CETI; Lomas et al., 1989) is an index of 16 daily situations in which the family member rates the partner's performance. ASHA's Functional Assessment of Communication Skills for Adults (Frattali, Thomson, Holland, Wohl, & Ferketic, 1995) is similar in scope to CETI. In addition, assessments may look at conversational interactions between partners using conversational discourse measures where not only is the client's discourse measured but also the partner's. Social Networks: A Communication Inventory for Individuals with Complex Communication Needs and their Communication Partners (Blackstone & Berg, 2003) is an inventory that assists clients and families in identifying their own everyday communication supports and contexts. There are three other published assessment tools that are useful for assessing the communication environment for individuals with severe developmental disabilities. The Communication Supports Checklist (McCarthy et al., 1998) includes a section about environmental support for communication, while Achieving Communication Independence (Gillette, 2003) and Analyzing the Communication Environment (Rowland & Schweigert, 1993) include items related to communication opportunities during daily routines.

FAMILY-CENTERED INTERVENTION IN COMMUNICATION DISORDERS

One of the guiding principles of ASHA's preferred practice patterns includes recognition that communication is an interactive process; the focus of intervention should include training of communication partners, caregivers, family members, peers, and educators. As with assessment, family-centered intervention implies that family members have key decision-making power in all aspects of intervention and that their personal styles, as well as linguistic, cultural, and traditional values, will be respected and incorporated into intervention. Styles of interaction between the family and the client may dictate, to a large extent, how directly involved with intervention the family may actually be. Within the framework of family-centered practice, there is a continuum of family involvement with intervention. On the one end, the family and the client identify communication goals and the mode of service delivery, but designated professionals provide intervention while family members focus indirectly on communication goals during daily interactions. On the other end, family members function directly as interventionists, assuming responsibility for intervention strategies and selecting techniques and materials according to collaboratively selected communication goals. For example, the family of a 33-month-old boy with a severe speech sound disorder chose to make the goal of the intervention for him to use family names, say "yes" and "no," and attempt to repeat some words of other family members. Through consultation with the clinician, the child's mother constructed specific pictorial material and games that were of particular interest to the child (e.g., his favorite animals and characters), and they reviewed these daily. After 3 months, the established objectives were achieved. Not all families are able and willing to assume this role, however. Some clients resist their families' efforts to assume the role of instructor. Some clients reject any activities that are structured and perceived as focusing directly upon their own difficulty. Between these two poles is a range of family involvement that includes both family-directed and client-directed activities along with clinician input.

Family-Centered Intervention with Infants, Toddlers, and School-Age Children

IDEA'04 provides mechanisms for parents and other family members to have direct input into the intervention process for children and adolescents, and young adults, ages 3–21. From birth to 3 years of age, the IFSP is family directed and the family states the specific outcomes that are the priority issues they wish to have addressed. Issues related to economic circumstance (i.e., education, employment, child care, respite, and housing), medical issues (i.e., health of the child or other family members) substance abuse, and/or behavioral health issues may be addressed on the IFSP. Communication outcomes are expected to project long-term goals and are generated by parents in their own words. Interim objectives for a specific period of time (e.g., 3–6 months) are developed by parents and the providing professionals. The materials and techniques included are chosen for their desirability and comfort for the parents as well as appropriateness.

There are a number of *parent programs* for communication skills available commercially, including Hickory Dickory Talk (Johnson & Heinze, 1990), HELP...at Home (Parks, 1990), Parent Articles (Schrader, 1988), It Takes Two to Talk (also in Spanish and French; Pepper & Weitzman, 2004), and Help Me Talk (Eichten, 2000). Paul (in press) included an extensive list and descriptions of programs, materials, and videos that can be used by parents in implementing family directed intervention. These tools provide family members with suggestions for activities and materials that can be adapted to suit the family's needs. Many families are eager to learn about various intervention approaches and techniques. Curricula and materials devised for overall early childhood education, such as included in *The Crosscultural, Language, and Academic Development Handbook* (Diaz-Rico & Weed, 1995), can provide ideas and sequences of activities that parents can implement and individualize to their own family context.

For school-age children, adolescents, and young adults, the planning and placement team is the mechanism that provides for parent input. Intervention is outlined through the IEP, which should be developed by all team members, including the student and his or her parents. Within the public schools, however, family-centered intervention may be difficult to achieve because of several obstacles: parent access to classrooms, availability of school staff and activities to working parents, and school accessibility to parents without transportation or child care services. In addition, service delivery often focuses on academic and social communication goals only in the school setting. School personnel must strive to have ongoing contact and flexible activities to be responsive to family needs.

In providing support for the adolescent or young adult with a communication disorder, clinicians can include family members. For example, in areas of articulation and fluency, family members can review lists of specific practice materials with the client. Carryover activities require the involvement of the family to provide contexts in which the client can practice new communication behaviors. The client, family, and clinician may devise specific contracts or procedures jointly. For higher-level language skills, a number of commercially available workbooks and computer-based programs can provide basic stimuli for client-family work sessions.

Family-Centered Intervention Among Adults

Although there is no legislated mechanism to ensure family input to intervention plans for adults with disabilities, many facilities follow a Patient Bill of Rights in administering adult care. This document provides for the patient's right to have his or her family involved with every case conference and aspect of planning, as well as family input on the services to be provided. A central issue relative to family involvement with an adult with disabilities is the willingness of the patient to have that involvement. This will be partially dependent upon preexisting family relationships, the degree of independence the patient had previously in self-care, and medical determination of whether the patient is capable of being responsible for his or her own decisions and future care. Family involvement cannot be mandated because the integrity of the adult's right to decide must be protected. This can present a challenge for the clinician when there is a disagreement between patient and family members about who is "in charge" of the patient's care. Often, when such conflicts exist, mediation may be needed to explore possible resolutions, and special personnel (e.g., a social worker) may need to take the lead in the situation.

The individual who experiences significant communication loss due to neurological illness or trauma presents a different challenge to the family. As an adult, the client has held a specific position and role in the family. A style of communication and interaction has developed between the person and his or her family, friends, and social or work associates. Loss of communication is devastating because it affects all of these areas. In addition, the client often experiences other medical difficulties, which may include loss of mobility, decrease in sensory or cognitive function, coronary and vascular fragility, and so forth. Communication disorders superimposed on preexisting medical conditions will significantly affect the person's overall function and degree of independence and quality of life, which has a consequent influence on the family. Still, much can be done to facilitate and broaden communication among the client, the family, and the community. For example, these individuals can participate in client-directed group therapy in which each client works on individualized goals but within a social context. At the same time, family members can participate in a parallel group therapy activity focused on family support and carry-over strategies (Johannsen-Horbach, Crone, & Wallesch, 1999).

Much of the information derived from the interview portion of the assessment may help establish goals related to activity and participation levels in collaboration with family partners. There are interventions that focus on family education, communication skills training for both the client and the partners, and counseling programs that offer support for the partners. The professional can work with families to develop realistic goals and match them to functional outcomes (Burns, 1996). Partners of people with acquired brain injury may not only participate in the therapy but may be the primary focus of therapy. Several authors have developed approaches that coach or co-construct conversation between the client and significant other. The spouse/partner serves as clinician while the clinician assumes the role of facilitator. Kagan's (1999) Supported Conversation for Adults with Aphasia (SCA) trains volunteers to interact with individuals with aphasia. The Family Based Intervention for Chronic Aphasia (FICA; Alarcon, Hickey, Rogers, Olswang, 1997) focuses on treating the disability within naturally occurring interactions. Sorin-Peters—who works with couples living with aphasia using adult learning approaches and incorporating education, skill training, and counseling within an experiential learning cycle—found that the result of his 2003 study "suggests a relationship in which the speech-language pathologist and couple are active collaborators in the process" (p. 415). Purdy and Hindenlang (2005) developed a family education and training program using these same adult learning principles, but rather than working with the couples individually, created classes of five to six couples. Benefits for both the client and partner included joint problem solving opportunities as well as a chance to view and discriminate different communication impairments. Ylvasaker and Feeney (1998) suggested collaboration within everyday contexts among all people who interact with individuals with disability caused by acquired brain injury. For individuals with a chronic disability and their families, the need for education and training is life long.

Professional Collaboration

To achieve a more comprehensive and family-centered approach, there are a number of areas in which collaboration is necessary. First, it is important that professionals become familiar with the cornerstones of each other's disciplines and how these relate to family-centered and transdisciplinary practice. Typically, when one discipline learns the scope of practice and professional language of another, the opportunities to collaborate expand. Second, it is helpful when each discipline is able to incorporate a broader perspective into evaluations and interventions. For example, the SLP who recognizes that a client has sensory issues can call upon the expertise of a colleague in occupational therapy. A psychologist may recognize that a client or his family experience challenges in treatment because of hearing impairments and will therefore consult with the audiologist. Collaborating professionals can offer a broader spectrum of insight and support to the family being served. This is particularly important when service is provided through a single transdisciplinary professional who must address a range of needs within the family as well as the client. Professionals can work together to assess the level and types of needs that exist in a family and then help families identify and secure community resources. In addition, professionals may find opportunities to partner with families to advocate for additional resources as a result of their joint assessment of the community.

Family-Centered Service Provision in Natural Environments

Family-centered service provision in natural environments (e.g., a home, a child or adult care center, a classroom, or a workplace) can immediately address the specific communication requirements of the context, including appropriate objectives and stimuli. Family members can be immediately part of communication services and help the client use skills in daily routines. There are, however, also challenges that the clinician may face in working within the natural environment. Distractions of a typical environment, such as noise, extraneous activity, and the comings and goings of the family members or other people, may be a factor. Natural environments may not always be safe, secure, healthy, supportive, or facilitative of development or rehabilitation. As the clinician-family relationship develops, it is likely that the family will confide in the clinician, at times revealing highly sensitive or complex situations and emotions. The clinician may also be affected by organizational or administrative issues. For example, services may be obstructed by the demands of time management, commuting from site to site, and managed care and economic realities (e.g., quotas on client contacts). In many states, consultation (i.e., the time spent conferring with other professionals, the family, or physicians that is not direct treatment time) is not compensated by insurance.

CONCLUSION

Family-centered practice is not merely a theoretical construct or philosophical position. Its practical implementation dictates collaboration among the family, the client, and the clinician in ways that are based on the needs and wishes of the family. For the clinician who embraces the notion that communication assumes immersion in human interactions, a family-centered approach to service provision will prove to be a vital element of practice.

REFERENCES

Alarcon, N., Hickey, E., Rogers, M., & Olswang, L. (1997, March). *Family-based intervention for chronic aphasia (FICA): An alternative service delivery model.* Paper presented at the Non-Traditional Approaches to Aphasia Conference, Yountville, CA.

Beach Center on Families and Disability. (1997). *Families and Disability Newsletter, 8*(2), 1. Lawrence: The University of Kansas.

Begun, A.L. (1996). Family systems and family-centered care. In P. Rosin, A.D. Whitehead, L.I. Tuchman, G.S. Jesien, A.L. Begun, & L. Irwin (Eds.), *Partnerships in family-centered care: A guide to collaborative early intervention* (pp. 33–63). Baltimore: Paul H. Brookes Publishing Co.

Blackstone, S., & Berg, M. (2003). *Social networks: A communication inventory for individuals with complex communication needs and their communication partners.* Monterey, CA: Augmentative Communication.

Burns, M. (1996). Use of the family to facilitate communication changes in adults with neurological impairments. *Seminars in Speech and Language, 17,* 115–122.

Bzoch, K., League, R., & Brown, V.L. (2003). *The Receptive-Expressive Emergent Language Scale, 3rd ed.* Austin, TX: PRO-ED.

Coplan, J. (1993). *Early Language Milestone Scale.* Austin, TX: PRO-ED.

Chapey, R. (2001). Assessment of language disorders in adults. In R. Chapey (Ed.). *Language intervention strategies in aphasia and related neurogenic communication disorders* (4th ed., pp. 55–126.) Philadelphia: Lippincott Williams & Wilkins.

Cress, C. (2004). Augmentative and alternative communication and language: understanding and responding to parents' perspectives. *Topics in Language Disorders, 24,* 51–61.

Diaz-Rico, L.T., & Weed, K.Z. (1995). *The crosscultural, language, and academic development handbook*. Boston: Allyn & Bacon.

Donahue-Kilburg, G. (1992). *Family-centered early intervention for communication disorders*. New York: Aspen Publishers.

Eichten, P. (2000). *Help me talk: Parent's guide to speech & language stimulation techniques for children 1–3 years* (2nd ed.). Richmond, VA: Pi Communication Materials.

Family Resource Coalition. (1996). *Guidelines for family support practice*. Chicago: Author.

Frattali, C., Thomson, C., Holland, A., Wohl, C., & Ferketic, M. (1995). *The American Speech-Language-Hearing Association functional assessment of communication skills for adults (ASHA FACS)*. Rockville, MD: American Speech-Language-Hearing Association.

Fenson, L., Marchman, V.A., Thal, D., Dale, P.S., Bates, E., & Reznick, J.S. (in press). *MacArthur-Bates Communicative Development Inventories: User's guide and technical manual, second edition*. Baltimore: Paul H. Brookes Publishing Co.

Gadow, S. (1981). Advocacy: An ethical model for assisting patients with treatment decisions. In C.B. Wong & J.P. Swazey (Eds.), *Dilemmas of dying: Policies and procedures for decisions not to treat*. Boston: GK Hall Medical Publishers.

Gillette, Y. (2003). *Achieving communication independence*. Eau Claire, WI: Thinking Publications.

Goldenberg, I., & Goldenberg, H. (2004). *Family therapy: An overview*. (6th ed.). Belmont, CA: Wadsworth Publishing.

Hammer, C.S. (1998). Toward a "thick description" of families: Using ethnography to overcome the obstacles to providing family-centered early intervention services. *American Journal of Speech Language Pathology 7*, 5–22.

Halpern, R. (1993). Poverty and infant development. In C.H. Zeanah (Ed.), *Handbook of infant mental health* (pp. 73–86). New York: The Guilford Press.

Hanson, M.J. (2004). Ethnic, cultural, and language diversity in intervention settings. In E.W. Lynch & M.J. Hanson (Eds.), *Developing cross-cultural competence: A guide for working with children and their families* (3rd ed., pp. 3–18). Baltimore: Paul H. Brookes Publishing Co.

Humphrey, R. (1995). Families who live in chronic poverty: Meeting the challenge of family-centered services. *American Journal of Occupational Therapy, 49*, 7.

Individuals with Disabilities Education Act Amendments of 1997, PL 105-17, 20 U.S.C. §§ 1400 *et seq*.

Individuals with Disabilities Education Improvement Act of 2004, PL 108-446, 20 U.S.C. §§ 1400 *et seq*.

Institute for Family-Centered Care (ND). *Patient- and family-centered care core concepts*. [Data file]. Available from the Institute for Family-Centered Care FAQ web site, http://www.familycenteredcare.org/faq.html

Jackson-Maldonado, D., Thal, D.J., Fenson, L., Marchman, V.A., Newton, T., & Conboy, B. (2003). *MacArthur Inventarios del Desarrollo de Habilidades Comunicativas: User's guide and technical manual*. Baltimore: Paul H. Brookes Publishing Co.

Johannsen-Horbach, H., Crone, M., & Wallesch, C. (1999). Group therapy for spouses of aphasic patients. *Seminars in Speech and Language, 20*(1), 73–82.

Johnson, B. (2000). Family-centered care: Four decades of progress. *Family Systems, and Health, 18*, 137–156.

Johnson, K., & Heinze, B. (1990). *Hickory dickory talk: A family approach to infant and toddler language development*. East Moline, IL: LinguiSystems.

Kagan, A. (1999). Supported conversation for adults with aphasia: Methods and resources for training conversation partners. *Aphasiology, 12*, 851–864.

Kreutzer, J., Leininger, B., Doherty, K., & Waaland, P. (1987). *General health and history questionnaire*. Richmond: Medical College of Virginia, Rehabilitation Research and Training Center on Severe Traumatic Brain Injury.

Lidz, C., & Pena, E. (1996). Dynamic assessment: The model, its relevance as a nonbiased approach, and its application to Latino American preschool children. *Language, Speech, and Hearing Services in Schools, 27*, 367–384.

Linder, T.W. (1993). *Transdisciplinary Play-Based Intervention: Guidelines for developing a meaningful curriculum for young children*. Baltimore: Paul H. Brookes Publishing Co.

Lomas, J., Packard, L., Bester, S., Elbard, H., Finlayson, A., & Zogharth, C. (1989). The communicative effectiveness index: Development and psychometric evaluation of a functional communication measure for adult aphasia. *Journal of Speech and Hearing Disorders, 54*(1), 113–124.

Lubinski, R. (2001). Environmental systems approach to adult aphasia. In R. Chapey (Ed.), *Language intervention strategies in aphasia and related neurogenic communication disorders* (4th ed., pp. 269–296). Philadelphia: Lippincott Williams & Wilkins.

Lund, N., & Duchan, J. (1993). *Assessing children's language in naturalistic contexts* (3rd ed.). Upper Saddle River, NJ: Prentice Hall.

McCarthy, C.F., McLean, L.K., Miller, J.F., Paul-Brown, D., Romski, M.A., Rourk, J.D., et al. (1998). *Communication supports checklist: For programs serving individuals with severe disabilities.* Baltimore: Paul H. Brookes Publishing Co.

Parks, S. (Ed.). (1990). *HELP . . . at Home.* Palo Alto, CA: VORT.

Paul, R. (in press). *Language disorders from infancy through adolescence* (3rd ed.). St. Louis: Mosby.

Paul, D., Frattali, C., Holland, A., Thompson, C., Caperton, C., & Slater, S. (2004). *Quality of Communication Life (ASHA QCL) Scale.* Rockville, MD: American Speech-Language-Hearing Association.

Pepper, J. & Weitzman, E. (2004). *It takes two to talk: A practical guide for parents of children with language delays.* Toronto, Canada: The Hanen Centre.

Purdy, M. & Hindenlang, J. (2005). Educating and training caregivers of persons with aphasia. *Aphasiology, 19*(35), 377–388.

Rini, D., & Whitney, G. (1999). Family-centered practice for children with communication disorders. In R. Paul (Ed.), *Child and adolescent psychiatric clinics of North America: Language disorders* (pp. 153–174). Philadelphia: W.B. Saunders.

Rosin, P., Whitehead, A.D., Tuchman, L.I., Jesien, G.S., Begun, A.L., & Irwin, L. (1996). *Partnerships in family-centered care: A guide to collaborative early intervention.* Baltimore: Paul H. Brookes Publishing Co.

Rossetti, L. (2005). *The Rossetti infant-toddler language scale.* East Moline, IL: LinguiSystems.

Rowland, C., & Schweigert, P. (1993). *Analyzing the communication environment.* Tucson, AZ: Communication Skill Builders.

Schrader, M. (1988). *Parent articles: Enhance parent involvement in language learning.* Tucson, AZ: Communication Skill Builders.

Sorin-Peters, R. (2003). Viewing couples living with aphasia as adult learners: Implications for promoting quality of life. *Aphasiology, 17*(4), 405–416.

Sparrow, S., Balla, D., & Ciccetti, D. (2005). *Vineland Adaptive Behavior Scales, second edition.* Circle Pines, MN: AGS Publishing.

Wahrborg, P., & Bornstein, P. (1989). Family therapy in families with an aphasic member. *Aphasiology, 3,* 93–98.

Wetherby, A.M., & Prizant, B.M. (2002). *Communication and Symbolic Behavior Scales: Developmental Profile™ (CSBS DP™).* Baltimore: Paul H. Brookes Publishing Co.

World Health Organization. (2001). *International Classification of Functioning, Disability and Health (ICF).* Retrieved June 20, 2006, from http://www.who.int/classifications/icf/en

Worrall, L. (1992). *Everyday communicative needs assessment.* Queensland, Australia: Department of Speech and Hearing,

Ylvisaker, M., & Feeney, T. (1998). *Collaborative brain injury intervention: Positive everyday routines.* San Diego: Singular Publishing Group.

STUDY QUESTIONS

1. What is family-centered practice?

2. What are the key concepts of family systems theory?

3. In what ways is family-centered practice different than traditional practice?

4. What are some ways in which assessment and intervention services can be provided in a family-centered manner?

5. What role does collaboration have in family-centered practice?

6. Name situations or professional demands that might pose challenges to providing true family-centered services

7. Name some issues that create different considerations between family-centered service delivery for adults and family-centered service delivery for children.

8. You have been asked to participate in an evaluation of a 2-year-old child from another country. You are not sure of the family's language, and you know you have no familiarity with it. When you arrive at the designated location, the family does not want to admit you to the premises, but expresses great concern about the child. A community member who is somewhat familiar with the family's language is present to serve as interpreter but has never participated in this type of professional activity before. What are some issues you might be facing? What questions need to be answered? What information should be provided to the family?

9. A child you have been seeing for intervention at home has begun making gains and attending to the activities in your sessions. The child's mother, who has been present for most of each session's duration, decided to begin to work at home part time. During your visit, she holds an exercise session in a neighboring room. There are eight women who come in and out of the home over the period of 90 minutes. Your client is naturally curious and restless and having difficulty remaining with you. What issues exist? What conversation, if any, should you have with the mother? What alternatives for intervention do you have?

10. A 50-year-old woman had a stroke 4 weeks prior to your evaluation of her in her home. She lives with her husband and 16-year-old son. Her daughter, age 20, is a sophomore at a college 3 hours away. During your first visit, you observed the client to be tired and easily frustrated. Her husband observed your visit; he said that he had been told by a speech-language pathologist in the hospital that his wife had global aphasia. During your second visit the following week, the client again appeared fatigued and was reluctant to participate in therapy. She also refused to have her husband present at the therapy session, and you observed her "yelling" at him. At the time the client had her stroke, she and her family were getting ready to take a trip to Florida to visit family. What issues exist? Who are the relevant stakeholders in this scenario? What information is needed and how might it be obtained?

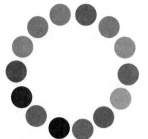

Glossary

activity limitations   Term used by the World Health Organization to describe difficulties experienced by an individual in executing one or more activities due to an impairment.

advocacy   Steps taken by individuals or groups to understand, implement, or influence public policy.

age equivalents   A derived score that expresses an individual's performance as the average performance for that age group. It is interpreted to mean that the individual's performance is equal to the average performance of an individual of that given age.

alerting devices   Devices for individuals with hearing impairment that convert sound into sight, different auditory signals, or vibration.

Alzheimer disease   A progressive disease of the brain that is characterized by impairment of memory and a disturbance in at least one other thinking function (e.g., language, perception of reality).

American Sign Language (ASL)   A symbolic communication system making use of manual signs, used by deaf people to communicate.

aphasia   A language disorder resulting from brain damage and characterized by impairment comprehension, formulation, and language use.

applied research   Research concerned with the impact of various intervention approaches.

appraisal   The process of collecting observations and measurements of a client's performance during assessment.

apraxia   A disorder characterized by difficulty in performing voluntary motor acts in the absence of paralysis.

artifacts   Data collected about an individual's performance, such as examples of written work, projects, and language samples.

assessment   The process of collecting and analyzing data about an individual in order to make clinical decisions.

assistive listening devices   Personal (e.g., hearing aids) or community (e.g., audio loops) enhancement systems for individuals with hearing impairment.

assistive technology (AT)   Tools that help an individual overcome limitations related to a disability by either enhancing the skills the individual has or by compensating for absent or nonfunctional skills.

asymmetry   Lack of symmetry between two normally alike parts.

atrophy   A wasting of tissues, organs, or the entire body.

auditory brain stem evoked response audiometry   A type of electrophysiologic testing designed to measure an individual's neural responses to sound. This is an objective hearing test that does not require the client's participation.

auditory brainstem response (ABR)   An electrophysiologic response to sound, consisting of five to seven peaks that represent neural function of auditory pathways.

augmentative and alternative communication (AAC) An area of practice that attempts to compensate temporarily or permanently for the impairment and disability patterns of individuals with severe communication disorders.

authentic assessment An alternative to standardized testing that emphasizes an individual's performance on real-life tasks in naturalistic situations.

baseline Frequency of a behavior or level of functioning prior to the initiation of treatment.

basic research Research that attempts to gain further knowledge of fundamental processes (e.g., speech, language, and hearing development).

behavior modification specialists The professional responsible for analysis and intervention surrounding the antecedents, responses, and reinforcement associated with challenging behavior.

behavioral audiologic tests Measures that pertain to the observation of the activity of a person in response to some stimuli.

behavioral objective Intervention goals that specify an action a client is to perform, the conditions under which the action will be performed, and how well the action must be performed for the objective to be achieved.

beneficence The promotion of interests and welfare of others.

benefit period Time defined by policy during which certain provisions of a policy are in force.

bifid A split or a cleft into two parts.

Blisssymbols A set of visual symbols developed to serve as an alternative communication system for individuals with severe speech disorders.

block A complete stoppage of the flow of speech, including air, voice, and articulators. One of the core behaviors in stuttering.

bound morphemes Units of meaning that do not appear unless attached to another morpheme (e.g., plural /s/, past tense -ed).

case conferences Formal meetings involving service providers, clients, and family members in which evaluation findings, treatment outcomes, and necessary support services are discussed.

case history questionnaire A written set of questions used as a tool to gather and organize information regarding the nature of a client's speech, language and hearing concerns, general developmental and health history, educational background, and history of related support services.

case law Court decisions regarding disputed interpretations of laws that influence how policies are implemented in the disputed case and that also set a precedent for future practice.

case series A collection of case studies in which several participants receive the same treatment and their outcomes are measured following the intervention.

case study design A single individual, event, or context is intensively studied using both qualitative and quantitative data to determine.

cerumen Earwax; the waxy secretion in the external auditory meatus.

cleft palate A cleft palate is an opening in the roof of the mouth in which the two sides of the palate did not fuse while the fetus was developing in utero.

closed questions Questions that elicit only a yes or no or a one-word answer (e.g., "Do you have a dog?" "What did you eat for lunch?").

cochlear implant Device that enables persons with profound hearing loss to perceive sound, consisting of an electrode array surgically implanted in the cochlea, which delivers electrical signals to the 8th cranial nerve and an external amplifier, which activates the electrodes.

code of ethics American Speech-Language-Hearing Association and American Academy of Audiology guidelines that define clinically acceptable conduct and conscientious judgement which members are expected to internalize and apply into clinical settings.

cognitive communication disorder Any aspect of communication (e.g., listening, speaking, reading, writing, pragmatic) that is affected by disruption of cognition.

cognitive impairments   When a client has difficulty with the collection of mental processes and activities used in perceiving, remembering, thinking, and understanding (e.g., attention, memory, executive functioning).

coherence   The relationship of the meaning or content of an utterance to the content of previous utterances and to the overall content of the discourse.

Commission of the Accreditation of Rehabilitation Facilities (CARF)   A regulatory body that oversees the quality of care provided to patients in rehabilitation facilities.

comorbidity   The co-occurrence of two disorders.

competent practice   Clinician actions including: effective diagnostic procedures, an accurate prognosis, appropriate therapy strategies for the particular disorder, and on-going analysis of client outcomes.

complex sentences   Sentences that contain more than one main verb phrase, including sentences containing conjoined, embedded, and subordinate clauses.

concurrent validity   The relationship between an individual's performance on a test and performance on a criterion measure.

confidence interval   The range of scores within which a person's true score will fall with a given probability.

confidentiality   The act of taking privileged client information and sharing it only with persons directly responsible for client management and care and only for purposes related to client welfare.

conflict of interest   A compromise in professional judgement in which a clinician loses their sense of objectivity because of personal or financial gains.

conjunctions   Linking words that tie ideas within and across sentences. Both coordinate (e.g., and, but, or) and subordinate (e.g., when, if, because) are included in this category.

construct validation   The way in which a test measures the theoretical trait or construct that it purports to measure.

consultative/collaborative   The provision of communication services through models of both direct and indirect formats.

content   Semantics, one aspect of language development.

content related validity   A measure of the extent to which a test represents an adequate sample of the domain being assessed.

continuing education   The act of updating clinical skills and keeping current of the latest trends and advances, achieved through reading textbooks and journal articles, attending workshops, shadowing professional colleagues, and participating in research activities.

continuum of care (COC)   Levels of rehabilitation through which patients pass based on need and intensity of services.

continuum of naturalness   The range of intervention activities, from the most highly structured to the most naturalistic.

conversation analysis   A type of qualitative research methodology used to analyze social interactions through conversation.

criterion-referenced tests   Tests or procedures that measure an individual's performance in terms of absolute levels of mastery.

criterion-related validity   A measure of the extent to which performance on a test can be correlated with performance on another instrument believed to measure the same skill or behavior.

Cronbach's coefficient alpha   A statistical procedure for calculating internal reliability of a test.

crossbite   An abnormal relation of one or more teeth of one arch to the opposing tooth or teeth of the other arch, caused by deviation of tooth position or abnormal jaw position.

cultural sensitivity   Attuning to and adjusting for the culturally determined characteristics of communication in various communities when engaging in interactions with culturally or linguistically different clients.

cut-off score   A predetermined score used to make pass/fail decisions in a screening.

cystic fibrosis   A genetic disease in which the body produces a thick, sticky mucus that clogs the lungs, leading to serious and life-threatening lung infections.

cysts   A small sac or pouch that contains fluid or semi-solid material.

decontextualized   Tasks, such as tests, which require language comprehension or formulation out of the context of naturally occurring events or activities.

dementia   Organically based deterioration of mental processes.

dependent variable   The particular outcome of a treatment.

descriptive-developmental model   An approach to assessment that emphasizes the client's current communication status.

developmental scales   Assessment instrument that samples behaviors from developmental stages.

developmental scores   Test scores that have been transformed into age or grade equivalents.

devices for telecommunications   An electronic aid that produces speech output.

diagnosis   Identification of a disease or disorder based on symptoms presented.

diagnostic   *See* evaluation.

diagnostic evaluation reports   A written report used to summarize information obtained in both audiological and speech-language evaluations. These reports serve as legal records of assessment findings, diagnoses, and recommendations.

dialect   Rule-governed and mutually intelligible forms of a language characterized by social, ethnic, and geographical differences in its speakers.

differential diagnosis   The process of distinguishing a disorder or condition from others with similar symptoms.

direct services   Working with a client in a hands-on format.

discharge summary   A written report of a client's cumulative progress from the initiation of therapy to their discharge from service.

dynamic assessment   Assessment process in which the examiner modifies interactions in order to achieve success for the client.

dysarthria   Motor speech disorder resulting from nervous system impairment.

dysfluency   An interruption in the smoothness of the flow of speech (e.g., stuttering).

dysphagia   Disorder of swallowing.

dysprosody   Disorders that affect the rate, loudness, intonation, and stress used in speech to modulate and enhance the meaning of words and sentences.

effect-size estimates   The magnitude of a treatment's effect in standard deviation units.

electrolarynx   A battery-operated instrument that makes a humming sound to help people who have lost their larynx to talk.

electronystagmography (ENG)   A method of measuring eye movements, especially nystagmus, to assess the integrity of the vesitibular mechanism.

electrophysiological test   Audiological testing procedure that measure involuntary responses to sound within the auditory nervous system.

endoscope   A device used for observing a bodily function through a body opening. It contains an optic device and a tube that can be inserted into the opening in order to view movements or structures otherwise not viewable.

entitlement program   Program of expected government benefits for selected groups who meet eligibility criteria defined by Congress, such as age, income, retirement, disability, or unemployment.

equivalent form reliability   Two forms of a test that measure the same skills and are standardized on the same population (also called alternate form reliability).

ethics   The moral and/or civil codes of conduct for a particular person, situation, community, religious group, organization, or society that evolve from a philosophy of human interaction that values behaviors personally or collectively regarded as good, honest, proper, and respectable.

Ethics Calibration Quick Test   A series of questions to enable clinicians to analyze the ethical propriety of a situation.

Ethnographic interviewing   Information gained from observations made of a family in context and told from a family's perspective.

ethnography   A qualitative method that provides an analytical description of a cultural scene.

etiology   Cause of a disorder or condition.

evaluation   The formal and informal procedures conducted as part of an assessment.

evidence-based practice (EBP)   The use of current high quality research-based data to make clinical decisions.

executive function   Skills that comprise the highest level of human cognition. Includes the ability to plan, sequence, and accomplish goal-directed activities in a flexible manner.

expository   Text that provides factual explanations, descriptions, argument, or opinion rather than narrative or stories.

facilitative play   A client-centered method of intervention in which the clinician provides indirect language stimulation by modeling language forms that are related to client-initiated actions.

false negatives   Errors in which clients are judged not have to problems when they really do.

false positives   Errors in which clients are judged to have problems when they do not.

family-centered practice   The provision of assessment and intervention from the family's point of view, taking into account family goals, dynamics, and circumstances.

fistula   An abnormal passage from one surface to another.

fluency   The smooth, uninterrupted flow that is typical of speech.

follow-up letter   Letters written to referral sources discussing the status of the individual referred for clinical services, evaluation finding, and/or treatment outcomes.

form   An aspect of language development that includes syntax, word order, morphology, phonology, and prosody.

formant analysis   Analysis of an acoustic signal through studying concentrated frequency bands of energy caused by resonance patterns produced by the speech production mechanism.

frenulum   *See* frenum.

frenum   The mucous membrane extending from the floor of the mouth to the midline of the undersurface of the tongue.

frequency modulation (FM) amplification system   An assistive listening device designed to enhance signal-to-noise ratio, in which a remote microphone/transmitter worn by a speaker sends signals via FM to a receiver worn by a listener.

functional assessment   An alternative to standardized testing that emphasizes an individual's performance on real-life tasks in naturalistic situations.

functional maintenance plans   A written plan developed by an SLP or other rehabilitation specialist working in a Medicare-funded healthcare facility outlining rehabilitation supports to be provided by non-certified support staff and other caregivers.

fundamental frequency   The tone produced by cyclic movements of the vocal folds, measured in cycles per second (hertz).

gag reflex   Retching or gagging caused by the contact of a foreign body with the mucous membrane of the throat.

generalization   Carry-over of trained behavior into settings other than the training context.

gloss   A clinician's interpretation of the intended meaning of a client's word or utterance.

grade equivalents   A derived score that expresses an individual's performance as the average performance for a particular grade. It is interpreted to mean that the individual's performance is equal to the average performance of a student in a given grade.

guidelines   Suggestions for implementing and monitoring public policies, which do not have the weight of law.

health maintenance organization (HMO)   A type of managed care organization that provides a range of care on a prepayment basis.

hearing conservation   A program designed to protect the ears from hearing loss due to exposure to noise.

home care services   Nursing and rehabilitation services provided to patients confined to their homes.

hypernasality   Speech produced with excessive resonance in the nasal cavity.

idiolect   Every individual's unique way of speaking.

immittance   An audiological procedure for assessing the mobility of the eardrum.

impairment   A disruption or abnormality in physiologic structure or function.

independent variable   A manipulated variable in an experiment or study whose presence or degree determines the change in the dependent variable.

indirect services   Consultation with family members, teachers, and/or medical personnel about a client's communication needs.

Individual Transition Plan (ITP)   An integrated component of an IEP for students ages 16 to 21 developed to facilitate their transition from an educational environment to an appropriate vocational or supported adult service setting.

Individualized Education Program (IEP)   A federally mandated written plan developed by an interdisciplinary educational team identifying services and supports for children ages 3 to 21 who have been determined eligible for special education services.

Individualized Family Service Plans (IFSPs)   A written plan outlining family centered supports and services for children birth to 3 years old who have be determined eligible for early intervention services based on the presence of significant developmental delays or disabilities.

infection control   The safeguarding of clients and clinicians from infectious diseases by maintaining universal precautions, including hand washing, the use of barriers (i.e., gloves and masks), disinfecting equipment, and procedures for the disposal of bodily fluids (i.e., saliva and blood).

informativeness   The degree to which a client's discourse is relevant, truthful, not redundant, and reflects plausible inferences and interpretations.

informed consent   Providing a client with information about their condition, and informing the client about the relative strengths, weakness and risks associated with a recommended plan of action or inaction.

inpatient rehabilitation   Therapy provided to patients who are staying in the hospital or rehabilitation center.

intelligibility   The degree to which a client's speech can be understood.

intensive care unit (ICU)   A specialized unit in a general medical hospital for patients in critical condition who require close monitoring.

interdisciplinary   A team approach in which professionals perform tasks within their own disciplines while sharing information and coordinating services with each other.

internal consistency   A measure of the degree to which items on a test correlate with each other.

interrater reliability   The extent to which two or more independent scorers are in agreement about a test score.

intervention   A planned clinical program to change client behavior.

interview   A process by which a clinician gathers information related to an individual's communication disorder through direct verbal exchange and through which a clinician begins to establish trust with a client while educating him or her about issues related to communication impairment.

intraoperative monitoring   Continuous assessment of integrity of cranial nerves during surgery.

intraoral   Within the mouth.

Joint Commission on the Accreditation of Health Care Organizations (JCAHCO)   A regulatory body that oversees the quality of care provided to patients in a variety of health care facilities.

language difference   Expected community variations in syntax, semantics, phonology, pragmatics, and the lexicon.

language disorders   Communication that deviates significantly from the norms of the community.

language interference   The influence of one language on another.

laryngectomy   A surgical procedure in which the larynx (and possibly connecting tissues) is removed, usually due to cancer. An individual who has undergone this procedure is referred to as a laryngectomee.

laws   Actions taken by legislative bodies, and signed into law by executive officials who are responsible for their implementation and enforcement of penalties for violations.

letters of justification   Written letters to other service providers, program administrators, insurance companies and other agents advocating for services, supports, and equipment needed for effective client management.

local norms   The administration of standardized tests to typically developing individuals in the community in which the clinician is working and noting the scores they receive and the quality of their responses.

long-term goals   The relatively broad changes in communicative behavior to be achieved during a course of therapy.

managed care   Approaches to the delivery of health care that attempt to control quality while containing costs.

managed care organization (MCO)   An agency that manages or controls health care expenditures by closely monitoring how service providers (e.g., hospitals and physicians) treat their patients and by evaluating the necessity, appropriateness, and payment efficiency of health services.

maze   A type of dysfluency involving repetitions, revisions and false starts in the flow of speech.

mean   The arithmetic average of scores.

measure of central tendency   Description of where the center of a distribution of scores lies. It is reported as the mean, median, and/or mode.

Medicaid   A program jointly funded by the states and the federal government that reimburses hospitals and physicians for providing care to qualifying individuals who cannot finance their own medical expenses.

Medicare   Prepaid hospital insurance (Part A) and optional additional medical insurance (Part B) available to individuals over age 65 who are eligible for benefits or disability based on their employment before retirement and administered by the federal Health Care Financing Administration (HCFA).

Medigap   Supplemental hospital insurance designed to cover what Medicare does not.

misrepresentation   A type of dishonesty that occurs when truth is distorted or falsified.

Möbius syndrome   A rare birth defect caused by the absence or underdevelopment of the 6th and 7th cranial nerves, which may result swallowing problems, crossed eyes, lack of facial expression, and speech difficulties.

modal verbs   Auxiliary verbs used to express the subjunctive mood or future tense (e.g., can, will, shall, may, could, would, should, must, might).

modifiability   The process of change through mediation or teaching.

morpheme   The smallest unit of meaning in a language and can be free-standing words, inflections (bound morphemes, such as plural /s/ or past tense -ed), prefixes (e.g., re-, un-) or suffixes (e.g., -ly, -ness).

morphology   The study of how morphemes or units of meaning are joined together to form words.

multidisciplinary   An approach to service provision in which professionals from different disciplines work independently and report to the team.

multiple sclerosis   A progressive inflamatory disease in which the myelin sheath of the nerves of the central nervous system (i.e., brain and spinal cord) degenerate resulting in problems with vision, speech, walking, writing, and memory.

narrative A form of connected discourse describing a temporally and causally ordered sequence of events, usually delivered in monologue form in the first or third person, in which animate characters attempt to confront and resolve some problem. Often conveys cultural values or mores.

nasal emission The sound of air flowing through the nose during speech.

nasogastric tube A feeding tube inserted through the nose and ends in the stomach.

neonatal intensive care unit (NICU) A specialized intensive care unit for newborn infants who need intensive medical management.

neurologist A physician who specializes in diagnosis and management of diseases of the nervous system.

nodule A small group of cells causing a knot or swelling on the edge of the vocal fold.

nondiscrimination The inclusion of clients in professional practice and avoiding clinical decisions based solely on a client's race, gender, ethnicity, religion, age, national origin, sexual orientation, or disability status.

nonmaleficence Deliberately avoiding the infliction of potential or actual harm or evil on others.

normal distribution A symmetrical bell shaped curve representing the scores of a normal population on a test. In a normal distribution, most scores fall in the middle and fewer scores are found at the high and low extremities.

norming sample The sample of individuals from a population to whom a test was administered to collect normative data.

norm-referenced Tests designed to compare a client's score results against a normed basis.

obturator A prosthesis used to close an opening of the hard palate.

odd-even reliability A way to measure internal consistency of a test. The degree to which odd and even numbered items on a test correlate with each other.

oncology A division of medicine specializing in diagnosis and management of cancer.

openbite A type of malocclusion characterized by the premature occlusion of posterior teeth and the absence of anterior occlusion.

open-ended question A remark that encourages an elaborated reply rather than a one-word answer (e.g., "Tell me more about that"); also called open-ended comment.

otoacoustic emissions (OAEs) Low level sounds produced by the cochlea that can be measured. Absence of OAEs suggests hearing loss.

otolaryngologist A physician who specialty in diseases of the ear, nose and throat.

otolaryngology Branch of medicine specializing in the diagnosis and treatment of diseases of the ear, nose, and throat.

otoscopic Inspection of the external auditory meatus and tympanic membrane with an otoscope.

ototoxic Having a poisonous action on the ear, particularly the hair cells of the cochlear and vestibular end organs.

outpatient facility Designated location where therapy can be provided to patients who live at home and are transported to a rehabilitation center.

overdiagnosis Labeling individuals with communication disorders who, instead, are typically developing.

paralinguistics Information that accompanies a speech signal to enhance its meaning, including tone of voice, facial expressions, and gestures.

paresis Weakness or partial inability.

Parkinson disease A neurological condition characterized by tremors, rigidity, a droopy posture, and mask-like faces.

participation restriction Term used by the World Health Organization to describe difficulties an individual may experience in involvement of life situations as a result of an impairment.

percentile ranks A derived score that indicates the percentage of individuals whose score fell at or below a given raw score.

performance assessment   An alternative to standardized testing that uses real-life tasks or projects that allow an individual to demonstrate competence or mastery.

personal ethics   One's own choices about moral behavior.

perturbation   The variance of consecutive cycles of an acoustic wave produced by the speaker. In some cases, these measures are related to vocal disorders. Variance between waves for intensity is called shimmer. Variance between waves for frequency is called jitter.

phonetic inventory   A list of all speech sounds (often restricted to consonant sounds) that are produced by a client in a speech sample.

phonology   Study of the rules which govern the way sounds are combined in a language.

PICO   Acronym standing for *patient, patient group*, or *problem; intervention* being considered; *comparison intervention;* and desired *outcome.* System for developing an appropriate clinical question.

planning and placement team (PPT)   An interdisciplinary team consisting of educators, therapists, family members, and educational support personnel charged with the development and implementation of an Individual Educational Plan (IEP) for students ages 3 to 21 who receive special educational services.

play audiometry   A technique used for testing the hearing of preschool children. The child is conditioned to perform an action, such as putting a block in a bucket, when he or she hears a sound.

polyp   A small growth with an attached stem.

portfolio   A collection of evidence, such as work samples, that demonstrates an individual's competence or mastery.

posttest   A pretest readministered after a course of therapy to assess client progress.

pragmatics   Study of the appropriate use of language in context.

predictive validity   A measure of the degree to which an individual's current test score can be used to estimate the individual's test score at a later date.

pretest   A baseline measurement taken before the initiation of treatment on a goal.

professional ethics   Right and wrong actions in the workplace.

professional relationships   Collegial behavior characterized by an open communication style and a climate of mutual respect and cooperation.

prognosis   A statement that describes the likelihood that a benefit will be gained from treatment.

prolongation   The maintenance of a speech sound or airflow during speech when the articulators have stopped. One of the core behaviors in stuttering.

prosody   The rhythm and melody of speech expressed by intonation, stress, pause, and juncture.

psychiatrist   A physician who specializes in the psychiatric needs of patients.

psychologist   A professional who evaluates and manages the psychological and/or psychosocial needs of the patient.

pull-out   Involve stopping a dysfluency in the middle of the stuttering moment, mentally rehearsing the intended word using an easier stuttering pattern, and then reproducing the word.

pure tone audiometry   Audiological testing procedures used to measure hearing thresholds.

quasi-experimental studies   A research design where the researcher does not randomly assign participants to different treatment groups.

radiologist   A physician specialized in radiology, the branch of medicine that uses ionizing and nonionizing radiation for the diagnosis and treatment of disease.

randomized clinical trial (RCT)   A research design in which the investigator assigns participants randomly to two or more groups who then receive systematic treatment (or, in some cases, no treatment) and the outcomes for each group are compared.

referral   Sending a client to another professional whose area of expertise better matches the client's needs.

referral letters   Letters written to doctors, therapists, or other service providers referring an individual for medical or clinical evaluation and/or treatment.

registers   The varieties of a language that depend on the context and conversational participants.

regulations   Detailed rules for interpreting and implementing a particular law.

Reinke's edema   Swelling along the superficial layer of the lamina propria of the vocal folds; also called polypoid degeneration.

reliability   The consistency of a test or a procedure over repeated administrations and by different examiners.

repetitions   A sound, syllable, or word repeated more than twice. One of the core behaviors in stuttering.

resonance   The modification of laryngeal tone by altering the shape of the oral and nasal cavities.

rubric   A set of criteria, including a scale, used to evaluate an individual's performance.

scaled score   A standard score, frequently having a mean of 100 and a standard deviation of 15.

scores of relative standing   Test scores that allow comparison among individuals of various ages and among scores on various tests taken by the same individual.

screening   Initial assessment procedure that allows individuals who require a complete evaluation to be identified.

self-contained classroom   A service provision model in which the speech-language pathologist is the primary educator, providing both academic and intense speech-language remediation.

semantics   Study of the way in which words and ideas are combined and expressed.

service delivery models   The systems that are used to organize speech-language and hearing programs.

SETT   Acronym standing for *student, environment,* the *tasks* a student needs to accomplish before attempting to determine what *tools* will be required. This framework assists a planning and placement team in goal setting and maintenance.

signal-to-noise ratio   The ratio of intensities of foreground to background noises, often used as a measure of vocal quality.

single-subject experimental design   A research design in which the investigator systematically manipulates variables so that a relationship between the treatment and the outcome can be inferred, usually on one or a small number of participants.

skilled nursing facility (SNF)   Previously known as a *nursing home.* Include a percentage of residents who require services from such trained professionals as nurses and rehabilitation specialists.

SOAP note   Acronym standing for *subjective, objective, assessment,* and *plan.* A commonly used format in medical and other service delivery settings to record and analyze data specific to a client's ongoing medical status and/or performance in therapy.

social workers   A professional who assists patients with management of psychosocial problems and to access various community resources.

specialization   The acquisition of advanced technical skills for a particular population, disorder and/or service delivery model, through in-depth experience, advanced knowledge, and training beyond the certificate of clinical competence credential.

spectral analysis   Analysis of an acoustic signal through the study of its charted band of wavelengths; also called spectrographic analysis.

speech audiometry   Audiological procedures used to determine speech detection levels, speech reception thresholds, and speech discrimination.

speech-generating device (SGD)   An electronic aid that produces speech output.

split-half reliability   A way to measure internal consistency of a test by calculating the degree to which scores from one half of a test correlate with scores from the other half.

standard deviation   Measure of the degree of variation in a distribution.

standard error of measurement (SEM)   The standard deviation of error around an individual's true score.

standard score   A derived score that has been transformed into a distribution with a known mean and standard deviation.

statistical significance   The probability that differences between groups observed over a course of treatment resulted from the manipulation of the independent variable.

stimulability   The degree to which a nonmastered skill or behavior can be elicited.

stridor   Breath noise on inhalation.

stuttering   A type of fluency disorder. Speech is usually marked by repetitions, prolongations and/or pauses in speech.

supplemental security income (SSI)   Benefits provided to qualified individuals that demonstrate financial need and meet the definitions of eligibility.

syntax   Study of the rules that govern the internal structure of language, including grammar and word order.

systems model   Model which emphasizes the importance of context in which an individual must function.

task analysis   The breakdown of an intervention goal into a series of prerequisite skills and the ordered steps that must be followed to achieve it.

task sequence   An ordered series of steps through which a clinician plans to help a client progress toward an intervention goal.

Telecommunication Access Program   Technology to improve public communication including captions, text and digital telephones, relay systems, and amplifier headsets.

Telecommunications for the Deaf, Inc.   A national advocacy organization focused on equal access issues in telecommunications and media for individuals with hearing impairment.

temporary assistance for needy families (TANF)   Government program that provides cash assistance and supportive services for qualified needy families with children under the age of 18.

test sensitivity   The extent to which a test identifies clients with real problems in the targeted area of communication.

test specificity   The extent to which a test correctly identifies clients who do not have real problems.

test-retest reliability   A measure of a test's consistency or stability over time.

tic   Repeated contraction of a muscle.

tinnitus   Sensation of ringing or other sound in the head, without an external cause.

transdisciplinary   A team approach in which members from different disciplines work collaboratively to focus on shared goals. Team members work together and may cross discipline lines.

tremor   Repetitive shaking involuntary movement.

T-scores   A standard score with a mean of 50 and a standard deviation of 10.

T-unit   Terminal units of production; used to segment utterances of school-aged children and adults. Consists of an independent clause and all the dependent clauses associated with it.

tympanometry   One type of immittance testing used to measure the compliance of the eardrum relative to changes in air pressure.

underdiagnosis   The process of not diagnosing a true communication disorder because all aspects of an individual's communication skills are believed to be dialect/second language features.

universal precautions   An approach to infection control in which all human blood, tissue, and certain fluids are treated as if known to be infectious for other blood-borne pathogens.

use   The function of language (pragmatics).

validity   The extent to which a test measures what it claims to measure.

verbosity   Excess speech; the use of more words than is necessary to convey an idea; often exhibited in acquired aphasia.

videoflouroscopic swallowing study (VFSS)   A radiographic examination of swallowing performed while the patient drinks liquids and eats solid food.

videostroboscopy   Instrumentation that allows visualization of vocal fold movement.

visual reinforcement audiometry   A technique for testing the hearing of very young children. The child is reinforced with lights or moving toys for looking toward a sound.

World Health Organization (WHO)   An international organization that developed the International Classification of Functioning, Disability and Health (ICF) that provides a model for evaluating the interaction between an individual's health condition, level of functioning, and contextual factors.

z-score   Standard score with a mean of 0 and a standard deviation of 1.

Index

Page references to figures and tables are indicated by *f* and *t*, respectively.

Norm-referenced tests
  administration procedures, 55
  derived scores, 53–55
  descriptive statistics, 51–53
  error, 53
  listed, 47*t*
  methods, 46–55
  reliability, 46–49
  standardization, 51
  validity, 49–50
Nose, assessing speech mechanism of, 96
Number of different words (NDW), 124
Nursing homes, 249

OAEs (otoacoustic emissions), 66
Observed effects, strength and consistency, 197*t*
Occlusions, types of, 104*f*
Odd-even reliability, 49
Office of Special Education and Rehabilitive
  Services (OSERS), 247
Older children, literacy of, 69
Oncology patient, 273
Open-ended question, 119
Operant conditioning procedures, 164
Oral mechanism
  cavity and adjacent structures, 100*f*, 101*f*
  concerns, syndromes and characteristics
    causing, 92–93*t*
  evaluation form, 87–89*f*
  examining, 64
  lingual frenulum, 105*f*
  screening instruments, 43*t*
Oral presentations, 204
Oral reports and conferences, 212–213
Oral Speech Mechanism Screening Exam, 43*t*
Oro-facial-digital syndromes, 92*t*
Orphans, 144*t*
Orthogaphy, 307*t*
OSERS (Office of Special Education and
  Rehabilitive Services), 247
Otolaryngology, 278
Oto-palatal-digital syndrome, 92*t*
Otoscopic examination, 275
Ototoxic effects of drug therapies, 277
Outcomes
  assessment, 13
  assistive technology (AT), measuring, 316–317
  documenting, 198–199
  speech-language pathology, Certificate
    of Clinical Competence (CCC) in, 16–17
Outpatient facility, 273
Outpatient rehabilitation centers, 271
Overdiagnosis, 292
Oxford Centre for Evidence-Based
  Medicine, 193

Oxford Centre for Evidence-Based
  Medicine levels, 193*t*

Palate, examining, 99–103
Paralinguistics, 113
Parallel talk, 165
Paraprofessionals, ethical competence and, 25*t*
Parental choice, 240
Parents
  assessment reporting tools, 330
  recording children's speech progress, 111
  role in new interventions, 179–180, 183–184
Participation restrictions, 41
Patient, Intervention, Comparison interven-
  tion, and Outcome (PICO), 188
Patterns, sound errors and, 140*t*
Pauses, 144*t*
Peabody Picture Vocabulary Test, 48*t*, 50*f*, 187
Peer interaction, 125
People, clients as, 2
Percentile ranks, 54
Performance assessment, 59
Personal ethics, 20
Personal qualities needed by clinicians, 2
Perturbation, 147
Phonemic awareness, 240
Phonetic inventory, 140
Phonics instruction, 240
Phonology, 43*t*, 47*t*, 56*t*, 63
  see also intelligibility
Photo Articulation Test, 140*t*
Photograph, 307*t*
Physical concomitants, 65
Physical context, naturalness of interven-
  tion, 163*t*
Physical disabilities, assessment challenges
  with, 73
Physical examination results, 94–95*t*
PICO (Patient, Intervention, Comparison
  intervention, and Outcome), 188
Picture communication symbols, 307*t*
Picture description, language sampling in
  adults with acquired disorders, 131
Picture Planner screen, 312*f*
Pierre-Robin sequence, 92*t*
Planning and placement team (PPT), 226
Play
  assistive technology (AT), 316
  audiometry, 65
  preschoolers, sampling language with, 118
  school-age children and adolescents, 125
Policy, 254
Political advocacy, American Speech-
  Langauge-Hearing Association
  (ASHA), 6